Examination Review for Ultrasound

Sonographic Principles and Instrumentation

Third Edition

Examination Review for Ultrasound

Sonographic Principles and Instrumentation

Third Edition

Traci B. Fox, EdD, R.T.(R)(ARRT), RDMS, RVT, FSVU

Program Director, Diagnostic Medical Sonography and Cardiovascular Ultrasound
Associate Professor, Department of Medical Imaging and Radiation Sciences
Jefferson College of Health Professions
Thomas Jefferson University
Philadelphia, Pennsylvania

Steven M. Penny, MA, RT(R), RDMS

Sonography Programs Director
Johnston Community College
Smithfield, North Carolina

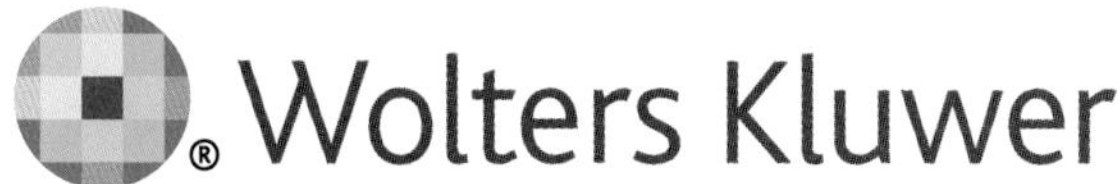

Philadelphia • Baltimore • New York • London
Buenos Aires • Hong Kong • Sydney • Tokyo

Acquisitions Editor: Matt Hauber
Development Editor: Eric McDermott
Editorial Coordinator: Priyanka Alagar
Marketing Manager: Kirsten Watrud
Senior Production Project Manager: Alicia Jackson
Manager, Graphic Arts & Design: Stephen Druding
Manufacturing Coordinator: Lisa Bowling
Prepress Vendor: Lumina Datamatics Ltd.

Third Edition

9 8 7 6 5 4 3 2 1

Printed in Mexico

Library of Congress Cataloging-in-Publication Data

ISBN-13: 978-1-9752-2210-9

Cataloging in Publication data available on request from publisher.

shop.lww.com

QUADM1024

Dedication

This book is dedicated to Thresa because it is her patience and support that give me the energy to keep going during my many projects, and to Cooper, my patient yet frustrated shorkiepoo, who doesn't get as much play time as he deserves. I also dedicate this book to my family as a thank you for their unwavering support, even though my mother says she doesn't understand a thing that I write.

—Traci B. Fox

To my mother Linda Penny. Thank you for always being such a loving and caring part of my life. I love you.

—Steven M. Penny

Preface

Examination Review for Ultrasound: Sonographic Principles and Instrumentation, 3rd ed.

Among the expansive list of resources offered for test preparation for the Sonography Principles and Instrumentation (SPI) examination offered by the American Registry for Diagnostic Medical Sonography (ARDMS), *Examination Review for Ultrasound: Sonographic Principles and Instrumentation* quickly became the most reliable resource for those pursuing ultrasound credentialing. Today it remains one of the most widely utilized registry review books for sonographic physics. And like the first and second editions of this text, this third edition continues to provide a clear-cut foundation needed to successfully pass the ARDMS SPI examination.

Objective

There is an inherent obligation for sonographers—and other professionals who utilize sound to create an image of the human body—to fully comprehend the physics behind this universally valued imaging technology. With a fundamental appreciation of ultrasound physics, one can gain deference for the prospective impact it can have on patient care. As we learn more about the creation of the image with sound, we tend to appreciate the benefits and potential (and theoretical) risks of ultrasound imaging for the patient. And through the deference gained by rigorous study, we learn how we can better serve the patient by efficiently utilizing this technology in our quest for a definitive diagnosis. There is a saying that the only certainty in life is change, and that is true with ultrasound physics and instrumentation. Technology existing at the time of writing this book is not in widespread use, and new technologies are continuously developing. At the time the author graduated ultrasound school, there was no microflow imaging, elastography, or virtual beamforming, and ultrasound contrast—as we know it today—was in its infancy. Consequently, *Examination Review for Ultrasound: Sonographic Principles and Instrumentation, 3rd ed.*, has been fashioned to provide an up-to-date basis for understanding more about ultrasound physics and to prepare those who plan to attempt the SPI exam offered by the ARDMS or questions on ultrasound principles and instrumentation offered by other credentialing bodies.

Organization

The material in this text is based on the current content outline (acquired prior to the publication date of this book) provided by the ARDMS for the SPI examination. Though only the essential points about the subject matter will be found in the following pages, each topic has been thoroughly researched. The format of this book ultimately leads to a review that is succinct and useful for the reader.

At the beginning of each chapter, key terms are provided for both a quick reference and to add clarity to the narrative. Again, the narrative provides a straightforward writing style that is easy to understand. Helpful figures, diagrams, and sonographic images are scattered throughout the text to provide a visual illustration of key concepts. Also supporting the text are *Sound Off* boxes. These boxes are used to highlight the information that is most significant about the preceding narrative. In September 2023, the ARDMS changed the SPI content outlines. Owing to the fluid nature of the SPI exam, this book contains items that are not currently listed on the ARDMS SPI content outlines. Material not included on the 2023 content outlines is highlighted where needed in the text. The reader is encouraged to review the current content outlines for the exam to ensure adequate preparation. At the end of each chapter, review questions allow for the subject matter assessment of the given chapter. Finally, at the end of this book, a 120-question registry review is provided with answers and rationale.

Additional Resources

As with the previous editions, the review associated with this book does not need to end with its conclusion. There are numerous online resources for this text, including a mock registry examination that can be attempted by using the code at the beginning of this book and visiting thePoint.lww.com/penny_spi2e. This exam simulator will provide the user with more intense "registry-like" questions, with topics that can be selected, and the answers that provide rationale. Instructors can use the faculty resources as well, which include an image bank and PowerPoint presentations.

Final Note

In the classroom setting, many instructors discovered that the use of the first and then second editions of this text was beneficial. This edition will also provide the instructor with a topic-based review that can identify subject matter weaknesses. And instructors that offer registry review courses will find that this book and its resources will offer them a focused tool for preparing their students for the national certification exam.

If you have chosen this book for personal preparation, we are thankful that you have done so, and it is our hope that this book serves you well. Though it is imperative to learn, sonographic physics is a topic in which not all people excel. However, we have tried to provide you with a means whereby you can assess your own knowledge in a concise manner prior to attempting this (often anxiety-inducing) examination. As you study, please keep in mind that the facts and information contained in this text are applicable to patient care. We hope that you are ultimately capable of applying the knowledge gained from this text not only to pass the SPI examination but also to utilize its principles throughout your daily practice as a credentialed sonographer.

Traci B. Fox and Steven M. Penny

Acknowledgments

I would like to thank Steven Penny for starting this review book and inviting me to be a part of it. I would also like to thank my Department Chair, Dr. Colleen Dempsey, for her constant support. In addition, many thanks to the research team in the Department of Radiology at Thomas Jefferson University, including Dr. Flemming Forsberg, Dr. John Eisenbrey, Dr. Ji-Bin Liu, and my colleagues, Maria Stanczak and Dr. Maureen McDonald, for all their support, knowledge, and images over the years. I would also like to thank Nate Pinkney, Dr. Fred Kremkau and Dr. Phil Bendick for their support, and others who have helped train and educate me. I stand on the shoulders of giants. Lastly, special shout-out to all the sonographers and former students who have encouraged me and who have bestowed upon me the moniker of The Physics Whisperer.

Traci B. Fox

Test-Taking Tips

"By failing to prepare, you are preparing to fail."
—Ben Franklin

The national certification examinations offered by the American Registry for Diagnostic Medical Sonography (ARDMS), CCI (cci-online.org/), and American Registry of Radiologic Technologist (ARRT) are not easy. These exams are difficult because they are created to test your knowledge of a vital imaging modality that can save people's lives. Consequently, preparing for and challenging these exams should not be approached dispassionately. There are many resources on test taking that you can access at your local library and online. Below are three essential steps that include tips for getting organized, studying, and preparing for these credentialing exams.

Step 1: Get Organized and Schedule the Exam

The ARDMS (ardms.org), CCI (cci-online.org/), and ARRT (arrt.org) provide content outlines for each of their certification examinations. The content of this book is based primarily on the content outlines of the SPI examination of the ARDMS. However, you can use these content outlines as a guide for focused study as well. Keep your study materials—which should include all the resources you obtained throughout your sonography education—organized by these content outlines. School lecture notes, note cards, quizzes, and tests should be organized well before you begin to study.

Once you have organized your study materials, you should apply for the exam and then try to consider the best time to attempt it. When scheduling the examination, consider all your other obligations (eg, family responsibilities, vacations, and job requirements) and allow for an ample amount of time to study so that you are thoroughly prepared on examination day. Do not postpone scheduling the exam. Scheduling the examination will provide you with a firm date, and it will hopefully help those of you who suffer from procrastination to focus on test preparation.

Step 2: Establish a Study Routine and Study Schedule

Next, since you have your deadline, find a quiet place to study and develop a study routine and schedule. Your study space should be quiet and free from distractions, like television and your cell phone. In fact, put your cell phone (and smart watch) in another room, turned to silent mode, to reduce the temptation to check it or reply to text messages. The study schedule that you create for yourself should be realistic—do not schedule 2 hours each night to study if you know that you will not be dedicated to that schedule. Instead, it may be best to schedule 1 solid hour each night. Also, studying in 45-minute increments with 15-minute breaks may work best for some. You can create your own deadlines on your schedule and strive to meet them. Be sure to study at least for a few minutes every day to maintain momentum going into the exam.

The amount of time one requires to study will vary per individual. Only *you* know how much time *you* need to study, so if you struggle with certain topics, then allow for extra time to focus more attention on those topics. It may be best to review those topics you are most familiar with first, and as the exam approaches, review the topics that you struggle with just before your attempt, with the hopes of making the challenging information more readily accessible.

Most people know what manner they prepare for an exam best. Some test takers find flashcards useful, either on paper or digital, and there is plenty of free software available to help you create them. Some create their own notes from class notes, whereas others may simply read and choose to gradually answer registry review questions. Studies have shown that *active recall* is a proven way to study, versus a passive activity like reading. When you are forced to recall things from your brain it creates permanent connections that will help you recall material later. A study group may be helpful for some as well, although these quickly may devolve into gab fests. Nonetheless, the main concern of your studies should be *learning* the material and not just *memorizing* it to pass the exam. By learning the information, you will most likely be successful on the exam, with the added benefit of being able to apply your knowledge in your daily clinical practice as a registered sonographer.

Step 3: Confidently Attempt the Exam

Test anxiety is a challenge for many people. Some tips for reducing anxiety include eating well, getting plenty of rest and exercise, keeping a positive attitude, and taking practice tests. The ARDMS offers tips for exam-day success, which include getting a good night's sleep before exam day, knowing how long it takes to get to the testing center (traffic included), being early to the testing center, and being familiar with all of the test center requirements, like testing day registrant identification specifications. Always check the exam information located on the credentialing body website as some exams may have multiple choice but there also may be hotspot questions or an interactive console.

Multiple choice questions consist of the stem—which is the question—and four possible answers (called *distractors*) to choose from. The correct answer is included along with three distractors, and you need to recognize which one is most likely to be correct versus which ones are not. There are three general types of exam questions:

1. *The Gimme Question:* This type of question will be more common the more prepared you are for the exam. For this question type, read the question first and try to answer the question before looking at the distractors. If your given answer is one of the options, select it and never return to that question. Individuals who do not pass the credentialing exams usually second guess themselves and change answers. Do not go back and review gimme questions or you will change correct answers to incorrect answers. Trust your gut.
2. *The Klingon Question:* This type of question looks like it is written in a language you do not understand, like Klingon (assuming you do not speak Klingon). Do not waste any time on a Klingon question, or you risk wasting valuable time for a question you are going to end up guessing anyway. Select a distractor (do not leave any blank), mark it for review, and go back later to review it again.
3. *The "Yes-No" Question:* This type of question is the most common type of exam question. With this question type you do not know the answer immediately, but you can review the distractors and eliminate the ones you know are wrong. The ones you know are wrong are the "no" answers; try to eliminate as many as you can to narrow down your options.

   Example: "What color is the sky?"

   A. Red
   B. Cyan
   C. Yellow
   D. Pink

   When you first read the question, you may think "blue" before reviewing the distractors. If blue had been there, it would have been a gimme question. Mark that distractor and never look back. However, "blue" is not there. So now go through each distractor and review which ones *cannot* be correct. The thought process might look like this, "Red and pink are the same hue, so they're probably not correct. The sky is yellow from pollution, but that's probably not what they're looking for. Hmm, cyan is a shade of blue, so that's probably correct."

You are allowed to mark questions and return to answer them later. You can also make changes before final submission. It is strongly recommended that you do not review the entire exam, and whether you review the entire exam or just the ones you mark for review, it may be best to not change any of your answers. You should only make changes to questions that you feel confident you have answered incorrectly because for many people the first thought is usually correct. Again, trust your gut. If you study and practice using this text, you will be well set up to have more "gimme" questions than ones seemingly written in a different language.

Suggested Readings

ARDMS.org. Review our tips for examination day success. Available at: http://www.ardms.org/get-certified/RDMS/Pages/Abdomen.aspx. Accessed March 16, 2017.

Fry R. *Surefire Study Success: Surefire Tips to Improve Your Test-Taking Skills.* Rosen Publishing Group; 2016.

Hill J. Test taking tips to give you an edge. *Biomed Instrum Technol.* 2009;43(3):223–224.

Mary KL. Test-taking strategies for CNOR certification. *AORN J.* 2007;85(2):315–332.

Medoff L. *Stressed Out Students' Guide to Dealing with Tests.* Kaplan Inc.; 2008.

Contents

1

Physical Principles

Outline

Introduction

This chapter focuses on units of measurement and the properties of sound. The purpose of this chapter is to provide a foundation for more complex material found in the following chapters.

Key Terms

absorption—the conversion of sound energy to heat

acoustic speckle—the interference pattern caused by scatterers that produce the granular appearance of tissue on a sonographic image

acoustic variables—changes that occur within a medium as a result of sound traveling through that medium

amplitude—the maximum or minimum deviation of an acoustic variable from the average value of that variable; the strength of the sound wave

attenuation—a decrease in the amplitude and intensity of the sound beam as sound travels through tissue (in dB)

attenuation coefficient—the rate at which sound is attenuated per unit depth (in dB/cm)

axial resolution—the ability to accurately identify reflectors that are arranged parallel to the ultrasound beam (in mm)

backscatter—scattered sound waves that make their way back to the transducer and produce an image on the display

beam uniformity ratio—the ratio of the center intensity to the average intensity across the transducer face; also referred to as the SP/SA factor or beam uniformity coefficient

capacitive micromachined ultrasound transducers—technology used to create comparable transducer technology to piezoelectric materials

compression—an area in the sound wave of high pressure and density

continuous wave—sound that is continuously transmitted

damping—the process of reducing the number of cycles of each pulse in order to improve axial resolution

decibels—a unit that establishes a relationship or comparison between two values of power, intensity, or amplitude

density—mass per unit volume

directly related—relationship that implies that if one variable decreases, the other also decreases, or if one variable increases, the other also increases; also referred to as directly proportional

distance—how far apart objects are; may also be referred to as vibration or displacement

duty factor—the percentage of time that sound is actually being produced

elasticity—see the key term "stiffness"

frequency—the number of cycles per second (in Hz)

half-intensity depth—the depth at which sound has lost half of its intensity (in cm)

half-value layer thickness—see the key term "half-intensity depth"

hertz—a unit of frequency

hydrophone—a device used to measure the output intensity of the transducer

impedance—the resistance to the propagation of sound through a medium (in rayls)

inertia—Newton's principle that states that an object at rest stays at rest and an object in motion stays in motion unless acted on by an outside force

intensity—the power of the wave divided by the area over which it is spread; the energy per unit area (in W/cm^2 or mW/cm^2)

intensity reflection coefficient—the percentage of sound reflected at an interface

intensity transmission coefficient—the percentage of sound transmitted at an interface

interface—the dividing line between two different media

inversely related—relationship that implies that if one variable decreases, the other increases, or if one variable increases, the other decreases; also referred to as inversely proportional

longitudinal waves—waves in which the molecules of the medium vibrate back and forth in the same direction that the waves are traveling

medium—any form of matter: solid, liquid, or gas

nonspecular reflectors—reflectors that are smaller than the wavelength of the incident beam

normal incidence—angle of incidence is 90° to the interface

oblique incidence—angle of incidence is less than or greater than 90° to the interface

parameter—a measurable quantity

particle motion—the movement of molecules owing to propagating sound energy

path length—distance to the reflector

period—the time it takes for one cycle to occur (in μs)

piezoelectric materials—a material that generates electricity when pressure is applied to it, and one that changes shape when electricity is applied to it; also referred to as the element or crystal

power—the rate at which energy is transferred/transmitted (in W or mW)

pressure—force per unit area or the concentration of force (in Pascals, Pa)

propagate—to transmit through a medium

propagation speed—the speed at which a sound wave travels through a medium (in m/s or mm/μs)

pulse duration—the time it takes for sound to be transmitted; the "on" time (in μs)

pulse repetition frequency—the number of pulses of sound produced in 1 s (in Hz)

pulse repetition period—the time taken for a pulse to occur, including the listening (or dead) time (in μs)

pulsed wave—sound that is sent out in pulses

rarefaction—an area in the sound wave of low pressure

Rayleigh scatterers—very small scattering reflectors, such as red blood cells

reflection—the echo; the portion of sound that returns from an interface

refraction—the change in the direction of the transmitted sound beam that occurs with oblique incidence angles and dissimilar propagation speeds

scattering—the phenomenon that occurs when sound waves are dispersed into different directions because of the small reflector size compared with the incident wavelength

Snell's law—principle used to describe the angle of transmission at an interface based on the angle of incidence and the propagation speeds of the two media

soft tissue—imaginary medium whose propagation speed is the average of propagation speeds of various tissues found in the human body

sound—a traveling variation through a medium

spatial pulse length—the length of a pulse (in mm)

specular reflections—reflections that occur when the reflector is larger than the size of the wavelength of the incident beam. Assumes a 90° angle of incidence

stiffness—the ability of an object to resist compression and relates to the hardness of a medium

total attenuation—the total amount of sound (in dB) that has been attenuated at a given depth

transverse waves—type of wave in which the molecules in a medium vibrate at 90° to the direction of travel

ultrasound—sound waves of frequencies exceeding the range of human hearing

wavelength—the length of a single cycle of sound (in mm)

FUNDAMENTALS AND UNITS OF MEASUREMENTS

A sonographer should be aware of the metric prefixes, their symbols, and their meaning (Table 1-1). Also, because ultrasound incorporates small units of measurements, sonographers must have a fundamental appreciation for fractions of whole numbers and their symbols (Table 1-2). Understanding the conversion of units is also significant. Figure 1-1 summarizes how to convert units.

TABLE 1-1 Metric whole numbers

Prefix	Symbol	Meaning	Value
Giga	G	Billion	10^9
Mega	M	Million	10^6
Kilo	k	Thousand	10^3
Hecto	h	Hundred	10^2
Deca	da	Ten	10^1

BASICS OF SOUND

What Is Sound?

Sound is a form of energy. It is *not* part of the electromagnetic spectrum, like radio waves, light, or x-rays. It is a pressure wave, created by a mechanical action, and is therefore referred to as a mechanical wave. Sound is produced when a vibrating source causes the molecules of a **medium** to move back and forth. This back-and-forth movement of the molecules creates waves of sound energy that travel, or **propagate**, through a medium. Therefore, although nothing physical is traveling through the medium, it is energy—in the form of sound—that is being moved from one point to another. A medium is any form of matter: solid, liquid, or gas. Sound requires a medium to propagate. Because the tissues of a human body are composed of different forms of matter, they provide a basis through which sound is able to propagate. Because a vacuum is devoid of matter, sound cannot travel in a vacuum.

When sound energy propagates through a medium, it does so in **longitudinal waves**, meaning that the molecules of the medium vibrate back and forth, parallel to the direction in which the wave is traveling (Figure 1-2). In summary, sound is a mechanical, longitudinal wave that propagates through a medium. Longitudinal waves should not be confused with **transverse waves**, where molecules in a medium vibrate at 90° to the direction of the traveling wave (Figure 1-3). Sound can be categorized

TABLE 1-2 Fractions of whole numbers

Prefix	Symbol	Meaning	Value
Nano	n	One-billionth	10^{-9}
Micro	µ	One-millionth	10^{-6}
Milli	m	One-thousandth	10^{-3}
Centi	c	One-hundredth	10^{-2}
Deci	d	One-tenth	10^{-1}

1000. mm ⟶ 1.000 m

Figure 1-1 Conversion of units. When the metric prefix gets larger (eg, mL to L, or mm to m), the number in front of the prefix gets smaller. To convert to a larger prefix, the decimal point will move to the left. (Notice that "larger" and "left" both begin with an "L.") In this example, a conversion is made from 1000 mm to meters. The prefix is getting larger, so the decimal point moves to the left. How much does one move the decimal point? The scientific notation for milli- is 10^{-3}, so the decimal point moves three places to the left. Therefore, 1000 mm is equal to 1 m. Converting from larger to smaller units would be the same idea, except the decimal point moves to the right.

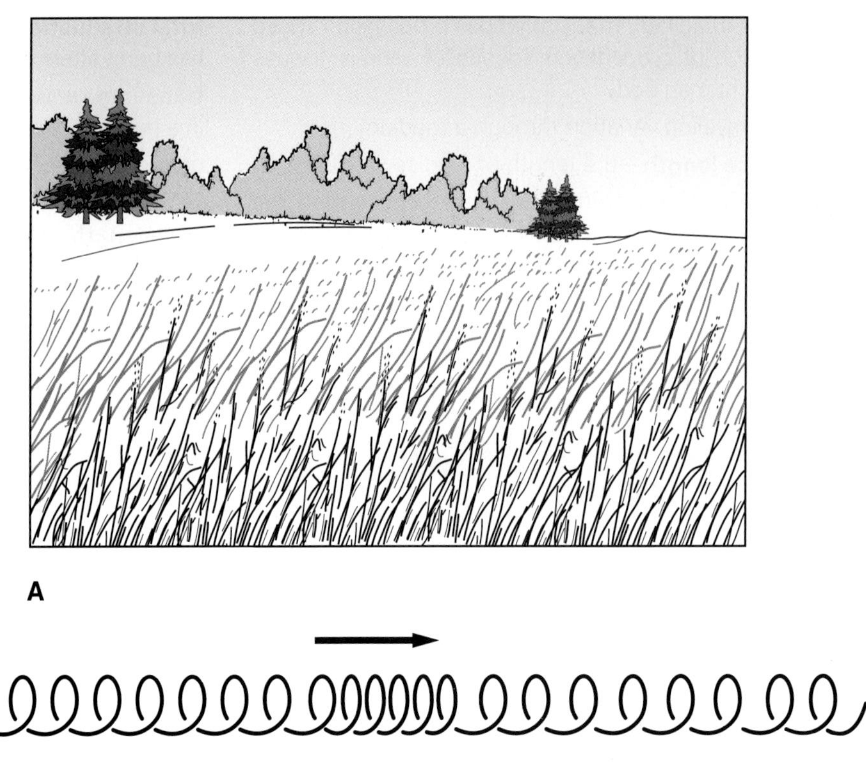

Figure 1-2 Example of longitudinal waves. If a gust of wind blows over a field of tall grass, the stalks bend back and forth in the same direction in which the wind is blowing **(A)**. If another gust of wind blows by, the longitudinal movement is repeated. The energy is traveling in the form of a longitudinal wave **(B)**. The movement of the grass is in the same direction parallel to the movement of the wave.

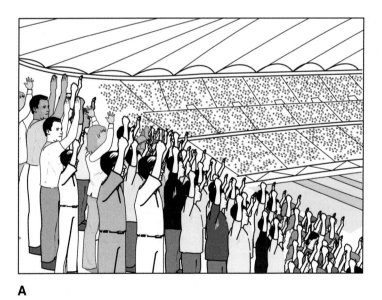

Figure 1-3 Example of transverse waves. **A.** When spectators in a stadium do "the wave," we are experiencing a transverse wave. The arms of the spectators move up and down at 90° to the direction of travel, which is horizontally around the stadium. **B.** The arms of the spectators do not move in the same direction in which the wave is moving, but rather in a direction perpendicular to the travel of the wave.

TABLE 1-3 Ranges of sound

Infrasound	<20 Hz
Audible sound	Between 20 and 20,000 Hz
Ultrasound	>20,000 Hz
Medical diagnostic ultrasound	Between 2 and 20 MHz (or higher)

as infrasound, audible sound, or **ultrasound** based on **frequency**. Frequency can be measured in **hertz** (Hz) (Table 1-3). Diagnostic medical sonography utilizes ultrasound, which ranges in megahertz (MHz), to image the body.

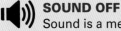

SOUND OFF
Sound is a mechanical, longitudinal wave.

Acoustic Variables

Acoustic variables are changes that occur within a medium as a result of sound traveling through that medium. The three primary acoustic variables are **pressure**, **density**, and **particle motion** (Table 1-4). As stated in the previous section, when sound energy propagates through a medium, it causes the molecules to move back and forth. Each back-and-forth movement completes one wave or one cycle of movement. Each cycle consists of two parts: a **compression**, where the molecules are pushed closer together, and a **rarefaction**, where they are spread wider apart (Figure 1-4). The molecules, as they are squeezed together and separated, cause changes in the pressure within the medium. Similarly, molecules undergoing compression and rarefaction show variations in density. Density is defined as mass per unit volume. **Particle motion** is the back-and-forth motion of the molecules in the medium, and its units are that of **distance**, in millimeters.

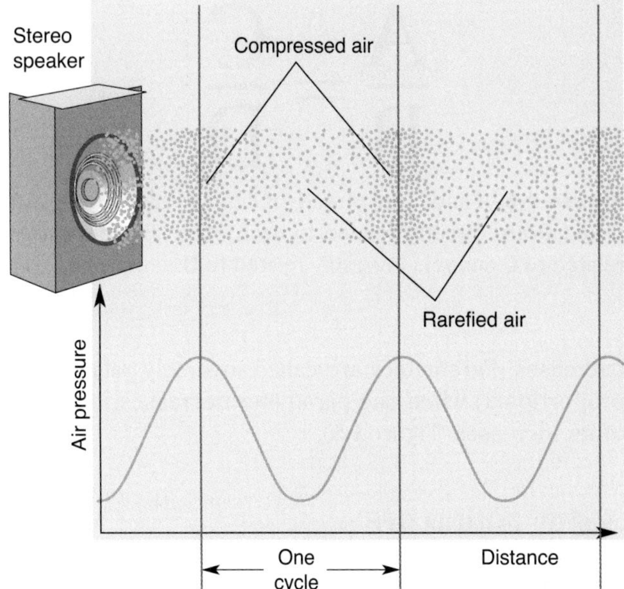

Figure 1-4 The production of sound by variations in air pressure. When the paper cone of a stereo speaker pushes out, it compresses the air, represented by peaks on the graph; when the cone pulls in, it rarefies the air, represented by troughs on the graph. If the push and pull are periodic, there is also a periodic variation in the air pressure, as shown in the graph. The distance between successive compressed (high pressure) patches of air is one cycle of the sound (indicated by the *vertical lines*). The sound wave propagates away from the speaker at the speed of sound.

TABLE 1-4 The three primary acoustic variables, their definitions, and their units

Acoustic Variable	Definition	Units
Pressure	Force per unit area or the concentration of force	Pascals (Pa) or pounds per square inch (lb/in^2)
Density	Mass per unit volume	Kilograms per centimeter cubed (kg/cm^3)
Particle motion	Distance molecules travel in a back-and-forth motion	Feet, inches, centimeters, or miles

SOUND OFF
Each cycle of movement consists of one compression (molecules pushed closer together) and one rarefaction (molecules spread wider apart).

PARAMETERS OF SOUND

A **parameter** is a measurable quantity. Sound waves have several parameters that may be utilized to describe them. Parameters of sound waves include the **period**, frequency, **amplitude**, **power**, **intensity**, **propagation speed**, and **wavelength**. As this chapter progresses, the relationships that these parameters of sound have with each other are discussed. For example, parameters may be described as **directly related** (directly proportional) or **inversely related** (inversely proportional) to each other. They are called directly related (or proportional) when one parameter decreases, then the other also

$$\frac{A}{B} = \frac{C}{D}$$

Figure 1-5 A and C are directly related to each other, and B and D are directly related to each other. B is inversely related to C and A is inversely related to D.

TABLE 1-5 Period

Term	Definition	Units
Period	The time it takes for one cycle to occur	Microseconds (μs), one-millionth of a second

decreases. Parameters are called inversely related (or proportional) when one parameter decreases, then the other increases (Figure 1-5).

> **SOUND OFF**
> Parameters are directly related when with decrease of one parameter, the other parameter also decreases. Parameters are inversely related when with decrease of one variable, the other increases and vice versa.

Period and Frequency

Period (*T*) is defined as the time it takes for one cycle to occur (Figure 1-6). Because period is measured in time units, it is most often described in microseconds (μs) or one-millionth of a second (Table 1-5). Frequency (*f*) is defined as the number of cycles per second (Figure 1-7). Frequency is measured in Hz, kilohertz (kHz), or MHz (Table 1-6). Frequency and period are inversely related. Therefore, as frequency increases, the period decreases, and as frequency decreases, the period increases (Table 1-7). Their relationship is also said to be reciprocal (Table 1-8). When two reciprocals are multiplied together, the product is 1. Consequently, period multiplied by frequency equals 1. Frequency and period are determined primarily by the thickness of the piezoelectric element used to generate the sound and, to a lesser extent, the propagation speed of the element itself (Table 1-9).

> **SOUND OFF**
> The main determinant of frequency (aka the operating frequency, center frequency, or resonating frequency) is the thickness of the piezoelectric element, sometimes described as just the "thickness of the element" (TotE).

Propagation Speed

Propagation speed (*c*) is defined as the speed at which a sound wave travels through a medium (Table 1-10). All sound, regardless of its frequency, travels at the same speed through any particular medium. Therefore, a 20-Hz sound wave and a 20-MHz sound wave travel at the same speed in a given medium (Figure 1-8). Propagation speeds tend to be the fastest in solids, such as bone, and slowest in gases or gas-containing structures, such as the lungs (Table 1-11; Figure 1-9). In the body, sound travels at slightly different speeds through the

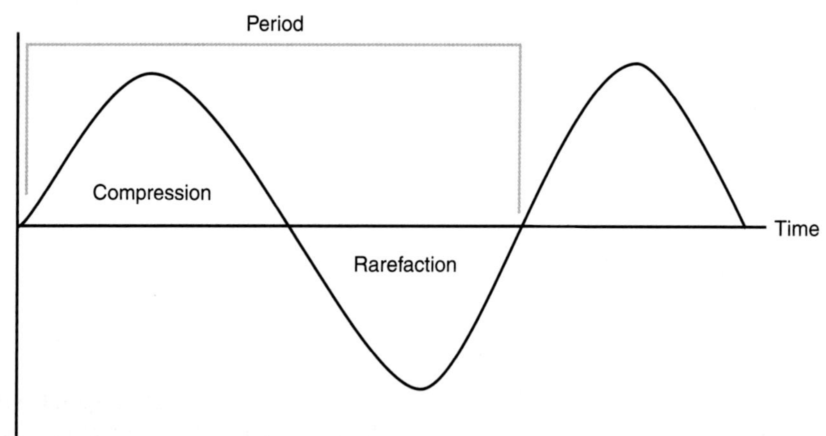

Figure 1-6 Period. Period is defined as the time it takes for one cycle to occur. One cycle consists of one compression and one rarefaction.

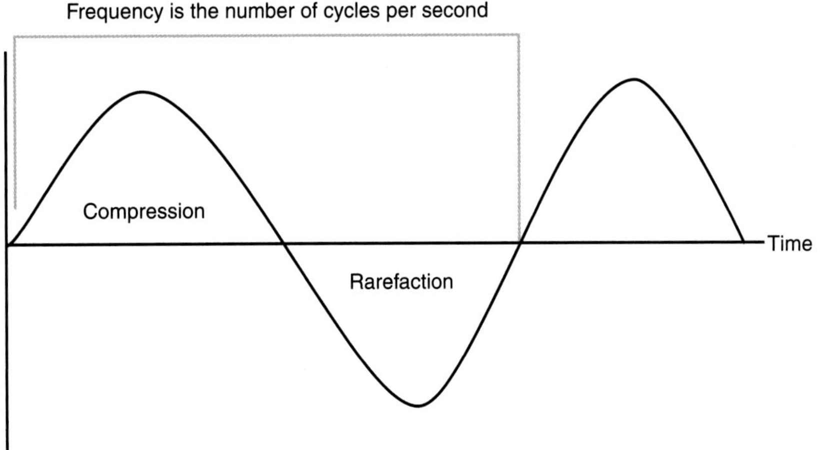

Figure 1-7 Frequency. Frequency is defined as the number of cycles per second.

TABLE 1-6 Frequency

Term	Definition	Units
Frequency	The number of cycles per second	Hertz (Hz), kilohertz (kHz), or megahertz (MHz)

TABLE 1-7 The relationship between frequency and period

Relationship
↑ Frequency ↓ period
↓ Frequency ↑ period

TABLE 1-8 Formula for period

Formula
$\text{Period} = \frac{1}{\text{Frequency}}$ $T = 1/f$

TABLE 1-9 Formula for frequency

Formula
$\text{Frequency} = \frac{\text{propagation speed of the element}}{2 \times \text{thickness of the element}}$ $f = \frac{c}{2 \times \text{TotE}}$

TABLE 1-10 Propagation speed

Term	Definition	Units
Propagation speed	The speed through which a sound wave travels through a medium	Meters per second (m/s) or millimeters per microsecond (mm/μs)

TABLE 1-11 A list of media and their propagation speeds

Medium	Propagation Speed (m/s)
Air	330
Water	1480
Soft tissue	1540 (average)
Liver	1555
Blood	1560
Muscle	1588
Bone	4080

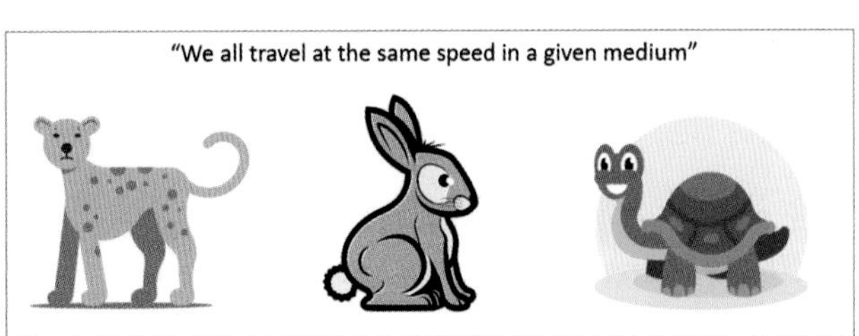
"We all travel at the same speed in a given medium"

Figure 1-8 Propagation speed. All sound, regardless of its frequency, propagates at the same speed through any particular medium. Cheetah, rabbit, or turtle: in a given medium they move at the same speed.

Slow----------------------------------Fast

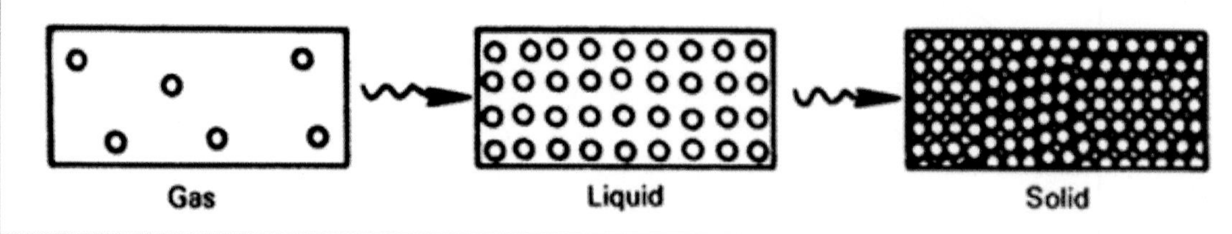

Figure 1-9 Sound propagation through different substances. Propagation speeds tend to be fastest in solids, such as bone, and slowest in gases or gas-containing structures, such as the lungs.

various organs and tissues. The units for propagation speed are meters per second (m/s) or millimeters per microsecond (mm/µs). The average speed of sound in all soft tissue is considered to be 1540 m/s or 1.54 mm/µs. This number was derived by averaging all the actual propagation speeds of the tissues in the body.

> **SOUND OFF**
> All sound, regardless of its frequency, travels at the same speed through any particular medium.

The propagation speed of sound in a medium is influenced by two properties: the **stiffness** (**elasticity**) and the density (**inertia**) of the medium (Table 1-12). Stiffness is defined as the ability of an object to resist compression and relates to the hardness of a medium. Stiffness and propagation speed are directly related: the stiffer the medium, the faster the propagation speed. Conversely, density, which can be defined as the amount of mass in an object, is inversely related to the propagation speed. As the density of a medium increases, the propagation speed decreases (Table 1-13). For example, lead is an extremely dense metal; however, pure lead is not very stiff, because it is quite flexible and, therefore, bends easily. Consequently, the propagation speed in lead is very slow. On the contrary, compact bone is not as dense as lead, but is much stiffer, resulting in a much faster propagation speed. Note that the relationship of stiffness and density to propagation speed is a gross oversimplification, but it is sufficient for performing diagnostic ultrasound exams.

TABLE 1-12 The relationship among stiffness, density, and propagation speed

Relationship
↑ Stiffness ↑ propagation speed
↑ Density ↓ propagation speed

> **SOUND OFF**
> The average speed of sound in "soft tissue" is 1540 m/s or 1.54 mm/µs.

Wavelength

The length of a single cycle of sound is called the wavelength (λ). It is the distance from the beginning of a cycle to the end of that cycle (Figure 1-10). Waves can be of any length, from several miles in some ocean waves to a few millimeters, as found in diagnostic ultrasound waves. In clinical imaging, the wavelengths are measured between 0.1 and 0.8 mm (Table 1-14). Like period, wavelength and frequency are inversely related (Table 1-15). If frequency increases, wavelength decreases and vice versa. However, the wavelength of a sound wave is also influenced by the propagation speed of the medium in which it is traveling. The faster the propagation speed, the longer the wavelength. So, according to our previous sample media, the wavelength of a given frequency would be very short in lead but much longer in bone. In diagnostic imaging, because the average propagation speed of sound in soft tissue is treated as a constant of 1540 m/s, any change in the wavelength would be related only to changes in the frequency. Wavelength is equal to the propagation speed divided by the frequency, $\lambda = c/f$, where $c = 1540$ m/s or 1.54 mm/µs (Table 1-16). It may be helpful to know that the wavelength of a 1- and 2-MHz transducer is 1.54 and 0.77 mm, respectively.

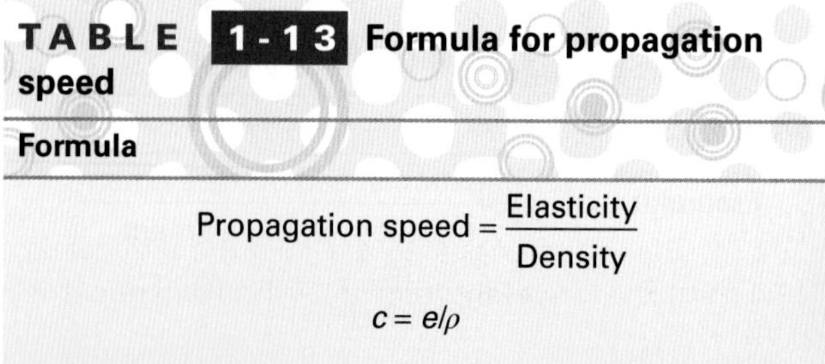

TABLE 1-13 Formula for propagation speed

Formula
$\text{Propagation speed} = \dfrac{\text{Elasticity}}{\text{Density}}$
$c = e/\rho$

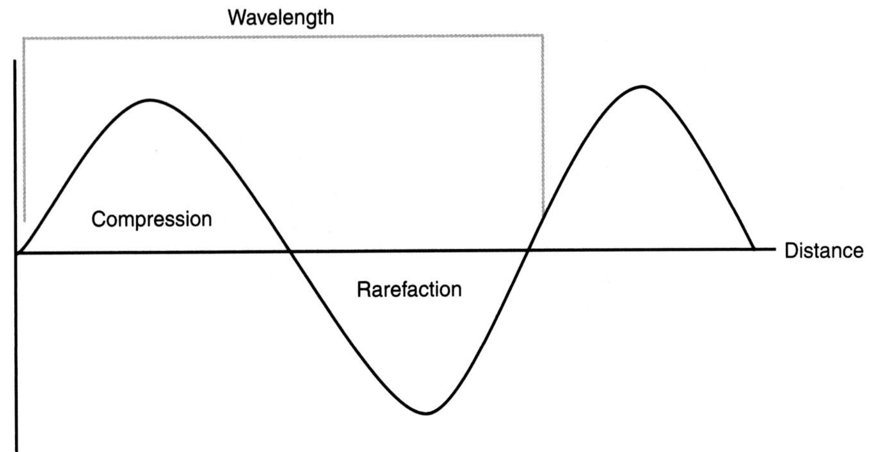

Figure 1-10 Wavelength. Wavelength is the distance from the beginning of a cycle to the end of that cycle.

TABLE 1-14 Wavelength

Term	Definition	Units
Wavelength	The distance over which one cycle occurs or the distance from the beginning of one cycle to the end of that same cycle	Millimeters (mm)

TABLE 1-15 The relationship between wavelength and frequency

Relationship
↑ Frequency ↓ wavelength
↓ Frequency ↑ wavelength

TABLE 1-16 Formula for wavelength

Formula
$\text{Wavelength} = \dfrac{\text{Propagation speed}}{\text{Frequency}}$
$f = c/\lambda$

SOUND OFF
The wavelength of a 1-MHz transducer is 1.54 mm. The wavelength of a 2-MHz transducer is 0.77 mm.

Amplitude, Power, and Intensity

Amplitude, power, and intensity all relate to the strength of the sound wave (Tables 1-17 and 1-18). Amplitude and intensity decrease as sound travels through a medium. Amplitude (*A*) is defined as the maximum or minimum deviation of an acoustic variable from the baseline value of that variable (Figure 1-11). For example, on a road trip, an average velocity may be 55 miles per hour (mph), but occasional increases in speed of up to 60 mph or decreases in speed down to 50 mph may occur. In this situation, the amplitude would be 5 mph, because that is the maximum and minimum variation from the average velocity. Note that the amplitude is not the difference between the maximum and the minimum extremes (aka peak-to-peak amplitude). As sound propagates through a medium, the acoustic variables (particle motion, density, and pressure) will increase and decrease. The amplitude of these changes can be measured. When amplitude is discussed in ultrasound physics, it is commonly the pressure amplitude that is being referenced. The units of pressure amplitude are pascals (Pa).

It is the transmit voltage (pressure) of the ultrasound machine that determines the amplitude, so amplitude can also be expressed in volts (V). The higher the driving voltage of the ultrasound machine, the higher the amplitude of the cycle. In a car stereo, increasing the amplitude of the signal would increase the volume of the sound, that is, make it louder. Figure 1-12 shows how a higher amplitude produces a higher volume.

SOUND OFF
Amplitude is not the difference between the maximum and minimum extremes but rather the deviation from the baseline.

TABLE 1-17 Sound wave strength descriptor and their units

Sound Wave Strength Descriptor	Definition	Units
Amplitude	The maximum value or minimum value of an acoustic variable minus the equilibrium value of that variable; the strength of the reflector	Pascals (Pa) for pressure amplitude
Power	The rate at which work is performed or energy is transmitted	Watts (W) or milliwatts (mW)
Intensity	The amount or degree of strength of sound per unit area or the energy per unit area	Watts per square centimeter (W/cm^2) or mW/cm^2

SOUND OFF
Another analogy for amplitude is to clap your hands softly. You applied a weak pressure, so you heard a weaker sound. Now clap your hands together with more force. You applied a stronger pressure, and the sound increased in amplitude.

SOUND OFF
If amplitude doubles, power is quadrupled. If amplitude triples, power is increased nine times. The reverse is true as well. If amplitude is halved, power is reduced by one-fourth.

Power (*P*) is defined as the rate at which work is performed or energy is transferred. The power of a sound wave is watts (W) or milliwatts (mW). Although amplitude often represents the pressure of the wave, power is the rate of energy transfer. However, power is proportional to the amplitude squared (Table 1-19). Therefore, if amplitude doubles, power quadruples. Figure 1-13 shows the relationship between power and amplitude. The important thing to remember is that they do not have a one-to-one relationship: if amplitude doubles, power is quadrupled. If amplitude triples, power is increased nine times. The reverse is true as well. If amplitude is halved, power is reduced by one-fourth.

TABLE 1-18 The relationships of the sound wave strength descriptors

Relationship
Power and intensity are proportional to amplitude squared
Intensity is proportional to power
Intensity is inversely related to area

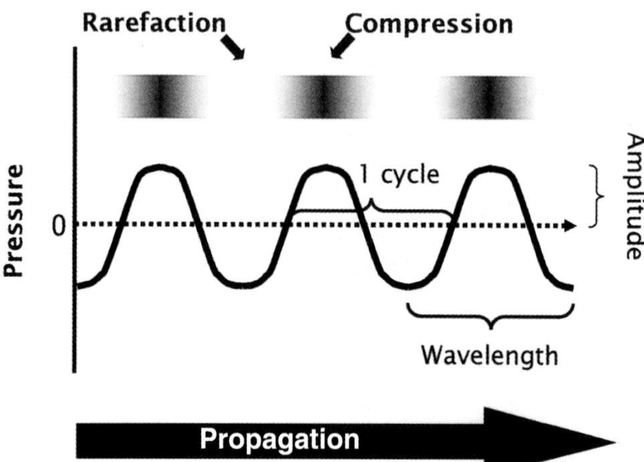

Figure 1-11 Amplitude. This schematic illustrates how sound can be depicted as a sine wave whose peaks and troughs correspond to areas of compression and rarefaction, respectively. The wavelength is the length of one cycle (one compression + one rarefaction) of sound.

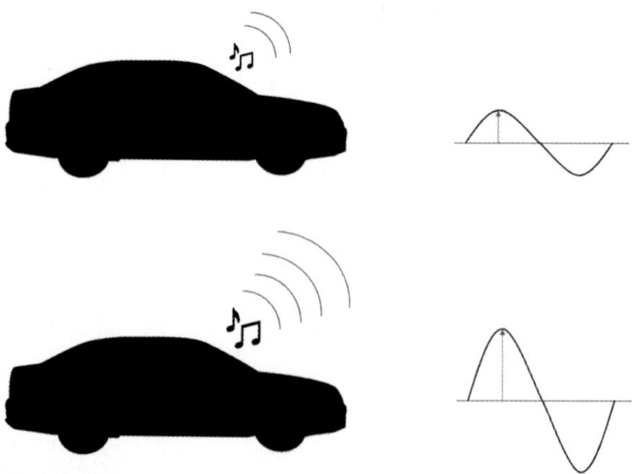

Figure 1-12 Amplitude is analogous to the volume of a stereo. Increasing the voltage (electrical pressure) to the car stereo increases the amplitude (acoustic pressure, or loudness).

TABLE 1-19 Relationship of power (*P*) and amplitude (*A*)

Relationship
$P \propto A^2$

The intensity (*I*) of a sound wave is defined as the power of the wave divided by the area (*a*) over which it is spread or the energy per unit area (Table 1-20). Our Sun produces an immense amount of power. However, one does not simply burst into flames when standing outside because that immense power is spread out over a very large area. However, if you hold a magnifying glass over an object with the Sun overhead, it bursts into flame. The power did not change, but the area decreased, thus increasing the intensity. Intensity is directly proportional to power ($I \propto P$) and also proportional to the amplitude squared ($I \propto A^2$). Intensity is measured in units of watts per square centimeter (W/cm^2) or milliwatts per square centimeter (mW/cm^2). Intensities typically range from 0.01 to 100 mW/cm^2 for diagnostic ultrasound. Intensity is discussed in more detail later in this chapter (see the "More about Intensity" section). Table 1-21 lists some sample problems of amplitude, intensity, and power.

SOUND OFF
The impedance of a medium depends on the density and the propagation speed of the medium.

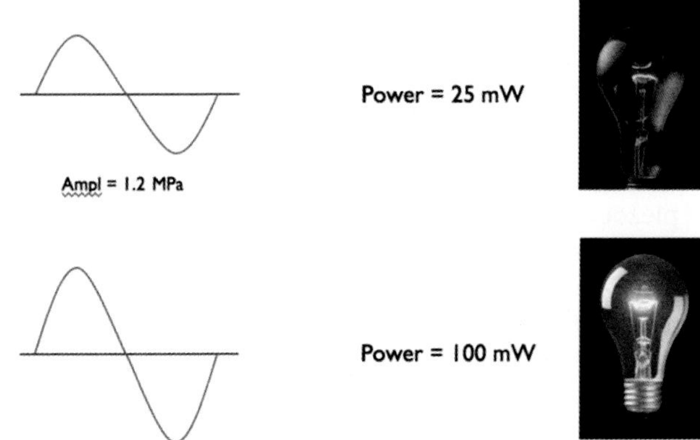

Figure 1-13 Relationship between power and amplitude. As seen here, if amplitude is doubled, then power is quadrupled.

TABLE 1-20 Formula for intensity (*I*)

Formula
$I = A = \dfrac{\text{Power (W)}}{\text{Area (cm}^2\text{)}}$

Impedance

Any medium sound is traveling through will offer some amount of resistance to the sound. For example, some of us can run fairly quickly on dry land. But trying to run at the same speed in 3 feet (ft) of water would be quite challenging. The water resists or impedes our movement. Acoustic resistance to the propagation of sound through a medium is called **impedance** (*z*). The amount of impedance depends on the density (ρ) and the propagation speed (*c*) of the medium. Density and stiffness are the controlling factors of the propagation speed; therefore, impedance has nothing to do with the frequency of the probe, the machine, or the transducer. Impedance is measured in units called rayls, named for Lord Rayleigh, an English physicist. Impedance is the product of the density of the medium and the propagation speed of sound in the medium (Table 1-22).

SOUND OFF
The larger the difference in impedances between two adjacent media, the stronger the return echo. The stronger the return echo, the brighter the "dot" displayed on the screen.

TABLE 1-21 Sample problems

Sample Problems

1. What is the change in intensity if the area is doubled?
   - Intensity is inversely related to the area. If the area is doubled, the intensity is halved.
2. What is the change in intensity if the power and the area of the wave are doubled?
   - Intensity is directly proportional to the power but inversely related to the area. If the power *and* the area increase, there is no change in intensity.

TABLE 1-22 Formula for impedance

Formula
$z = \rho c$

c, propagation speed; *ρ*, density; *z*, impedance.

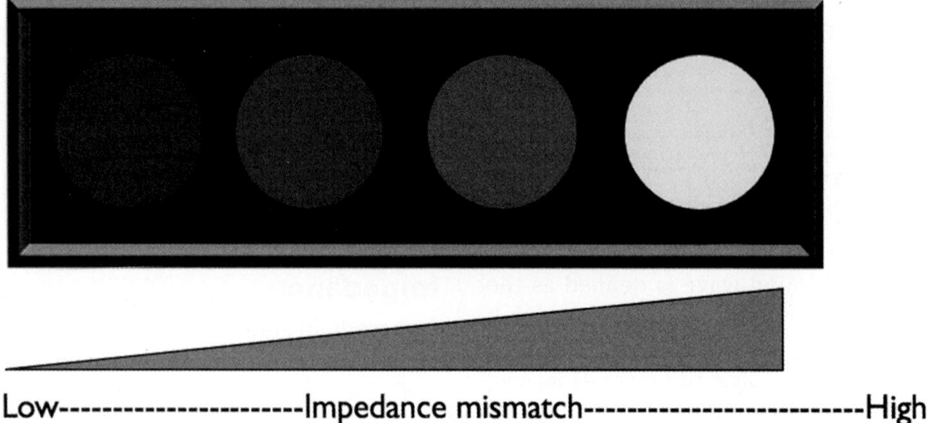

Figure 1-14 The greater the impedance mismatch, the stronger the return echo. The stronger the return echo, the brighter the dot on the screen.

There are slight variations in the density of the various tissues in the body just as there are slight variations in the propagation speed. Recall that 1540 m/s is used as the *average* speed of sound in all soft tissues. As a result, many tissues will have different impedance values. It is these variations in impedance that help create reflections at the **interface** between adjacent tissues. Assuming the beam strikes the interface at a 90° angle, and there exists a large impedance difference between two tissues, there will be a strong **reflection** and a well-defined boundary displayed on the imaging screen. If the impedance difference between two media is more subtle, there will be a weaker reflection. If impedances are the same, no reflection occurs. Figure 1-14 illustrates the concept that the bigger the impedance mismatch, the stronger the return echo. The stronger the return echo, the brighter the dot on the screen. The principle of reflection is described in more detail in the "More About Reflection" section.

CONTINUOUS-WAVE ULTRASOUND

Thus far in this chapter, we have been describing general properties of sound waves, with a special focus on ultrasound wave transmission. Ultrasound equipment can produce sound either in pulses or continuously. Sound that is continuously transmitted is termed **continuous-wave** (CW) ultrasound. CW ultrasound equipment requires the use of two piezoelectric elements at a minimum because piezoelectric elements can transmit and receive, but not at the same time. One element is tasked with transmitting sound, and the other element is constantly receiving the sound. No part of the machine is timing how long it takes sound to propagate, so an image is not obtained image using CW ultrasound. CW ultrasound is only used for spectral Doppler studies, either as part of an imaging transducer or a dedicated CW probe. CW devices are discussed further in Chapter 4 of this book.

PULSE-ECHO TECHNIQUE AND PARAMETERS OF PULSED SOUND

Pulse-Echo Technique

For an image to be created using sound, not only must the sound waves be sent into the body, but the sound returning from the body must be timed to determine the reflector's distance from the transducer; this describes the pulse-echo technique or principle (Figure 1-15). After a pulse is sent out, the machine waits for the sound to come back, calculating the time that it takes for the pulse to return to the transducer. This waiting time is the listening or dead time. As a result of waiting for the pulse of sound to come back and timing its travel, the machine can plot the location of the reflectors on the display. As the reflections come back, a scan line is created. As the scan lines are placed side by side, an image, or frame is created. This will be described in more detail in Chapter 3.

Transducers have materials within them that, when electronically stimulated, produce ultrasound waves. These materials are referred to as **piezoelectric materials** and most likely consist of some form of lead zirconate titanate (PZT). PZT operates according to the principle of piezoelectricity, which states that pressure is created when voltage is applied to the material, and electricity is created when a pressure is applied to the material (Figure 1-16). "*Piezo*" is from the Greek language (πιέζω) and means to squeeze or press. Although PZT is the predominant transducer material used today, newer technology and materials may also be used, which are described in more detail in Chapter 2. Within the transducer, when electricity is applied to the element, a pressure wave (in the form of a sound wave) is produced by the vibration of the piezoelectric material. Diagnostic ultrasound uses

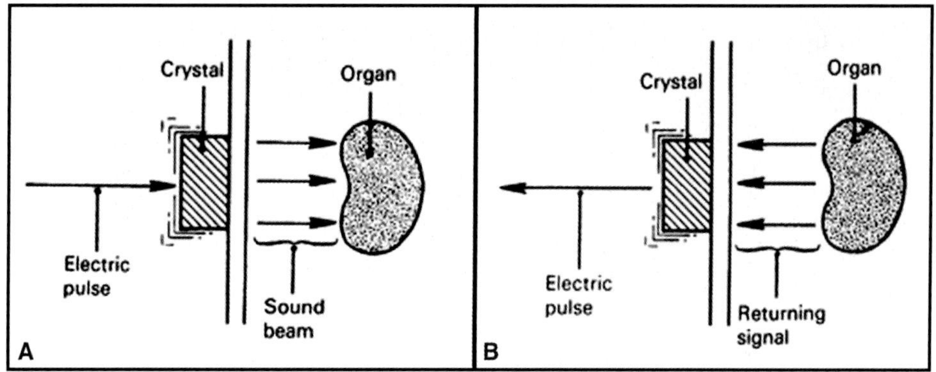

Figure 1-15 Pulse-echo principle. **A.** When an electrical pulse is provided to the crystal, the crystal vibrates, and a pulse of sound is produced and sent into the body. **B.** The sound wave hits a reflector and is then returned to the crystal, causing the crystal to vibrate again, generating the electrical pulse comparable to the strength of the returning echo.

high-frequency sound waves that are sent into the body by the transducer (transmission), and then the transducer momentarily listens for returning echoes (reflection). The characteristics of the returning echoes are utilized by the ultrasound machine to create an image. The process by which sound waves are produced and received by the machine is described in detail in Chapter 3.

Table 1-23 presents all the cycle parameters discussed thus far in this chapter.

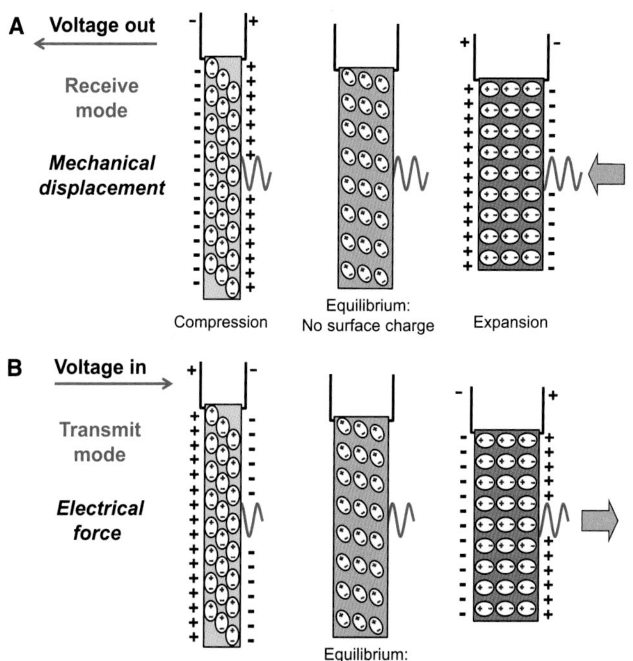

Figure 1-16 Piezoelectric crystal. **A.** When a pressure is applied across the crystal, the highly polarized molecular dipoles rotate, causing the crystal to expand and contract, producing electricity. **B.** Conversely, when a voltage is applied, sound wave is produced. Reprinted with permission from Bushberg JT, Seibert JA, Leidholdt Jr. EM, Boone JM. *The Essential Physics of Medical Imaging*. 4th ed. Wolters Kluwer; 2020:559. Figure 14-7.

Parameters of Pulsed Sound

Pulsed-wave (PW) sound has several specific parameters as well. Parameters of PW sound include the **pulse repetition frequency** (PRF), **pulse repetition period** (PRP), **pulse duration** (PD), **duty factor** (DF), and **spatial pulse length** (SPL).

Pulse Repetition Frequency

Remember that the operating frequency, also called the center frequency or resonating frequency, (in Hz, typically MHz), is defined as the number of cycles of sound produced in 1 s. The number of pulses of sound produced in 1 s is called the PRF. Frequency and PRF are not the same. In fact, they are not related in any way. Think of a train made up of five coaches. These represent five pulses. The people on the train represent frequency. Whether there are 2 people (2 Hz) in each coach or 200 (200 Hz), the number of coaches (pulses) stays the same. Therefore, a transducer may produce sound at a frequency of 2 MHz, but it sends out five pulses of this sound every second. Here, the *frequency* is 2 MHz, but the *PRF* is 5 Hz. If the machine sends out 15 pulses per second, the PRF changes to 15 Hz, but the frequency of the sound is still 2 MHz. In diagnostic imaging, the PRF has typical values between 1000 and 10,000 Hz (1 to 10 kHz) (Table 1-24). It is critical

TABLE 1-23 Parameters of sound

Parameter	Units	Formula (Where Applicable)
Frequency (f)	Hz	1/thickness of the element
Period (T)	μs	$1/f$
Wavelength (λ)	mm	c/f
Propagation speed	m/s or mm/μs	$c \propto \varepsilon/\rho$
Impedance	rayls	$z = \rho c$

TABLE 1-24 Pulse repetition frequency

Term	Definition	Units
Pulse repetition frequency	The number of ultrasound pulses emitted in 1 second	Kilohertz (kHz)

TABLE 1-25 Relationship between imaging depth and pulse repetition frequency (PRF)

Relationship
↑ Imaging depth, ↓ PRF
↓ Imaging depth, ↑ PRF

that the pulse term "PRF" is not confused with the cycle term "operating frequency" or just "frequency." Despite sounding similar, the two terms have no relation to each other, and the PRF is completely independent of the operating/transducer frequency.

SOUND OFF

Do not confuse the cycle term "operating frequency" or just "frequency" with the pulse repetition frequency (PRF). These two terms have no relation to each other, and the PRF is completely independent of the operating/transducer frequency.

The PRF changes whenever the sonographer adjusts the depth control on the ultrasound machine. Recall that when a pulse of sound is emitted, the machine waits for echoes to return before sending out another pulse. If the imaging depth is shallow, echoes return quickly. If the area of interest is deep, it will take a longer time for echoes to get back to the transducer. Therefore, the deeper the area of interest, the slower the PRF (Table 1-25). Depth and PRF are inversely related to each other: as the imaging depth increases, the PRF decreases, and as the depth decreases, the PRF increases. Figure 1-17 demonstrates this principle with a person bouncing a basketball against the wall. If

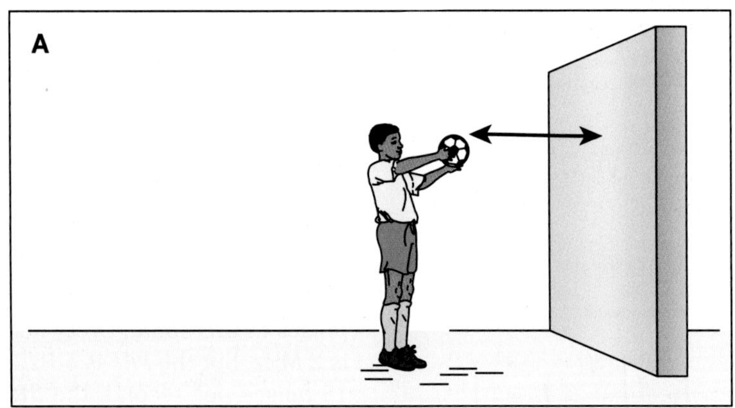

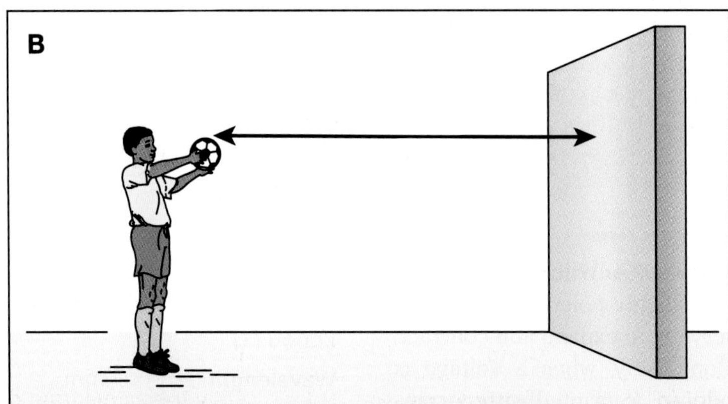

Figure 1-17 Pulse repetition frequency (PRF). A simple comparison for PRF is the act of bouncing a ball against a wall. **A.** If the distance (depth) from the wall is decreased, the bounce repetition rate is increased (↑ PRF). **B.** If the distance from the wall is increased, the bounce repetition rate decreases (↓ PRF).

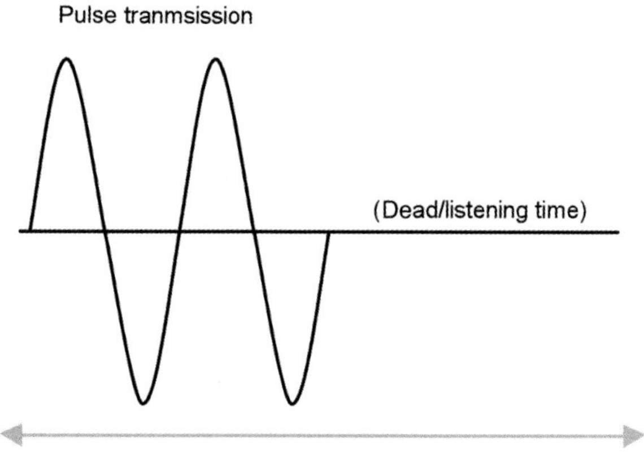

Figure 1-18 Pulse repetition period (PRP). PRP is the time of the pulse including the listening time. It is measured from the beginning of one pulse to the beginning of the next pulse.

the person is standing close to the wall (Figure 1-15 A), the ball will strike the wall and return rapidly because of a short distance. Therefore, with a short distance (depth), the bounce repetition rate will be high. If the person moves farther away from the wall (Figure 1-15 B), the distance (depth) increases, and the bounce repetition rate will decrease because the distance increased, and it takes longer for the ball to reach the wall and return.

SOUND OFF
The PRF is altered by adjusting the depth control on the machine. Depth and PRF are inversely related.

Pulse Repetition Period

Previously, it was noted that the period (time of one cycle) is inversely related to frequency (number of cycles per second). Similarly, the time it takes for a pulse to occur plus the listening/dead time (PRP) is inversely related to the frequency of the pulses (PRF). The time taken for a pulse to occur plus the listening/dead time is called the pulse repetition period or PRP (Figure 1-18). The PRP is the time from the start of one pulse to the start of the next pulse, and, therefore, it includes the "on" (or transmit) and "off" (or listening) times (Table 1-26). The relationship between the PRP and the PRF is similar to that between the period and frequency: when the PRP increases, the PRF decreases and vice versa (Table 1-27).

When imaging of superficial structures is performed, echoes from each pulse return to the transducer quickly, so the time between pulses (PRP) is short. Because the machine is receiving the echoes quickly, it can emit pulses at a faster rate (PRF). Imaging deeper in the body takes a longer time for the echoes to return to the transducer, so the time between pulses, the PRP, increases. Consequently, the transducer is unable to emit pulses as often, so the PRF decreases.

TABLE 1-26 Pulsed repetition period (PRP)

Term	Definition	Units
PRP	Time from the beginning of one pulse to the beginning of the next pulse	Milliseconds (ms)

TABLE 1-27 Relationship between pulse repetition frequency (PRF) and pulse repetition period (PRP)

Relationship
↑ PRF ↓ PRP
↓ PRF ↑ PRP

Pulse Duration

Whereas the PRP refers to the time from the beginning of one pulse to the beginning of the next, the PD relates only to the time during which the sound is actually being transmitted, or simply stated, the "on" time (Table 1-28; Figure 1-19). The duration of the "on" time depends on how many cycles are there in the pulse and the period of each cycle. The PD is equal to the number of cycles in the pulse (n) multiplied by how long each cycle lasts (period, T) (Table 1-29).

When the crystal in a transducer vibrates or "rings," it produces long pulses with several cycles in each pulse, that is, a long PD. For imaging purposes, a short PD is preferable. To do this, the vibrations of the crystal are damped by a special backing material inside the transducer. The backing or **damping** layer reduces the long "ring" of a vibrating crystal to two or three cycles per pulse. This decrease in the number of cycles in a pulse (n) helps to improve the image by decreasing the

TABLE 1-28 Pulse duration (PD)

Term	Definition	Units
PD	Only the active time or "on" time that a transducer is pulsing	Microseconds (μs)

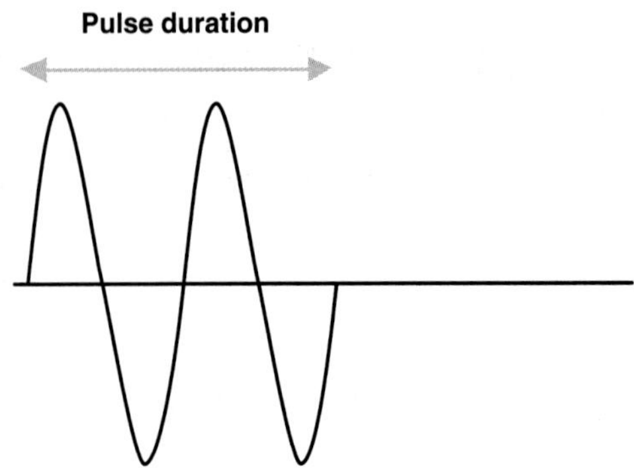

Figure 1-19 Pulse duration (PD). PD is the time of the pulse only during pulse transmission. It is measured from the beginning of one pulse to the end of that pulse.

length of the whole pulse, the SPL, thus improving the **axial resolution**. This is further discussed in Chapter 2. The PD is determined when the transducer is manufactured and cannot be changed by the sonographer.

> **SOUND OFF**
> PD is determined by the transducer manufacturer and cannot be adjusted by the sonographer.

Duty Factor

The percentage of time that sound is being produced is called the duty factor (DF), or duty cycle, and it is equal to PD/PRP (Tables 1-30 and 1-31). If the time between pulses (PRP) is 10.0 μs and the "on" time of the pulse lasts for 5.0 μs, then sound is being produced 50% of the time from one pulse to another. If the "on" time is reduced to 2.0 μs, then sound is being made only 20% of the time between pulses. An ultrasound system with a DF of 100% is CW ultrasound, as it is transmitting 100% of the time. Pulsed ultrasound will always have a DF less than 100% because the machine must wait for all echoes to return before transmitting a new pulse. In clinical PW imaging, the DF is typically 1% or less (Figure 1-20). Table 1-32 has sample problems related to PD, PRP, and DF.

> **SOUND OFF**
> The typical DF for PW imaging is less than 1%.

TABLE 1-29 Formula for pulse duration (PD)

Formula
PD = number of cycles × period PD = nT or n/f

TABLE 1-30 Duty factor (DF)

Term	Definition	Units
DF	The percentage of "on" time only	No unit

TABLE 1-31 Formula for duty factor (DF)

Formula
$DF = \frac{PD}{PRP}$

TABLE 1-32 Example of questions on PD, PRP, and DF

1. What happens to the duty factor if the depth is increased?
   - Duty factor (DF) = pulse duration (PD) divided by the pulse repetition period (PRP). It is important to remember that depth is inversely related to PRF and that PRF is inversely related to PRP. Therefore, depth is directly related to PRP. If the depth increases, the PRP increases, and the DF will decrease.
2. What is the change in duty factor if the frequency increases?
   - This is where it helps to take an equation down to the DNA. Remember that PD = n/f. If the frequency increases, PD decreases. $DF = \frac{PD}{PRP}$. If the PD decreases, the DF decreases. In summary, if the frequency goes up, the DF goes down.

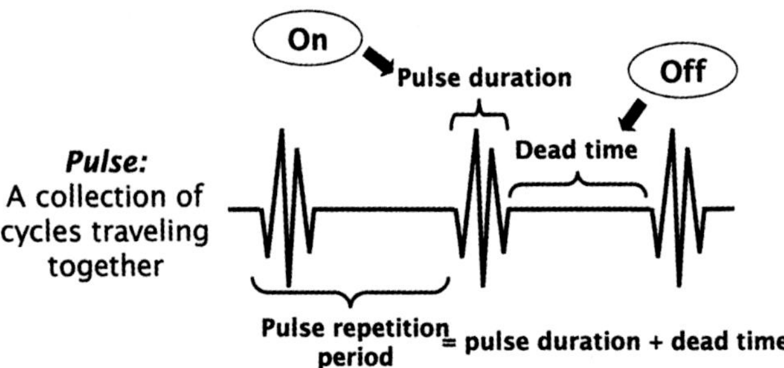

Figure 1-20 Duty factor. Comparison between PD, DF, and PRP. Ultrasound energy is usually emitted from the transducer in a series of pulses, each one representing a collection of cycles. Each pulse has a transmission duration and is separated from the next pulse by the dead time. DF, duty factor; PD, pulse duration; PRP, pulse repetition period.

SOUND OFF
Damping reduces the SPL by reducing the number of cycles of each pulse. This damping reduces the PD and SPL and consequently improves axial resolution.

Spatial Pulse Length

SPL is defined as the length of a pulse (Table 1-33). The length of the pulse depends on the wavelength of each cycle and the number of cycles in each pulse (Table 1-34). Therefore, the SPL equals the number of cycles (n) in the pulse multiplied by the wavelength (λ). If the wavelength increases, the SPL increases and vice versa. If the number of cycles in the pulse increases, then the SPL also increases. Either of these would result in a longer lasting pulse or a long PD. SPL, like PD, can be controlled with damping or backing material. Damping reduces the SPL by reducing the number of cycles of each pulse (n). This damping reduces the PD and SPL and consequently improves axial resolution. To expand on this concept, remember that the wavelength is inversely related to the frequency of the sound in a given medium. So, higher frequencies have shorter wavelengths, and shorter wavelengths result in shorter SPLs. Shorter SPLs mean shorter PDs, and therefore better axial resolution and improved image quality. Table 1-35 has a sample question on SPL.

TABLE 1-33 Spatial pulse length (SPL)

Term	Definition	Units
SPL	The length of a pulse from beginning to end	Millimeters (mm)

TABLE 1-34 Formula for spatial pulse length (SPL)

Formula
SPL = number of cycles × wavelength $SPL = n\lambda$

TABLE 1-35 Examples of questions relating to SPL

1. During the manufacturing process, the frequency of a transducer is changed from 2.0 to 4 MHz. What is the resultant change in the spatial pulse length?
   - By looking at the SPL equation, which is $SPL = n\lambda$, it does not appear that frequency is part of the equation. However, you can further break the equation down to be written as: $SPL = \frac{c}{f}n$. Now, you see that frequency is inversely related to SPL. If the frequency increases, the pulse gets shorter.

THE SOUND SOURCE AND THE MEDIUM

Parameters of sound can be determined by the sound source, the medium through which the sound is traveling, or a combination of both. The sound source means the device that is creating the sound. The medium is the tissue through which the sound waves are traveling. Tables 1-36 and 1-37 provide a summary.

TABLE 1-36 Sound wave parameters

Determined by Sound Source	Determined by Medium	Determined by Sound Source and Medium
• Period • Frequency • Amplitude, power, and intensity	• Propagation speed • Impedance	• Wavelength

TABLE 1-37 Pulsed sound wave parameters

Determined by Sound Source	Determined by Sound Source and Medium
• Pulse duration • Duty factor • Pulse repetition period • Pulse repetition frequency	• Spatial pulse length

INTERACTIONS OF SOUND WITH TISSUE

Attenuation

Attenuation is a decrease in the amplitude and intensity of the sound beam as sound travels through tissue. There are three mechanisms of attenuation: **absorption**, reflection, and **scattering**. When evaluating two intensities, powers, or amplitudes, the units of **decibels** (dB) are used. Decibels imply that one thing is being compared with another, such as the initial intensity and the end intensity. If an intensity or power doubles, it changes by 3 dB. Similarly, if an intensity or power

TABLE 1-38 Decibel (dB) chart for intensity/power

Increasing Intensity/ Power		Decreasing Intensity/ Power	
0	No change	−0	No change
3	Double	−3	One-half
6	Quadruple	−6	One-fourth
10	10 times	−10	One-tenth
20	100 times	−20	One-hundredth

decreases by half, it has changed by −3 dB. Table 1-38 provides a summary of dB changes. This chart is suitable only for intensity or power because amplitude uses a different equation.

Absorption, the conversion of sound energy to heat, is the greatest contributor to attenuation in tissue. It is also a potential source of thermal bioeffects, as will be discussed in further detail in Chapter 6. The amount of attenuation that occurs as sound travels is related to the frequency of the beam. As the frequency increases, attenuation increases (Table 1-39). Thus, it is important to remember that high-frequency transducers do not penetrate the body as well as lower frequency transducers.

SOUND OFF
There are three mechanisms of attenuation: absorption, reflection, and scattering.

SOUND OFF
Absorption (production of heat) is the greatest contributor to attenuation in tissue.

The **attenuation coefficient** (in dB/cm) is the rate at which sound is attenuated per unit depth. It is equal to one-half of the frequency ($f/2$) in soft tissue. **Attenuation** is the total amount of sound (in dB) that has been attenuated at a given depth. To determine the total amount of attenuation, one needs to know the **rate of attenuation** and the **path length**. The path length is the distance to the reflector. As the path length increases, attenuation increases (Table 1-40). Note that the rate of attenuation,

TABLE 1-39 Relationship between frequency and attenuation

Relationship
↑ Frequency ↑ attenuation

TABLE 1-40 Relationship between path length and attenuation

Relationship
↑ Path length ↑ attenuation

the attenuation coefficient, does not change with depth. Only the total amount of attenuation changes with path length.

SOUND OFF
Attenuation is the total amount of sound (in dB) that has been attenuated at a given depth:

Attenuation (dB) = attenuation coefficient (A_c − in dB/cm) × path length (L − in cm).

The act of traveling on a toll road can be used to demonstrate the attenuation of the sound beam. For example, let's take an imaginary road trip on I-95 from Philadelphia to Washington, D.C. On this imaginary road, there is a toll booth every mile. The toll, or price that a car pays to travel, is $1.00 per mile, and it does not change with distance. If someone traveled 103 miles to stop off at Inner Harbor, Baltimore, MD, the total toll paid would be $103 ($1 toll × 103 miles = $103). At the end of the trip of 137 miles, the total toll paid would be $137 ($1 toll × 137 miles). Instead of dollars per mile, sound must pay a toll in dB for every centimeter (cm) it propagates through soft tissue. The toll that sound pays is called the **attenuation coefficient** (A_c), which is measured in dB/cm. The total amount of sound lost at the end of the path is called **attenuation,** or sometimes "total attenuation" (Figure 1-21).

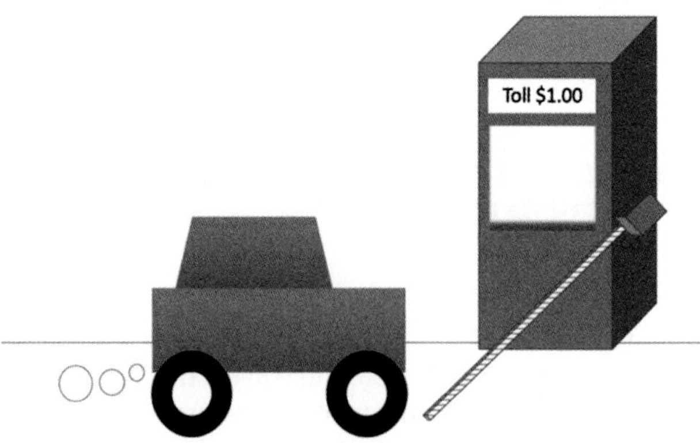

Figure 1-21 Attenuation. When taking a road trip, imagine paying $1.00 for every mile of travel. Note that the toll does not change regardless of where on the highway you are: it's always $1.00/mile. Now imagine traveling 100 miles. How much was the total toll paid? $100.

TABLE 1-41 Formula for attenuation coefficient

Formula	Example
Attenuation (dB) = Attenuation coefficient (A_c) × path length (L) $\text{Atten} = \frac{f}{2} \times L$ or $\text{Atten} = A_c$	If a 10-MHz sound travels through soft tissue, how much attenuation has occurred at a depth of 5 cm? Attenuation coefficient = $f/2$ = 10 MHz/2 = 5 dB/cm Attenuation = $f/2 \times L$ = 5 dB/cm × 5 cm = 25 dB

The A_c is the same as the highway toll in the example above. It is the rate at which sound is lost in dB per unit distance (cm) and is equal to one-half the frequency ($f/2$) in soft tissue. If the A_c, or toll, is known and the path length (L, the distance of the trip, in cm) is known, the attenuation (total toll paid in dB) can be calculated (Table 1-41). The average rate of attenuation in soft tissue is 0.7 dB/cm/MHz, although authors vary between 0.5 and 1.0 dB/cm/MHz.

Sample question: A 6-MHz transducer produces a beam that propagates to a depth of 10 cm. What is the attenuation coefficient at 10 cm depth?

Did you say 30 dB? If you did, it is incorrect. Read the question again: the question is asking for the attenuation coefficient (the "toll"), which does not change with depth. It is a constant at all depths because it is only based on ½*f*. If the question writer had asked for the "attenuation of 6 MHz sound at 10 cm," then an attenuation of 30 dB would be correct because attenuation is ½*f* multiplied by the path length (L).

Another term related to attenuation is **half-intensity depth** (HID) or **half-value layer thickness**. This term describes the depth at which sound has lost half (–3 dB) of its intensity. In soft tissue, the HID is equal to 6/*f*. Therefore, for a 1-MHz transducer, the HID is 6/6 or 1 cm. For a 12-MHz transducer, the HID is 6/12 or 0.5 cm. Tip: when taking the examination, if an attenuation question asks you to solve for a depth, it may be the HID equation. Table 1-42 has sample questions related to attenuation.

SOUND OFF
In soft tissue, the HID is equal to 6/*f*. Therefore, for a 1-MHz transducer, the HID is 6/6 or 1 cm. For a 12-MHz transducer, the HID is 6/12 or 0.5 cm.

Specular and Nonspecular Reflectors

An interface is the dividing line between two different media. At the interface, the sound may be absorbed, reflected, scattered, transmitted, or refracted. Reflectors in the medium are often referred to as being either specular or **nonspecular reflectors**.

Specular reflections occur when the sound impinges upon a large, smooth reflector at the 90° angle. (Specular is Latin for "mirror.") A specular reflector is one in which the size of the reflector is larger than the

TABLE 1-42 Examples of questions related to attenuation

1. 3-MHz sound propagates for 60 mm in soft tissue. What is the total attenuation of sound at that depth?
   - First, solve for the attenuation coefficient:
     $$\text{Attenuation coefficient } (A_c) = \frac{1}{2}f = (0.5)(3\text{ MHz}) = 1.5\text{ dB/cm}.$$
   - Then, solve for attenuation:
     $$\text{Attenuation} = A_c \times \text{path length (AcL), so attenuation} = 1.5\text{ dB/cm} \times 6\text{ cm} = -9\text{ dB}.$$
2. What is the frequency of the transducer if the attenuation coefficient is 4 dB/cm?
   - $A_c = \frac{f}{2} \rightarrow f = A_c \times 2 \rightarrow f = 4\text{ dB/cm } (2) = 8\text{ MHz}.$
3. At what depth is the intensity of sound reduced by half (–3 dB) if the frequency is 12 MHz?
   - $\text{HID} = \frac{6}{f} = \frac{6}{12} = 0.5\text{ cm or 5 mm}.$

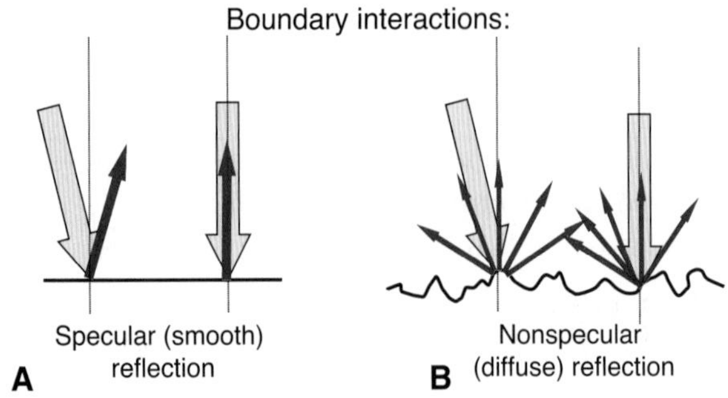

Figure 1-22 Reflection and scattering. The interaction between an ultrasound wave and its target depends on several factors. **A.** A specular reflection occurs when ultrasound encounters a target that is large relative to the transmitted wavelength. Specular reflections only occur when the beam is at normal incidence, which is perpendicular to the boundary between two adjacent tissues. The amount of ultrasound energy that is reflected to the transducer by a specular reflector is proportional to the impedance difference or mismatch. At an oblique angle of incidence, sound does not return to the transducer. **B.** Reflectors that are small relative to the transmitted wavelength produce a scattering of ultrasound energy, resulting in a small portion of energy being returned to the transducer. This type of interaction results in "speckle" that produces the texture within tissues. Scattered sound that returns to the transducer is called backscatter.

wavelength of the incident beam (Figure 1-22). Examples of specular reflectors are the diaphragm, the capsules of organs, and the wall of the aorta (Table 1-43). Specular reflections are highly angle dependent, that is, if the sound strikes a reflector at an oblique angle, the reflection will not return to the transducer. Therefore, the best two-dimensional (2D) images come from striking a reflector perpendicular to the interface.

SOUND OFF
The best 2D images come from striking a reflector perpendicular (90°) to the interface.

TABLE 1-43 Specular versus nonspecular reflectors

Specular Reflectors	Nonspecular Reflectors
Smooth surface	Rough surface
Border is larger than the incident wavelength (λ)	Border is smaller than the incident wavelength (λ)
Angle dependent	Not angle dependent

Nonspecular reflectors are the ones in which their size is smaller than the wavelength of the incident beam. The parenchyma of an organ is an example of nonspecular reflectors. Nonspecular reflectors scatter sound in many different directions. Some of this sound, termed **backscatter**, makes it back to the transducer and produces an image on the display. The intensity of a backscatter is much lower than that from specular reflectors, although nonspecular reflectors are not angle dependent compared with specular reflectors. A scatter permits the imaging of the parenchyma, whereas specular reflectors are the boundaries. When sound strikes a number of scatterers, the scatter waves interact with each other (constructively and destructively) and send the result of these interactions back to the transducer. This interference pattern is termed **acoustic speckle** and appears as "parenchyma" on the screen. In other words, when imaging a liver, the tiny dots on the screen that represent liver tissue do not actually represent the liver cells but are the result of all of the scattering reflectors interfering with each other (Figure 1-23). Manufacturers have employed "speckle reduction" algorithms to try to smooth out the appearance of speckle in the image and create a smoother appearing image (Figure 1-24).

With higher frequency transducers, there is a higher intensity of scatter. For this reason, higher frequency transducers are limited to shallower depths. If the energy of the beam is scattered, there is a reduction in the amount of sound that remains to be transmitted through the tissue. Extremely small reflectors, like red

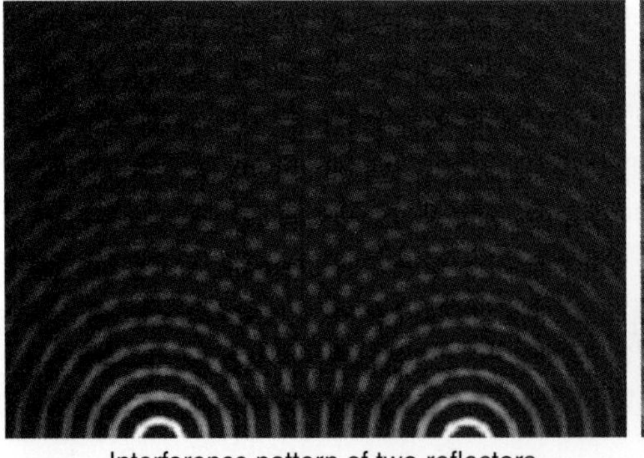
Interference pattern of two reflectors

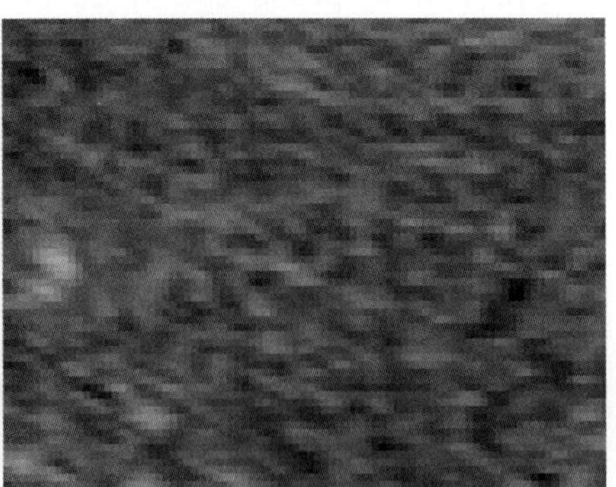
Parenchyma, magnified

Figure 1-23 Acoustic speckle. Acoustic speckle is formed as a result of the interference pattern from multiple interfering scatterers. This gives parenchyma its characteristic look on a sonogram.

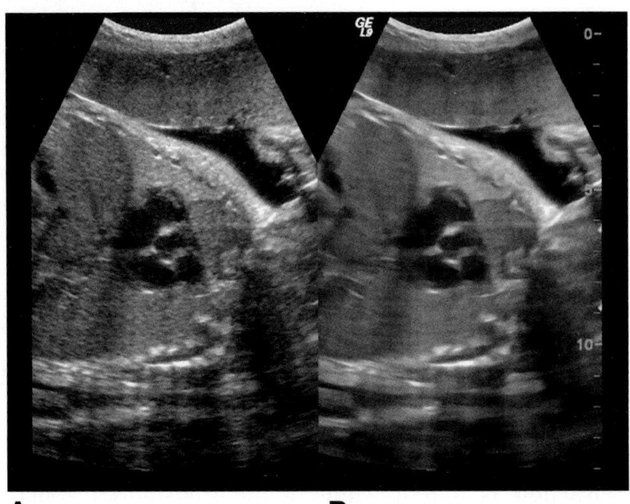

Figure 1-24 Speckle reduction. Speckle reduction algorithms to try to smooth out the appearance of speckle in the image **(A)** and create a smoother-appearing image **(B)**.

blood cells, are termed **Rayleigh scatterers**. Rayleigh scatterers scatter sound equally in all directions (omnidirectional). With Rayleigh scatterers, as the frequency increases, the intensity of scatter increases proportional to the fourth power of the frequency.

SOUND OFF
When sound strikes a number of scatterers, the scatter waves interact with each other (constructively and destructively) and send the result of these interactions back to the transducer. The result appears as what we call "parenchyma."

SOUND OFF
With higher frequency transducers, there is a higher intensity of scatter.

More about Reflection

A reflection is formed when two criteria are met: there is **normal incidence** and the two media have different impedances (Figure 1-25). Synonyms for normal incidence include orthogonal, right angle, perpendicular, and 90°. If there is no change in impedance, then there is no reflection, and all of the sound is transmitted through the tissue. Sound that is transmitted travels through the tissue in the same direction as it was transmitted, and reflected sound returns to the source. That is to say, the angle of reflection equals the angle of incidence.

With **oblique incidence**, which is when the incident sound strikes the interface at a nonperpendicular angle, any sound that is reflected does not return to the transducer and therefore does not produce an image on the display. However, as with normal incidence, the angle of reflection equals the angle of incidence ($\theta_r = \theta_i$). Two types of oblique angles are acute (<90°) and obtuse (>90°). The intensity of sound reflected at an interface depends on the intensity of the transmitted sound and the difference in impedances (aka impedance mismatch) between the two media. The bigger the impedance mismatch, the stronger the reflection. The percentage of sound transmitted at an interface, or **intensity transmission coefficient** (ITC), is equal to 1 minus the percentage of sound reflected at an interface, or **intensity reflection coefficient** (IRC) (Table 1-44). The IRC plus the ITC must equal 100%. If the impedances of the media are the same, then there is no reflection, and the ITC is equal to 100%.

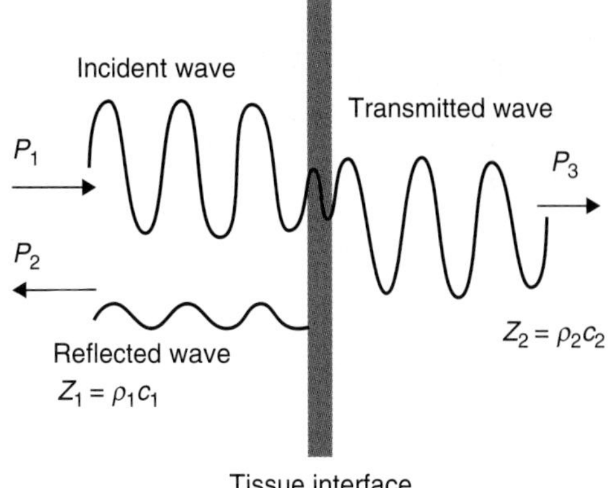

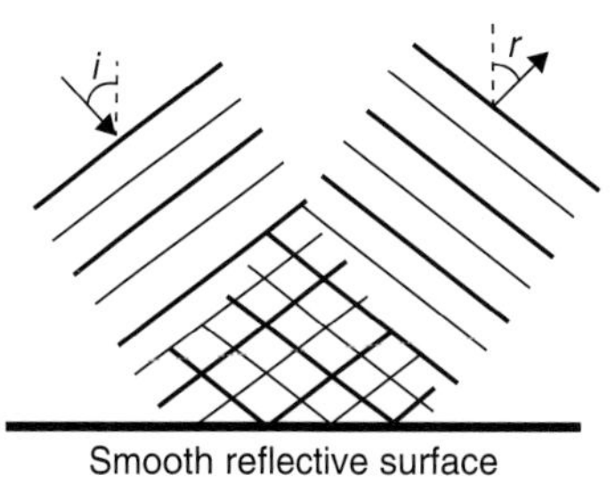

Figure 1-25 Reflection. **A.** The reflection of ultrasound at a flat interface between two media of different acoustic impedance. **B.** The reflection of ultrasound at a smooth interface. *P*, pulse; *Z*, impedance; *ρ*, density; *c*, speed; *I*, incident angle; *r*, reflected angle.

TABLE 1-44 Intensity transmission coefficient (ITC)

Formula	Example
ITC = 1 – IRC	Sound travels through an interface at normal incidence, and 40% of the sound is reflected back to the transducer. How much sound was transmitted at the interface? ITC = 1 – 40% = 60%

TABLE 1-45 Intensity reflection coefficient (IRC)

Formula
$$IRC = \frac{I_r}{I_i} = \left[\frac{Z_2 - Z_1}{Z_2 + Z_1}\right]^2$$

I_i, incident intensity; I_r, reflected intensity; Z_1, impedance one; Z_2, impedance two.

Table 1-45 provides the equation used to calculate the percentage or intensity of the reflected sound. Table 1-46 has examples of questions related to reflection.

SOUND OFF
The intensity of sound reflected at an interface depends on the intensity of the transmitted sound and the difference in impedances between the two media.

SOUND OFF
The angle of reflection always equals the angle of incidence.

SOUND OFF
Another name for the IRC could be the "what percent is reflected?" coefficient. Another name for the ITC could be the "what percent is transmitted?" coefficient.

TABLE 1-47 Reflection versus refraction

Reflection	Refraction
• Normal (perpendicular) incidence • Impedance mismatch • Percentage or intensity of sound reflected and transmitted at an interface	• Oblique incidence • Propagation speed mismatch • Angle of transmitted sound

Refraction

Refraction is a redirection of the transmitted sound beam. Refraction should not be confused with reflection (Table 1-47). With normal incidence, the transmitted beam angle is equal to the incident angle. When sound strikes an interface with an oblique angle of incidence, the transmitted beam angle will equal the incident angle only if the propagation speeds are identical. If there is oblique incidence and a propagation speed mismatch, the transmitted angle will be different from the incident angle. If the propagation speed of medium 2 is *less than* the propagation speed of medium 1, then the angle of transmission will be *less than* the angle of incidence. Likewise, if the propagation speed of medium 2 is *greater than* the propagation speed of medium 1, then the angle of transmission will be *greater than* the angle of incidence (Figure 1-26). **Snell's law** describes the angle of transmission at an interface based on the angle of incidence and the propagation speeds of the two media (Table 1-48). Figure 1-27 is a demonstration of the principle of refraction with light, which is similar to refraction with sound. Table 1-49 has examples of questions related to refraction.

TABLE 1-46 Examples of problems related to reflection

When answering reflection questions, make sure that there is a normal (nonoblique) angle of incidence and different impedances. Otherwise, there will be no reflection, and all sound will be transmitted.

1. Sound travels at normal incidence from medium A, which has an impedance of 800k rayls into medium B, which has an impedance of 800k rayls. What is the intensity reflection coefficient?
   - It is 0%. In order for reflection to occur at an interface, there must be a normal/perpendicular angle of incidence (there is) and an impedance mismatch (which is absent). With no difference in impedances, all sound is transmitted (ITC = 100%) and none of the sound is reflected (IRC = 0%).
2. If sound strikes an interface at a 45° angle? What can be said of the angle of reflection?
   - The angle of reflection is 45° because the angle of reflection *always* equals the angle of incidence, whether the angle of incidence is 0° or oblique.
3. Sound travels through medium A into medium B at normal incidence. The IRC is 40%. If the incident intensity (I_i) is 100 mW/cm^2, what is the transmitted intensity (I_t)?
   - First, solve for I_r, the reflected intensity.
     i. The reflected intensity equals the Incident intensity × IRC = I_i(100 mW/cm^2) × IRC (0.4) = 40 mW/cm^2.
   - Then $I_t = I_i$(100 mW/cm^2) − I_r(40 mW/cm^2) = 60 mW/cm^2.

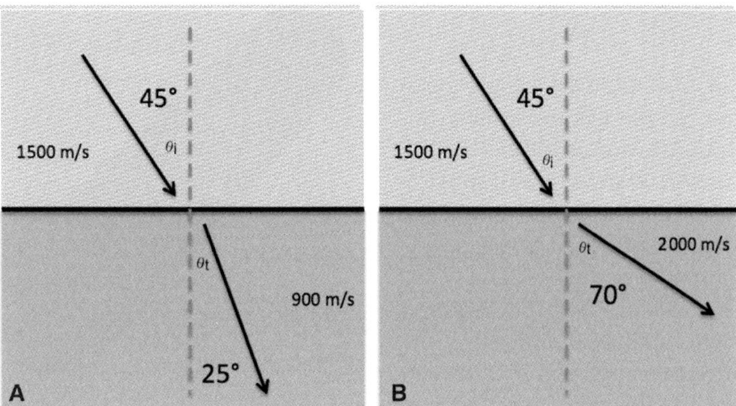

Figure 1-26 Refraction. **A.** If the propagation speed of medium 2 is less than the propagation speed of medium 1, then the angle of transmission will be less than the angle of incidence, or $\theta_t < \theta_i$ if $c_2 < c_1$. **B.** Likewise, if the propagation speed of medium 2 is greater than the propagation speed of medium 1, then the angle of transmission will be greater than the angle of incidence, or $\theta_t > \theta_i$ if $c_2 > c_1$.

SOUND OFF
When sound strikes an interface with an oblique angle of incidence, the transmitted beam angle will equal the incident angle only if the propagation speeds are identical.

SOUND OFF
Be careful not to mix up reflection and refraction. Reflection, which requires normal incidence and a difference in impedances, calculates *how much* sound (what percentage or what intensity) is reflected and/or transmitted at an interface. Refraction, which requires an oblique angle of incidence and a difference in propagation speeds, only provides information on the *angle* of transmitted sound.

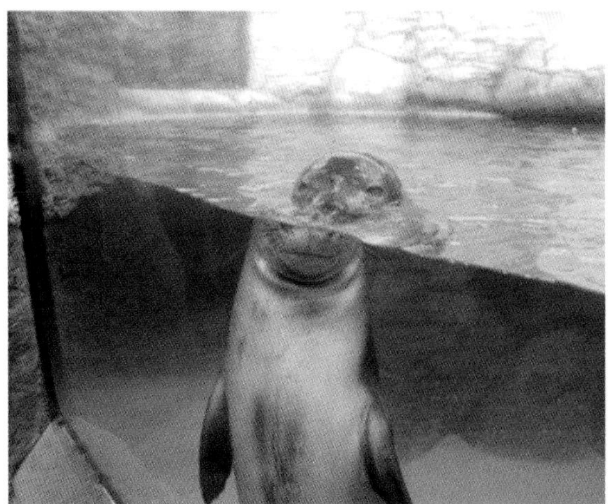

Figure 1-27 Refraction with light. Light and soundwaves have similar wave properties. This photo of a seal shows refraction of light, and the seal's head appears separate from its body.

TABLE 1-48 Snell's law

Formula
$\sin \theta_t = \sin \theta_i \frac{c_2}{c_1}$

c_1 and c_2, the propagation speed of medium 1 and medium 2, respectively; θ_t, the angle of reflection; θ_i, the angle of incidence.

TABLE 1-49 Examples of problems related to refraction

When answering questions about refraction, be sure that there is an oblique (non-90°) angle of incidence and differing propagation speeds.

1. Sound strikes a boundary between two media at a 30° angle. The propagation speed of medium A is 2700 m/s and the propagation speed of medium B is 2700 m/s. What is the angle of refraction?
   - Although there is an oblique angle of incidence, there are identical propagation speeds. Therefore, no refraction occurs, and the angle of transmission is the same as the angle of incidence, that is, 30°.
2. Sound strikes a boundary between two media at a 45° angle. The propagation speed of medium A is 4700 m/s and the propagation speed of medium B is 2700 m/s. What is the angle of refraction? Will it be less than 45°, greater than 45°, or equal to 45°?
   - In this case, the two conditions for refraction are met. There is an oblique angle of incidence and different propagation speeds, so there cannot be an angle of transmission that is identical to the angle of incidence – refraction must occur. Since the propagation speed in medium B is *less than* the propagation speed of medium A, the angle of transmission will be *less than* the angle of incidence. The answer is "less than a 45° angle."

MORE ABOUT INTENSITY

With PW sound operation, the intensity of the beam varies with space and time. Simply acknowledging that the intensity of an ultrasound beam is 100 mW/cm^2 is not always enough information. Many times, it must be specified as to *where* and *when* the sound beam was measured. The spatial intensities, spatial average (SA), and spatial peak (SP) refer to *where* the beam was measured. The SP intensity is measured at the center of the beam. Often, a flashlight analogy is utilized. If one were to look at a flashlight with a single bulb in the center, they would notice that the center of the flashlight yields the brightest light or the most intense light. This is similar to how the ultrasound beam is shaped, that is, the strongest intensity is in the center of the beam and gradually reduces as the beam spreads out. The SA intensity is the average intensity across the face of the entire beam. The **beam uniformity ratio**, also referred to as the SP/SA factor or beam uniformity coefficient, is the ratio of the center intensity to the average spatial intensity (Table 1-50). Because the edge intensity is always less than the center intensity, the SP/SA factor is usually greater than 1. Figure 1-28 depicts the SP and SA of a transducer using a flashlight as an analogy.

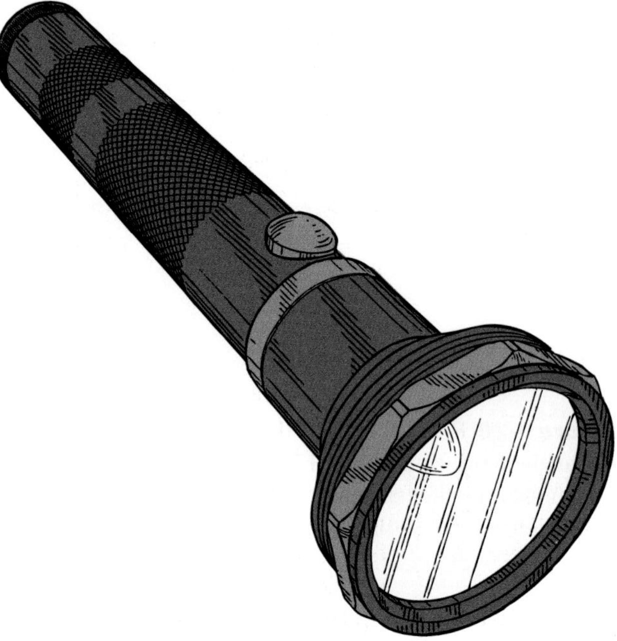

Figure 1-28 The transducer can be thought of as a single-bulb flashlight, with the strongest intensity at the center of the beam (SP) and the average of the intensities (SA) getting weaker toward the edges.

> **SOUND OFF**
> Ultrasound beams are similar to the light produced by a single-bulb flashlight, in that the beam is strongest is in the center of the beam and decreases in brightness as the beam spreads out.

> **SOUND OFF**
> When the transducer is waiting for the pulse to come back, the intensity is zero because the sound is produced only during the transmission phase.

The temporal intensities depict when the beam was measured. The temporal peak (TP) is the intensity measured at the highest intensity, or peak, of the pulse and is, therefore, the highest of all the temporal intensities. The temporal average (TA) is the average of all the intensities during both transmission and the listening period. Note that when the transducer is waiting for the pulse to come back, the intensity is zero, because the sound is produced only during the transmission phase. Because the beam is transmitting only less than 1% of the time in PW operation, the TA is the lowest of all the temporal intensities. This means that 99% of the time, the intensity is zero. The pulse average (PA) is measured only during beam transmission. PA and TA are analogous to PD and PRP in that one is only during sound transmission and the other is during sound transmission and the listening period. As the DF relates PD to PRP, it also relates PA to TA. The formula for TA is provided in Table 1-51. The TA is equal to the PA times the DF. With CW operation, where the DF is equal to 1, the TA is equal to the PA because there is no listening time.

When grouped together, the spatial and temporal intensities provide a specific explanation for the measurement of the intensity of the sound beam in both

TABLE 1-50 Beam uniformity ratio (BUR)

Formula
BUR = SP/SA

The BUR is derived from dividing the spatial peak (SP) by the spatial average (SA).

TABLE 1-51 Temporal average (TA) formula

Formula
TA = PA × DF

The TA is equal to the pulse average (PA) multiplied by the duty factor (DF).

TABLE 1-52 The list of intensities from lowest (SATA) to highest (SPTP)

Intensities from Lowest to Highest
SATA < SPTA < SAPA < SPPA < SATP < SPTP

SA, spatial average; SP, spatial peak; TA, temporal average; PA, pulse average; TP, temporal peak.

space and time. For example, the spatial average-temporal average (SATA) intensity signifies that the beam was measured using the SA and TA intensities. Table 1-52 lists the order of intensities from the lowest to highest. It is most important to note that SATA is the lowest of the intensities, spatial peak-temporal peak (SPTP) is the highest, the spatial peak-temporal average (SPTA) intensity is used when describing thermal bioeffects, and the spatial peak-pulse average (SPPA) intensity is used when describing mechanical bioeffects. Intensity, and its association with bioeffects, will be discussed further in Chapter 6 of this book.

SOUND OFF
SATA is the lowest of the intensities, whereas SPTP is the highest. The SPTA intensity is used when describing thermal bioeffects. The SPPA intensity is used when describing mechanical bioeffects.

The **hydrophone**, or microprobe, is a device used to measure the output intensity of the transducer (Figure 1-29). It can be a needle-type device or a broad, disk-shaped device. Both types of hydrophones consist of a transducer that is placed in the path of the beam to measure PRP, PD, and period. From these measurements, other parameters, such as frequency, wavelength, SPL, PRF, and DF, can be derived. The hydrophone is also used to determine pressure amplitude and intensities, which are important for patient safety.

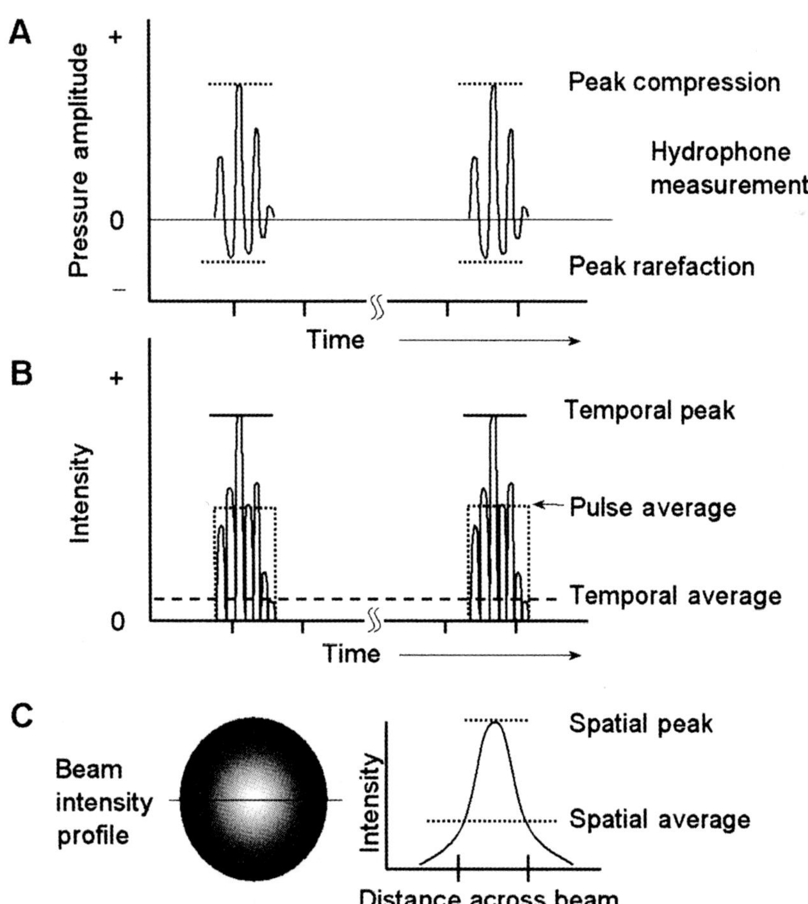

Figure 1-29 Intensities. **A.** Pressure amplitude variations are measured with a hydrophone and include peak compression and rarefaction variations with time. **B.** Temporal intensity variations of pulsed ultrasound vary widely, from temporal peak and temporal average values; pulse average intensity represents the average intensity measured over the pulse duration. **C.** Spatial intensity variations of pulsed ultrasound are described by the spatial peak value and the spatial average value, measured over the ultrasound beam.

REVIEW QUESTIONS

1. Which of the following is described as the ability of an object to resist compression and relates to the hardness of a medium?
   a. Stiffness
   b. Density
   c. Pressure
   d. Inertia

2. An increase in PRF would lead to:
   a. An increase in DF
   b. A decrease in PD
   c. An increase in the number of cycles
   d. A decrease in resolution

3. Which of the following would have the highest propagation speed?
   a. Air
   b. Bone
   c. Soft tissue
   d. Water

4. Which of the following would have the lowest propagation speed?
   a. Water
   b. Soft tissue
   c. Bone
   d. Lung tissue

5. As imaging depth increases, the PRF must:
   a. Not change
   b. Increase
   c. Decrease
   d. PRF does not relate to imaging depth

6. Which of the following describes refraction at an interface?
   a. Bernoulli's law
   b. Poiseuille's law
   c. Law of reflection
   d. Snell's law

7. Pressure is typically expressed in:
   a. Frequency
   b. Pascals
   c. Decibels
   d. Kilograms per centimeter cubed

8. The typical range of frequency for medical diagnostic ultrasound imaging is:
   a. 20 to 20,000 Hz
   b. 2 to 20 MHz
   c. 2 to 15 kHz
   d. 12 to 100 MHz

9. The attenuation coefficient in soft tissue is equal to:
   a. One-half of the operating frequency
   b. Two times the operating frequency
   c. Frequency times path length
   d. The total decibels

10. Micro denotes:
    a. One-millionth
    b. One-hundredth
    c. One million
    d. One-thousandth

11. Which of the following is described as the distance over which one cycle occurs?
    a. PD
    b. DF
    c. Period
    d. Wavelength

12. Which of the following requires an oblique interface and a propagation speed mismatch?
    a. Reflection
    b. Refraction
    c. Normal incidence
    d. Damping

13. Areas of high pressure and density are referred to as:
    a. Compressions
    b. Rarefactions
    c. Diffractions
    d. Refractions

14. SPL can be calculated by:
    a. Multiplying the number of cycles by the frequency
    b. Dividing the period by the frequency
    c. Multiplying the number of cycles by the wavelength
    d. Dividing the number of cycles by the wavelength

15. Density is typically measured in:
    a. Kilograms per centimeter cubed
    b. Millimeters
    c. Watts per square centimeter
    d. Pascals

16. As a sound wave travels through the human body, the intensity of the sound wave decreases as a result of:
    a. Attenuation
    b. Elevational resolution
    c. Huygen's principle
    d. Refraction

17. What is the amount of attenuation that occurs if a 6-MHz sound beam travels through 4 cm of soft tissue?
    a. –24 dB
    b. –12 dB
    c. –6 dB
    d. –1.5 dB

18. As imaging depth increases, PRP:
    a. Remains constant
    b. Increases
    c. Decreases
    d. Doubles

19. What are the units of DF?
    a. dB
    b. dB/cm
    c. Hz
    d. Unitless

20. The percentage of time that the ultrasound system is producing pulses of ultrasound describes the:
    a. Pulse repetition period
    b. Pulse duration
    c. Duty factor
    d. Pulse repetition frequency

21. Density and propagation speed are:
    a. Inversely related
    b. Directly related
    c. Directly proportional
    d. Unrelated

22. Which of the following is true when discussing power?
    a. As amplitude increases, power decreases
    b. Power is proportional to amplitude squared
    c. Intensity is inversely related to power
    d. Power is measured in mW/cm^2

23. Which of the following accurately describes wavelength?
    a. It is determined by both the medium and the sound source
    b. It is equal to the period divided by the frequency
    c. It is directly related to frequency
    d. It is the time it takes for one cycle to occur

24. Which of the following is determined by the medium only?
    a. Propagation speed
    b. Frequency
    c. Period
    d. Wavelength

25. Which of the following is defined as the number of ultrasound pulses emitted in 1 second?
    a. PRP
    b. DF
    c. PRF
    d. SPL

26. Which of the following is defined as only the time of transmission?
    a. DF
    b. PRF
    c. Period
    d. PD

27. A doubling of the amplitude results in what change to the intensity of the beam?
    a. The intensity is doubled
    b. The intensity is halved
    c. Amplitude and intensity are unrelated
    d. The intensity is quadrupled

28. Which of the following is determined by the sound source only?
    a. Frequency
    b. Wavelength
    c. SPL
    d. Propagation speed

29. The prefix "centi" denotes:
    a. One-thousandth
    b. One-hundredth
    c. One-billionth
    d. Hundreds

30. If the angle of incidence is 40°, what is the angle of transmission at the interface if medium 1 has a propagation speed of 1320 m/s and medium 2 has a propagation speed of 1700 m/s?
    a. 0°
    b. >40°
    c. <40°
    d. Cannot tell the angle of transmission

31. The change in the direction of a transmitted sound wave that occurs when sound interacts with two different tissue types that have a different propagation speed is referred to as:
    a. Wavelength
    b. Scattering
    c. Refraction
    d. Absorption

32. Which of the following is an appropriate unit of measurement for propagation speed?
    a. millimeters per microsecond (mm/µs)
    b. watts per square centimeter (W/cm^2)
    c. microseconds (ms)
    d. kilohertz (kHz)

33. The major component of attenuation is:
   a. Scatter
   b. Absorption
   c. Transmission
   d. Refraction

34. In clinical imaging, the wavelength typically measures between:
   a. 1 and 10 Hz
   b. 1540 and 2000 m/s
   c. 0 and 1
   d. 0.1 to 0.8 mm

35. The DF for CW ultrasound is:
   a. 1.0%
   b. 100%
   c. 20,000 Hz
   d. 8 Pa

36. All of the following relate to the strength of the sound wave except:
   a. Amplitude
   b. Wavelength
   c. Intensity
   d. Power

37. What is the change in intensity if the power decreases by half?
   a. Intensity doubles
   b. Intensity is halved
   c. Intensity is one-fourth
   d. Intensity does not change

38. Damping of the sound:
   a. Reduces the SPL
   b. Increases the SPL
   c. Increases the PD
   d. Has no impact on SPL or PD

39. Adding damping to the transducer improves which type of resolution?
   a. Transverse resolution
   b. Temporal resolution
   c. Axial resolution
   d. Elevational resolution

40. What time is defined as the beginning of one pulse to the beginning of the next pulse and, therefore, includes both the "on" and "off" time?
   a. PRP
   b. PD
   c. DF
   d. PRF

41. What are the units for pressure?
   a. feet, inches, centimeters, or miles
   b. pascals or pounds per square inch
   c. kilograms per centimeter cubed
   d. hertz, kilohertz, or megahertz

42. What term is defined as "the power of a wave divided by the area over which the power is distributed?"
   a. Amplitude
   b. Power
   c. Intensity
   d. Absorption

43. Transducers have material within them that when electronically stimulated produces ultrasound waves. This is most likely some form of:
   a. Tungsten acetate
   b. Dilithium zirconium
   c. Lead zirconate titanate
   d. Barium sulfate

44. The amplitude in a wave is doubled. What effect does this have on the power of the beam?
   a. It doubles
   b. It triples
   c. It quadruples
   d. It is quartered

45. The portion of the sound beam where the molecules in the medium are farther apart describes an area of:
   a. Compression
   b. Rarefaction
   c. Refraction
   d. Amplitude

46. If only the density of a medium is increased, then the propagation speed will:
   a. Increase
   b. Decrease
   c. Double
   d. Stay the same

47. Sound is technically a:
   a. Transverse and longitudinal wave
   b. Mechanical and transverse wave
   c. Electromagnetic and pressure wave
   d. Mechanical and longitudinal wave

48. The maximum or minimum value of an acoustic variable from the baseline to the peak describes the:
   a. Power
   b. Intensity
   c. DF
   d. Amplitude

49. Which of the following would be considered ultrasonic?
    a. 10 Hz
    b. 18 kHz
    c. 0.5 MHz
    d. 200 Hz

50. Which of the following is considered the speed of sound in soft tissue?
    a. 1.54 m/s
    b. 0.77 m/s
    c. 100 mW/cm^2
    d. 1540 m/s

SUGGESTED READINGS

Bushberg J, Seibert JA, Leidholdt EM, Boone JM. *The Essential Physics of Medical Imaging.* 4th ed. Wolters Kluwer; 2021.
Case T. *A Primer in Ultrasound and Vascular Physics.* Lippincott Williams & Wilkins; 2007.
Edelman SK. *Understanding Ultrasound Physics.* 4th ed. ESP Inc.; 2012.
Kremkau FW. *Diagnostic Ultrasound: Principles and Instruments.* 10th ed. Saunders; 2020.
Liu J, Xu J, Forsberg F, Liu J. CMUT/CMOS-based Butterfly iQ: A portable personal sonoscope. *Adv Ultrasound Diagn Ther.* 2019;3(3):115.
Miele F. *Ultrasound Physics and Instrumentation.* 6th ed. Miele Enterprises; 2022.
Rosen J. *Encyclopedia of Physics.* Facts on File Inc.; 2004.
Sanders R, Hall-Terracciano B. *Clinical Sonography: A Practical Guide.* 5th ed. Wolters Kluwer; 2016.
Szabo TL. *Diagnostic Ultrasound Imaging: Inside Out.* Elsevier; 2014.

2

Ultrasound Transducers

Outline

Introduction

This chapter will describe the way in which sound is produced by a transducer, including the construction of a transducer, its care and maintenance, and image resolution.

Key Terms

aperture—the diameter of the piezoelectric element(s) producing the beam

array—a transducer with multiple active elements

automatic scanning—same as real-time ultrasound

axial resolution—the ability to accurately identify reflectors that are arranged parallel to the ultrasound beam (in mm)

backing material—the damping material of a transducer assembly that reduces the number of cycles produced in a pulse

bandwidth—the range of frequencies present within the beam

connector—the part of a transducer cable that connects to the ultrasound machine

constructive interference—occurs when in-phase waves meet; the amplitudes of the two waves are added to form one large wave

contrast resolution—the ability to differentiate tissues with similar shades of gray

crystal—a synonym for the active element of a transducer, the piezoelectric part of a transducer assembly that produces sound

Curie point—the temperature at which an ultrasound transducer will gain its piezoelectric properties and also the temperature at which a transducer will lose the ability to produce sound if heated again above this temperature

curved sequenced array—a transducer commonly referred to as a curvilinear or convex probe

damping—the process of reducing the number of cycles of each pulse in order to improve axial resolution

damping material—the same as the backing material; the part of the transducer assembly that reduces the number of cycles produced in a pulse

depth ambiguity—the inability to determine the depth of the reflector if the pulses are sent out too fast for them to be timed

destructive interference—occurs when out-of-phase waves meet; the amplitude of the resultant wave is smaller than either of the original waves

divergence—spreading of the beam that occurs in the far zone

element—the piezoelectric part of the transducer assembly that produces sound

elevational plane—*see* the key term "slice-thickness plane"

elevational resolution—the resolution in the third dimension of the beam; the slice-thickness plane

far zone—the diverging part of the beam distal to the focal point

focal depth—the depth of the focal point/focal zone. It is the same as the depth of one near-zone length

focal point—the area of the beam with the smallest beam diameter

footprint—the size of the face of the transducer; the portion of the transducer that is in contact with the patient's skin

four-dimensional ultrasound—three-dimensional ultrasound in real time

frame—one complete ultrasound image

frame rate—the number of frames per second (FPS, in Hz)

Fraunhofer zone—*see* the key term "far zone"

frequency—the number of cycles per second (in Hz)

Fresnel zone—*see* the key term "near zone"

housing—the plastic outside of a transducer that surrounds the electronics of the transducer and electrical shielding/insulation

Huygen's principle—waves are the result of the interference of many wavelets produced at the face of the transducer

in-phase—waves whose peaks and troughs overlap

lateral resolution—the ability to accurately identify reflectors that are arranged perpendicular to the ultrasound beam (in mm)

lead zirconate titanate—the man-made ceramic of which many transducer elements are made; abbreviated PZT

linear sequenced array—a transducer commonly referred to as a linear probe or transducer

matching layer—the component of a transducer that is used to step down the impedance from that of the element to that of the patient's skin

matrix array transducer—a 2D array transducer that acquires real-time volumes utilizing over 90,000 elements compared with the 128 to 512 elements used in standard 1D array transducers

mechanical scanheads—transducers with a motor for steering the beam

near zone—the part of the beam between the element and the focal point

near-zone length—the length of the region from the transducer face to the focal point

out-of-phase—waves that are 180° opposite to each other; the peak of one wave overlaps the trough of the other and vice versa

phased array—a transducer that uses phasing; shocking the elements in a pattern with small time differences, to steer and focus the beam

phasing—the method of focusing and/or steering the beam by applying electrical impulses to the piezoelectric elements with small time differences between shocks

piezoelectric—the ability to convert pressure into electricity and electricity into pressure

quality factor (Q-factor)—a measure of beam purity; the operating frequency of the transducer divided by the bandwidth

range resolution—the ability to determine how far away a reflector is so it can be displayed on the screen; without range resolution, there is depth ambiguity

real time—live ultrasound, also known as automatic scanning

resonate—the action of the crystal that produces sound

scan lines—created when one or more pulses of sound return from the tissue containing information related to the depth and amplitude of the reflectors

section-thickness plane—*see* the key term "slice-thickness plane"

sensitivity—the ability of a system to display low-level or weak echoes

sequenced array—transducer elements in an array that are shocked in sequence to produce the beam; contrasts with the key term "phased array"

slice-thickness plane—the "third dimension" of the beam

spatial pulse length—the length of one pulse (in mm)

spatial resolution—the ability of the system to distinguish between closely spaced objects; refers to axial, lateral, contrast, and elevational resolution

strain reliever—flexible sheath that connects the cable to the transducer and is a potential shock hazard if damaged

temporal resolution—ability to display moving structures in real time; also known as the frame rate

three-dimensional ultrasound—allows the user to see width, height, and depth; may also be referred to as volume scanning and multiplanar scanning

transducer—any device that converts one form of energy into another; may also refer to the part of the ultrasound machine that produces sound

tungsten—component of the backing material

wavefront—the leading edge of a wave that is perpendicular to the direction of the propagating wave; formed as a result of Huygen's principle

wavelet—a small wave created as a result of Huygen's principle

THE PIEZOELECTRIC ELEMENT AND THE PRODUCTION OF SOUND

The Piezoelectric Element

A **piezoelectric** material, as mentioned in Chapter 1, is an element that generates electricity when pressure is applied to it and that changes shape when electricity is applied to it. It produces diagnostic ultrasound. Piezoelectric materials may be man-made or natural, such as quartz and tourmaline. A piezoelectric material that is commonly used in current ultrasound transducers is a man-made ceramic called **lead zirconate titanate** (PZT). The PZT is the actual **transducer** inside the scan head. It may also be referred to as the **crystal**, the **element**, or simply, the transducer. Newer technologies for transducer material includes silicon-based capacitive micromachined ultrasound transducers (CMUTs), polyvinylidene fluoride (PVDF), and single crystal transducers made with lead magnesium niobate/lead titanate (PMN-PT) and lead zirconate niobate/lead titanate (PZN-PT). Figure 2-1 is an image of the Butterfly (Butterfly Network, Inc., Burling MA), which is a transducer that uses CMUT technology.

> **SOUND OFF**
> An ultrasound transducer should not be heat sterilized, because once a ceramic is taken to its Curie point, it must never return to that temperature again or the material will lose its piezoelectric properties forever.

Man-made piezoelectric materials like PZT must undergo a process to obtain their piezoelectric properties. First, the PZT is placed into an oven that is used to heat the material to the **Curie point**. The Curie point, which is around 328° C to 365° C, is the temperature at which the material will obtain piezoelectric properties. While being heated, the PZT is placed into a magnetic field. This causes magnetically charged molecules, which are located within the material and referred to as dipoles, to align themselves in relation to the magnetic field. Once the material is cooled, it is functional as a piezoelectric element. Unfortunately, once a ceramic is taken to its Curie point, it must never return to that temperature again or the material will lose its piezoelectric properties forever. For this reason, ultrasound transducers must never be heat sterilized.

When high-level disinfection is necessary, a disinfection method must be used that does not exceed the Curie point, such as a room-temperature bath using either a glutaraldehyde solution, such as Cidex or Metricide, or a non–glutaraldehyde-based solution, such as *ortho*-phthalaldehyde. Cold-disinfection solutions can be dangerous if they get in the eyes, on the skin, or are inhaled. Personal protective equipment must be worn while handling these solutions. Sonographers should be familiar with the appropriate safety data sheets for these solutions. Another method of high-level disinfection uses

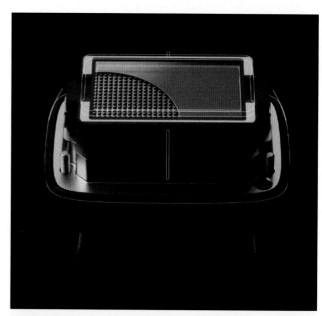

Figure 2-1 An image of the Butterfly (Butterfly Network, Inc., Burlington, MA), which is a transducer that uses CMUT technology.

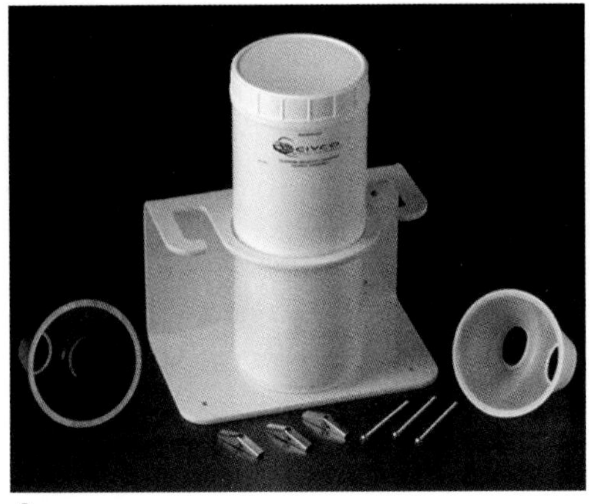
A

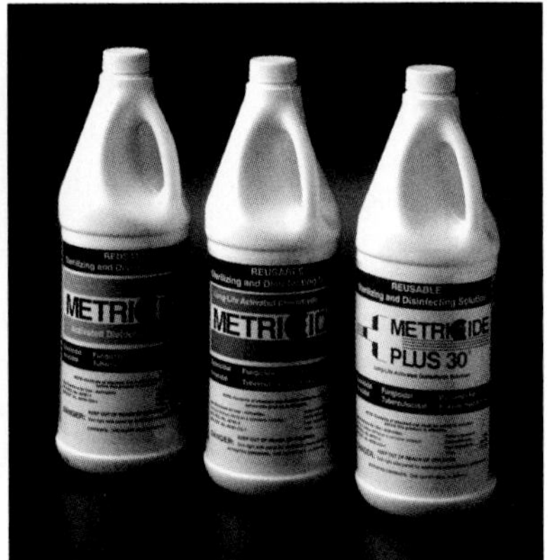

B

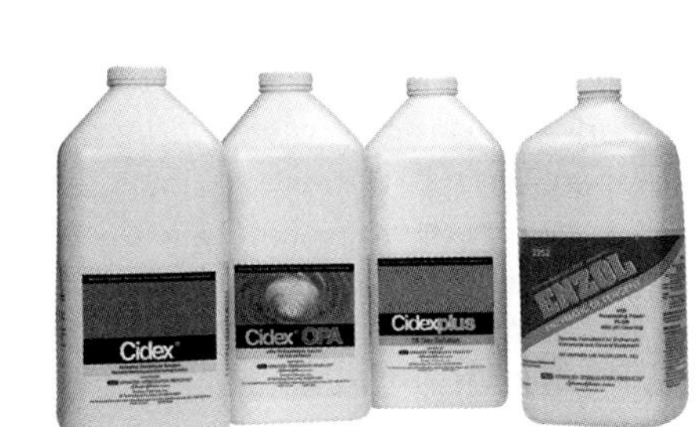

C

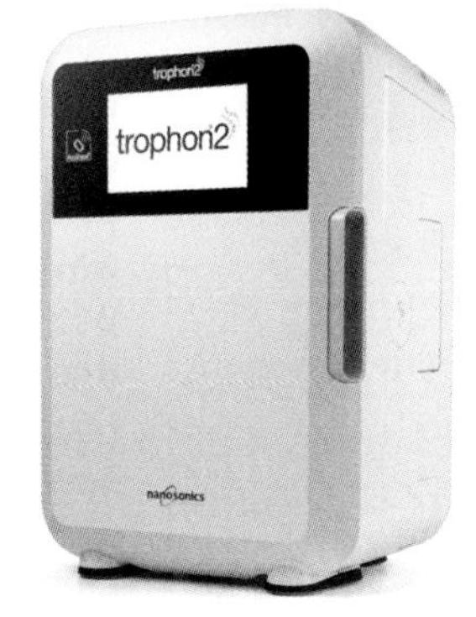

D

Figure 2-2 Ultrasound transducers may be placed in a container **(A)** and can be soaked in a cold sterilization chemical **(B, C)**. A newer method involves sterilization using a hydrogen peroxide solution **(D)**.

a warmed hydrogen peroxide mist, commonly used for endocavity transducers. (Figure 2-2).

> **SOUND OFF**
> In pulsed-wave (PW) operation, the thickness of the element is the primary determinant of the resonating frequency of the transducer. A thicker element will produce a lower frequency, whereas a thinner element will produce a higher frequency.

Production of Sound

One or more piezoelectric elements are attached to a wire in the transducer. Applying electricity to the element causes it to **resonate**, or alternatively expand and contract. Refer back to Figure 1-14 for an illustration of this process. The **frequency**, or the rate at which the material resonates, is related to two factors: the thickness of the piezoelectric element and the propagation speed of the element itself (Table 2-1). In PW operation, the thickness of the element is the primary determinant of the resonating frequency of the transducer. A thicker element will produce a lower frequency, whereas a thinner element will produce a higher frequency (Figure 2-3). The operator cannot change the resonating frequency of a piezoelectric element.

The resonating element produces a pressure wave within the medium. This wave consists of alternating areas of high pressure and low pressure, or compressions and rarefactions, respectively. The resonating frequency, also known as the center or operating frequency, of a medical diagnostic ultrasound transducer is typically between 2 and 20 MHz. The expansion and contraction of the element produce a propagating ultrasound wave that travels into the human body. Imaging ultrasound transducers use pulses of sound, called PW ultrasound.

> **SOUND OFF**
> Rarefaction is a fancy word for "low pressure." Note that it is *rare*faction, not refraction. Think of a rare steak. Refraction was discussed in Chapter 1.

A unique property of ultrasound piezoelectric elements is that they can send and receive ultrasound,

TABLE 2-1 Formula for the frequency of the transducer for pulsed-wave operation

Formula
$F_o = c/2 \times \text{thickness}$

The operating frequency (F_o) is equal to the propagation speed (c) of the element divided by the thickness of the element multiplied by 2.

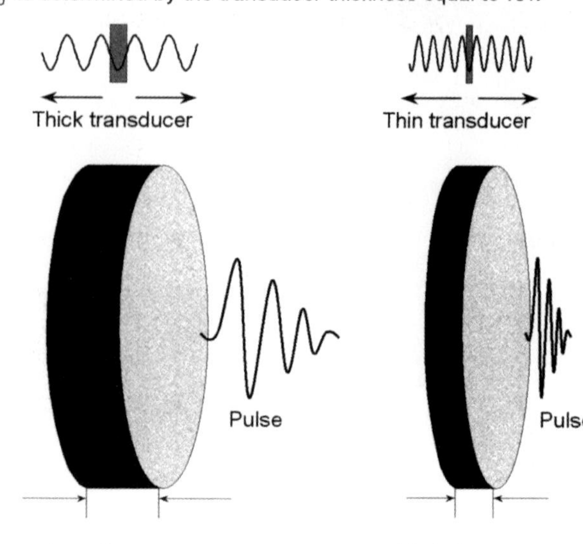

Figure 2-3 Transducer elements. The thicker the element, the lower the frequency, and the thinner the element, the higher the frequency.

though not at the same time, that is, a single element can emit sound, but it must wait for that sound to return before it can send out the next pulse. The machine must time how long it takes for a pulse of sound to reach the reflector in order to appropriately display anatomy on the monitor. If the transducer sends out a pulse before it receives the last one, it is unable to recognize where the echo originated and therefore cannot display the received echo correctly on the monitor. This is referred to as **depth ambiguity** or range ambiguity.

> **SOUND OFF**
> The resonating frequency, also known as the center or operating frequency, of a medical diagnostic ultrasound transducer is typically between 2 and 20 MHz.

Wave Interference and Huygen's Principle

As stated in Chapter 1, sound travels as a wave. These waves may interact with each other. Subsequently, these waves may be described further as **in-phase** waves or **out-of-phase** waves. In-phase waves are waves that, when overlapped, have matching peaks and troughs. When in-phase waves meet, they undergo **constructive interference**. This means that their amplitudes are added together, and they ultimately become one big wave. Out-of-phase waves, when overlapped, are 180° opposite to each other. When out-of-phase waves meet, they undergo **destructive interference**. With destructive interference, the resultant wave is smaller. Also, if the out-of-phase waves have identical amplitudes, they will completely cancel each other out (Figure 2-4). Active noise-canceling headphones use the principle of destructive interference to reduce outside ambient noise.

> **SOUND OFF**
> When in-phase waves meet, they undergo constructive interference (wave gets bigger). When out-of-phase waves meet, they undergo destructive interference (wave gets smaller).

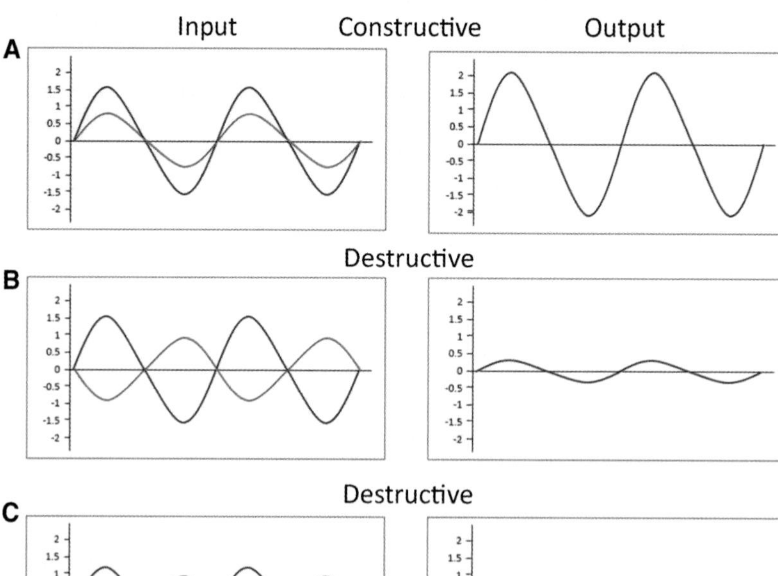

Figure 2-4 Demonstration of wave interference. **A.** The amplitudes of the two waves are added together, which results in one large wave. **B.** With out-of-phase waves that are nonidentical in amplitude, the resultant wave has a smaller amplitude than the two initial waves. **C.** With out-of-phase waves that are identical in amplitude, they cancel each other out.

Ultrasound Transducers

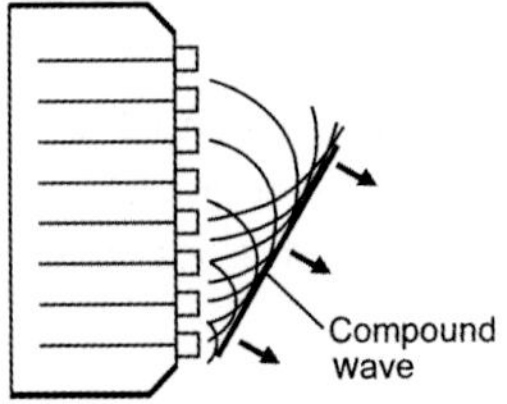

Figure 2-5 Huygen's principle. The beam starts out as small wavelets at the face of the transducer. The interference of the wavelets produces a propagation sound beam. The direction in which the beam travels is perpendicular to the wavefront.

The surface of a transducer is made up of many tiny point sources of sound. Each tiny point on the transducer produces a **wavelet**. All of the wavelets that are created undergo either constructive or destructive interference. The result is a propagating sound wave whose direction of travel is perpendicular to the **wavefront**, which is the line tangential to all the wavelets (Figure 2-5). This is referred to as **Huygen's principle**. The principle simply claims that waves are the result of the interference of many wavelets produced at the face of the transducer.

CONSTRUCTION OF A TRANSDUCER

The various components of a transducer can be seen in Figure 2-6 and are summarized in Table 2-2 and further discussed in detail in the following sections.

Transducer Housing and the Cable

Diagnostic ultrasound instruments use electricity to generate an image. Inside the transducer housing are electrical wires used to transmit the signals from the machine to the piezoelectric elements and vice versa (Figure 2-7). The ultrasound machine produces between 10 and 500 V in order to drive the piezoelectric elements. If a crack occurs in the transducer housing, there is a potential risk for an electrical shock to either the practitioner or the patient. Consequently, the ultrasound transducer has electrical shielding (insulation) not only to protect the image from outside electrical

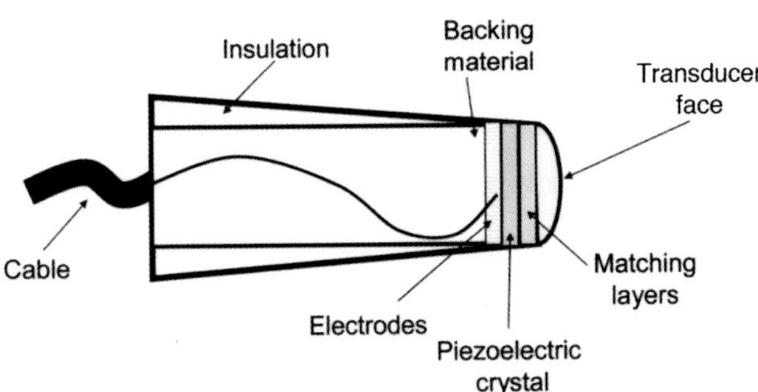

Figure 2-6 Simplified construction of a transducer.

TABLE 2-2 Summary of the transducer assembly

Transducer Part	Purpose
Backing material	Shortens the length of the pulse by decreasing the number of cycles in the pulse
Crystal	Material that produces diagnostic ultrasound. Composed of piezoelectric material, most commonly lead zirconate titanate. Converts electrical energy into acoustic energy during transmission and acoustic energy into electrical energy during reception
Housing	Provides electrical insulation to reduce radiofrequency (RF) interference and protection from electrical shock
Matching layer	Used to minimize the impedance mismatch between that of the element and that of the patient's skin. Improves sound transmission efficiency
Cable	Used to transfer electrical signals to and from the transducer

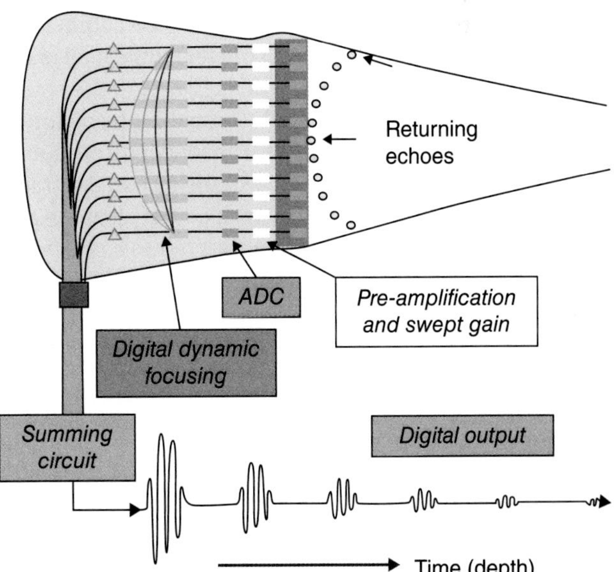

Figure 2-7 Electronic wiring of a transducer. Modern ultrasound transducers often contain more than a hundred individual transducer elements, each of which is supplied with electrical energy via a wire. The wire also transmits the received echo amplitude information to the machine for processing.

radiofrequency (RF) interference but also to protect the user and the patient from the shock.

> **SOUND OFF**
> Modern conventional scan heads often contain more than a hundred individual transducer elements, each of which is supplied with electrical energy via a wire.

An electrical connection to the ultrasound machine is achieved via a cable, also called the wire or cord. Modern scan heads often contain hundreds of individual transducer elements, each of which is supplied with electrical energy via the cable. This cable also transmits the received echo amplitude information to the machine for processing. A flexible strain reliever holds the cable to the transducer. The importance of this strain reliever is to allow the flexibility of the cord and prevent damage to the cable where it connects to the transducer. This flexible sheath is a potential point of failure with extended use. On the opposite end of the cable is the connector, which connects the transducer to the ultrasound machine (Figure 2-8).

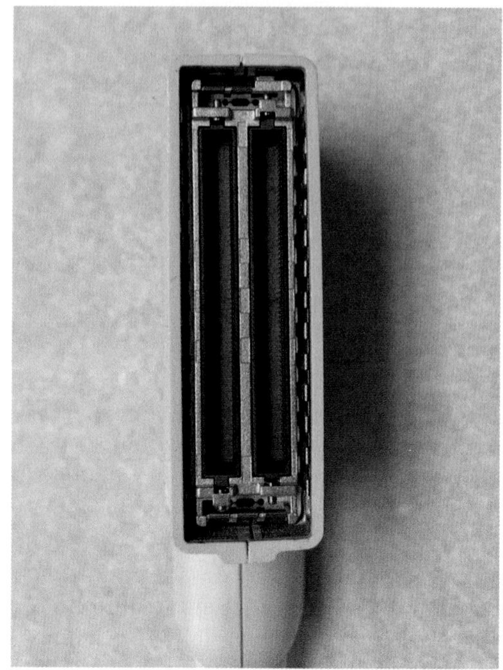

Figure 2-8 An image of modern transducer connector.

Matching Layers

Remember from Chapter 1 that the bigger the impedance mismatch, the stronger the reflection at an interface. The more sound that is reflected from the skin interface, the less sound there is to be transmitted into the tissue. The impedance of the piezoelectric element is significantly different from that of the patient's skin. If no action were taken, this large mismatch would prevent almost all of the sound from entering the patient. In fact, 80% of the sound would be reflected, and only 20% would be transmitted into the patient. Therefore, the transducer is equipped with a **matching layer**, which is also the face of the transducer, that lies between the piezoelectric element and the patient's skin. Although often referred to as if it were a single layer, the matching layer is composed of multiple layers (Figure 2-9). The purpose of the layers is to step down the impedance from that of the element to that of the patient's skin. The matching layers improve the efficiency of transmitting sound into the patient by decreasing this impedance mismatch. An additional "matching layer," although one employed by the sonographer, is a coupling medium or gel. In addition to removing air between the transducer and the patient, the gel is especially formulated to have an impedance value between that of the matching layer and the patient's skin to further enhance the transmission of sound.

> **SOUND OFF**
> The matching layer improves the efficiency of transmitting sound into the patient by decreasing this impedance mismatch.

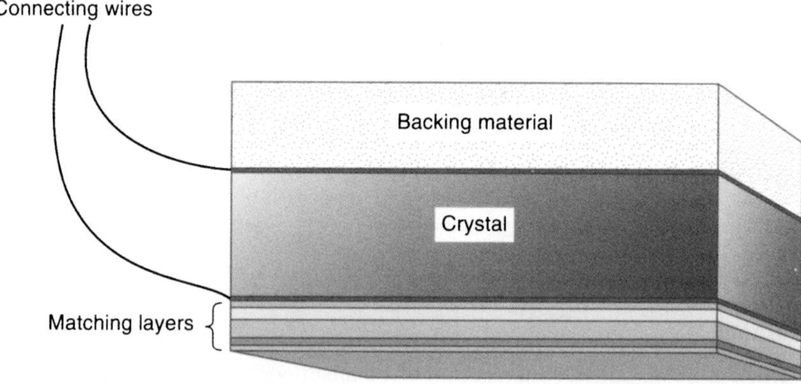

Figure 2-9 Enlarged diagram of the construction of the transducer. This diagram depicts the multiple layers that create the matching layer.

TABLE 2-3 Advantages of damping

Decreases the number of cycles in a pulse
Decreases spatial pulse length
Improves axial resolution

TABLE 2-4 Side effects of damping

Decreases sensitivity of the transducer
Increases the bandwidth
Reduces the quality factor (Q-factor or "purity" factor)

Backing Material and Damping

The **backing material**, as the name implies, sits on the back of the transducer, behind the elements (Figure 2-9). The purpose of the backing material, also referred to as the **damping material**, is to provide **damping** of the piezoelectric element. The damping material serves to shorten the length of the pulse by decreasing the number of cycles in the pulse. This material is composed of an epoxy resin containing **tungsten**.

There are several advantages of damping (Table 2-3). The element can be compared to a bell. When a bell is struck, it will keep ringing until it eventually slows to a stop. Grab a bell while it is ringing, or wrap it in a heavy blanket, and it decreases the length of the ringing of the bell. In PW ultrasound, short pulses are very desirable; anything that will decrease the length of the pulse improves the **axial resolution** of the image (Figure 2-10). Damping decreases the number of cycles in a pulse, effectively decreasing the **spatial pulse length** (SPL). Damping shortens the pulse to two or three cycles per pulse.

SOUND OFF
The damping material serves to shorten the length of the pulse by decreasing the number of cycles in the pulse.

SOUND OFF
In PW ultrasound, short pulses are very desirable; anything that will decrease the length of the pulse improves the axial resolution of the image. SPL = λn, so adding more damping or increasing the frequency (which decreases wavelength) while building a transducer shortens the length of the pulse.

Other Effects of Damping

Damping is needed to decrease the number of cycles in the pulse to shorten the pulse. As a result of adding this tungsten-containing backing material, some of the sound energy is lost in the damping material (Table 2-4). Therefore, one of the side effects of damping is the decreased **sensitivity** of the transducer. Another side effect of damping is the production of other frequencies in the beam in addition to the operating frequency. Although the piezoelectric element is resonating at the operating frequency, the beam itself will contain a range of frequencies. **Bandwidth** is the range of frequencies present within the beam. Continuous-wave (CW) transducers do not have any damping. Therefore, if a sample of the beam of a 4.0-MHz CW transducer is taken, only a 4.0-MHz beam will be discovered. However, PW transducers have damping, so there is always a range of frequencies present within the beam. Therefore, it can be said that damping produces a "less pure," or heterogenous beam, than the "pure," or heterogenous beam of CW ultrasound (Figure 2-11). Figure 2-12 demonstrates that, compared to a CW probe with an identical operating frequency, if a sample of the beam of a 4.0-MHz PW transducer were obtained, many frequencies would be present in addition to the 4.0-MHz center frequency. This wide range of frequencies is the bandwidth of the transducer. These additional frequencies present within the beam are the reason why PW ultrasound machines have a "frequency" button that makes it appear that you can change the transducer's frequency. You cannot—it is determined (primarily) by the thickness of the element—but you select any frequency present with the bandwidth. To determine the bandwidth of the transducer, subtract the lowest frequency present within the beam by the highest frequency, and that the number is the bandwidth. For example, if you have a 5-MHz center

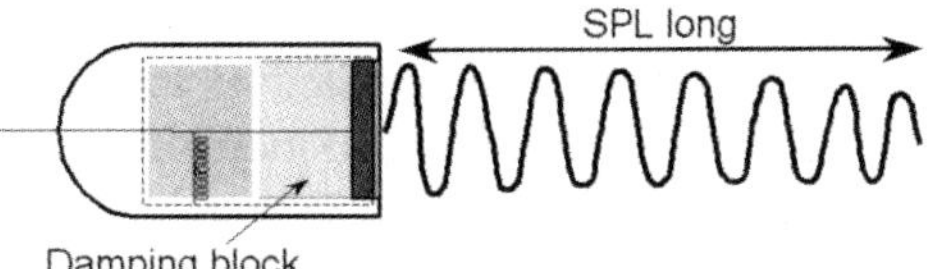

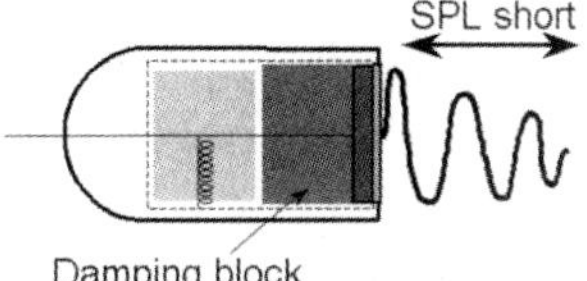

Figure 2-10 Damping. **A.** Ultrasound pulse with less damping produces many cycles in a pulse. **B.** With more damping, the number of cycles in the pulse is reduced, shortening the pulse.

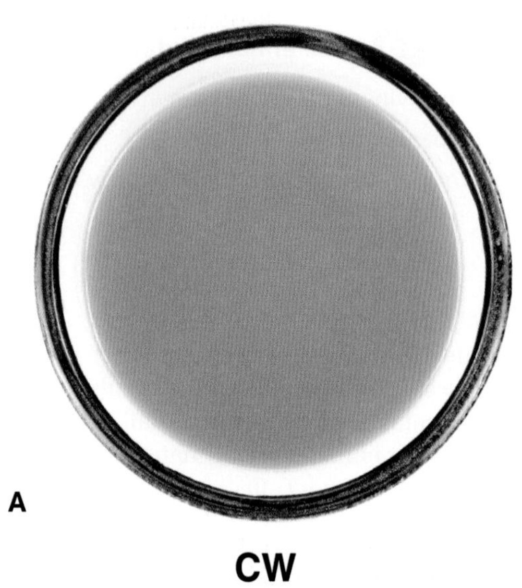

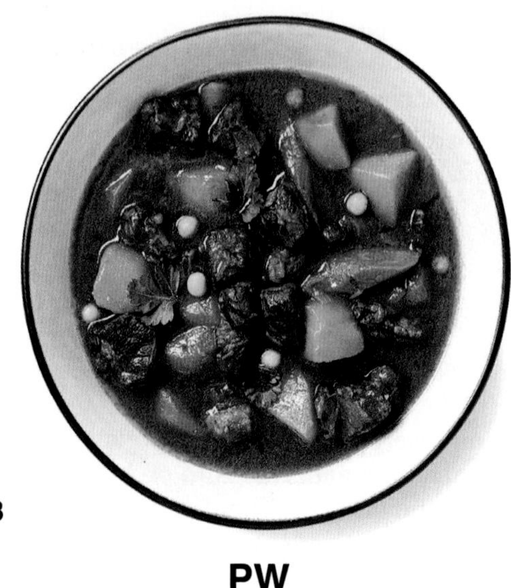

Figure 2-11 Purity of the beam. The beam from CW probes is like broth – it is homogenous, or "pure." The beam from PW probes, in contrast, is like stew; it is heterogeneous, with a lower "purity" than CW. CW, continuous wave; PW, pulsed wave.

frequency transducer with anywhere from 3 to 7 MHz present within the beam, subtract 3 from 7 and you get a 4-MHz bandwidth. Transducers that have a bandwidth are also called "broadband" transducers.

> **SOUND OFF**
> CW transducers do not have damping because they transmit continuously. It is the damping/backing material in PW transducers that causes additional frequencies to be present within the beam. Therefore, PW transducers have a wide bandwidth.

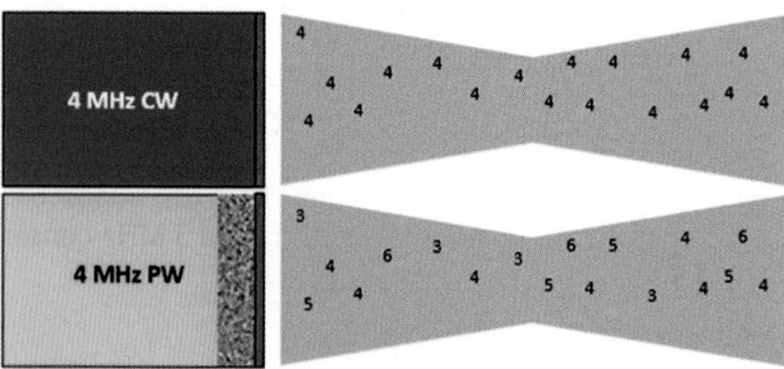

Figure 2-12 Damping and bandwidth. Both transducers have the same center frequency (4 MHz). The CW transducer, which has no damping, only has a pure, or homogeneous 4 MHz frequency present within the beam. The PW transducer is less pure, or heterogeneous, and has a range of frequencies present within the beam. These frequencies make it possible to have multi-hertz transducers. CW, continuous wave; PW, pulsed wave.

Q-Factor

The Quality-factor, or, as it will be called here, Q-factor, should be thought of as the "purity" of the beam. So instead of the "Q" word, think of purity. The **quality factor (Q-factor)** is a term used to quantitate the purity of the beam. The Q-factor is the operating frequency of the transducer divided by the bandwidth (Table 2-5). PW transducers typically have low Q-factors because they need damping to make the pulse shorter (ie, decrease the SPL). CW transducers have a narrow bandwidth with subsequent high Q-factors because of the absence of a backing material to provide damping (Figure 2-13 and Table 2-6). Therefore, although the "Q" in Q-factor indeed stands for "quality," it is not the resolution of the image that is being referred to there but rather the purity of the beam. Table 2-7 has sample problems related to damping, bandwidth, and Q-factor.

> **SOUND OFF**
> Q-factor relates to the purity of the ultrasound beam.

TABLE 2-5 Formula for the quality factor

$$\text{Q-factor} = \frac{F_o}{\text{Bandwidth}}$$

Q-factor is determined by dividing the operating frequency (F_o) by the bandwidth.

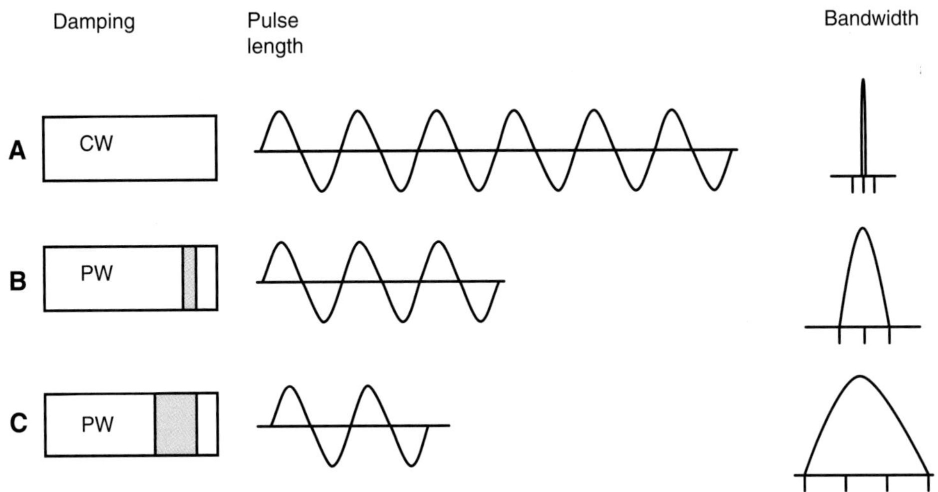

Figure 2-13 Quality factor (Q-Factor). CW probes are not damped, so they have a high Q-factor **(A)**. With PW probes **(B, C)**, the more damping there is (signified by the gray boxes within the transducers shown in **(B)** and **(C)**), the shorter the pulse, and therefore, the wider the bandwidth and lower the Q-factor. CW, continuous wave; PW, pulsed wave.

TABLE 2-6 Summary of the effects of damping on the pulse

↑ Damping = ↓ Spatial pulse length = ↑ Bandwidth = ↓ Q-factor = Better axial resolution

TABLE 2-7 Examples of questions on damping, bandwidth, and Q-factor

1. You want to use a linear transducer that has a 10-MHz center (operating) frequency and a 4-MHz bandwidth. Can you operate this transducer at 7 MHz?
   - No. If the bandwidth is of 4 MHz, the range is of 8 to 12 MHz (determined by one-half of the bandwidth, or in this case, 2 MHz, on either side of the center frequency). You could select frequencies between 8 and 12 MHz but not outside of that range.
2. You are building an ultrasound transducer and want to build a probe with a wide bandwidth. Which of the following would be best? (A) a CW probe, (B) a PW probe with no damping, (C) a PW probe with more damping, or (D) a CW probe with damping
   - (C) Only PW transducers have a wide bandwidth. CW transducers have no backing material, so they do not have additional frequencies in the beam.
3. You build the transducer from the previous question. Did you build a transducer with a relatively high Q-factor? Or relatively low Q-factor?
   - PW transducers have always low Q-factor because of damping, and CW transducers have always high Q-factor.

The aim of damping is to decrease the SPL to provide the best axial resolution, thus resulting in the optimal diagnostic image. The more damping is there, the shorter the pulse (because of the decreased "n" or the number of cycles in a pulse), and therefore the better the axial resolution, and the wider the bandwidth (Figure 2-14).

SOUND OFF
Real-time imaging offers the sonographer instant viewing of internal structures of the body.

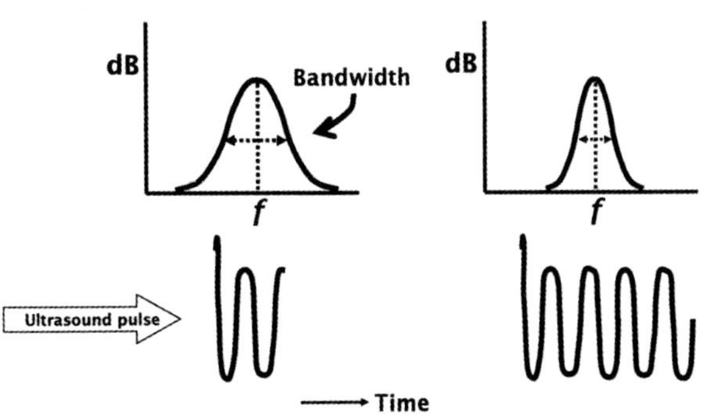

As pulse length increases, the frequency spectrum narrows
∴ Longer pulse length ⇒ narrower bandwidth ⇒ lower resolution

Figure 2-14 Bandwidth. This diagram demonstrates the relationship between pulse duration, or length, and bandwidth. With increasing pulse length, the bandwidth becomes narrower, thereby reducing resolution. Therefore, to improve axial resolution, a short pulse length is optimal.

REAL-TIME SCANNING

Modern ultrasound equipment utilizes **real-time** or **automatic scanning** to obtain diagnostic images of the body. With real-time scanning, the transducer is responsible for creating sound that is sent into the body and receiving echoes that are turned into images. For a sonographer, real-time imaging offers the ability to instantly view internal structures of the body. Pulses of ultrasound are sent out and produce scan lines. All of the scan lines, when placed next to each other, form an image that is called a **frame**.

TYPES OF TRANSDUCERS

There are two methods of sending out scan lines to form an image using real time: mechanical scanning (via mechanical transducers) and electronic scanning (via electronic transducers). Both methods provide a means for sweeping the ultrasound beam through the tissue repeatedly and rapidly. Although electronic scanning is most often the method used today, a brief review of mechanical transducers will be provided in the following section.

Mechanical Transducers

Mechanical scan heads with an element attached to a motor are mostly gone from everyday scanning. Modern-day's equivalent versions of mechanical transducers are three- (3D) and four-dimensional (4D) transducers. These transducers consist of an entire array transducer mounted on a motor and enclosed within a housing. Some similar specialty transducers, like endorectal and intravascular transducers, may also use a single element mounted on a motor, although this older technology is quickly being replaced by CMUT scan heads. More information about intravascular technology can be found in Chapter 6 of this book.

> **SOUND OFF**
> Modern examples of mechanical transducer technology include some that are used to perform 3D/4D, endorectal, and intravascular imaging.

> **SOUND OFF**
> An array is formed by taking a single slab of PZT and slicing it down into multiple subelements.

Electronic Transducers

Electronic scanning is performed with transducers that have multiple active elements. This is referred to as an **array**. An array is formed by taking a single slab of PZT and slicing it down into multiple subelements. Each subelement is connected to a wire, so it may fire independently. The system can selectively excite the elements as needed to shape and steer the beam. With most array transducers, no motors are needed for beam steering. Arrays may be either **sequenced** or **phased** and can produce various image shapes. Sequencing means that the elements are fired in sequence—one after another. Phased transducers can shock the elements individually or more than one at a time but use a pattern that determines the direction and shape of the beam.

Linear Sequenced Array

The **linear sequenced array**, also referred to as the linear sequential array or linear array, is a transducer that is often used in vascular or high-resolution imaging (Figure 2-15). This transducer produces a rectangular-shaped image

A

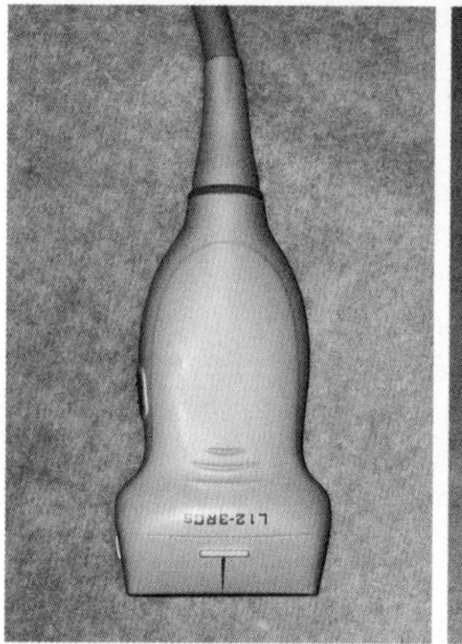

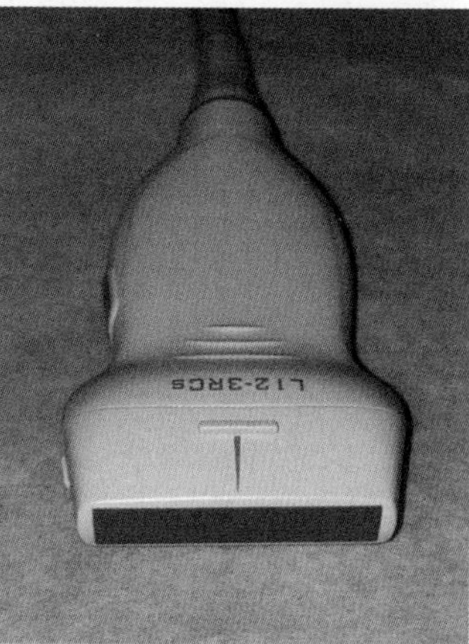

B

Figure 2-15 Linear sequenced array transducer. **A.** The rectangular image shape of the linear sequenced array transducer. **B.** Image of a linear sequenced array transducer.

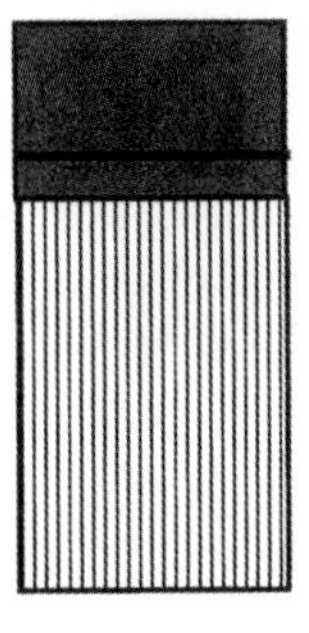

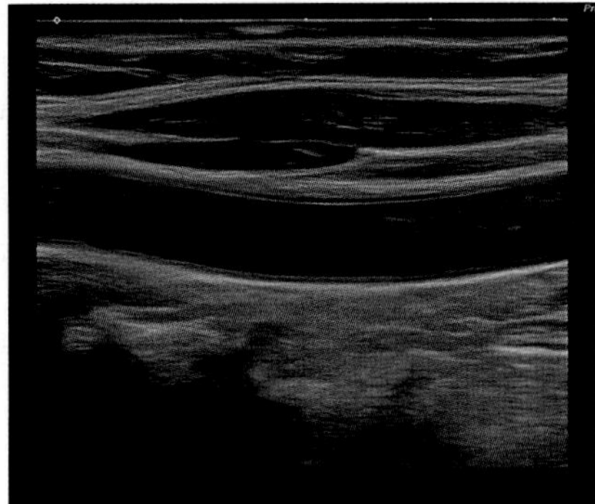

A B

Figure 2-16 Linear sequenced array transducer format **(A)** and image **(B)**.

(Figure 2-16). With the linear sequenced array, the elements are arranged in a line, next to each other, but are shocked in small groups in sequence. For example, the elements are not shocked in this pattern: 1–2–3–4–5, but are shocked in this pattern: (1–2–3) ... (4–5–6) ... (7–8–9) are shocked. Linear sequenced arrays do not need any beam steering to produce a rectangular image. However, should beam steering be needed, whether for Doppler or to create a vector image, the beam can be electronically steered via phasing (Table 2-8).

> **SOUND OFF**
> The image from a linear sequenced array is produced by shocking the elements in groups, in sequence.

Curved Sequenced Array

The **curved sequenced array** transducer, also referred to as a convex, curvilinear, or curved sequential array, is based on the same technology as that of the linear sequenced array but with a curved face (Figures 2-17 and 2-18). As with the linear sequenced array, the elements are fired in groups, in sequence (Table 2-9).

Phased Arrays

The **phased array** is more commonly known as a sector or vector transducer (Figure 2-19). The sector/vector transducer typically has a small footprint, also referred to as the "face" of the transducer, and it may be used for cardiac imaging, neonatal brain imaging, with some endocavity transducers, and any other application where a sector or vector image shape is desired (Figure 2-20).

TABLE 2-8 Linear sequenced array

- Also referred to as linear sequential array or linear array
- Rectangular-shaped image
- Elements shocked in sequence
- Electronic steering available via phasing
- Electronically focused via phasing
- Used for vascular and high-resolution imaging

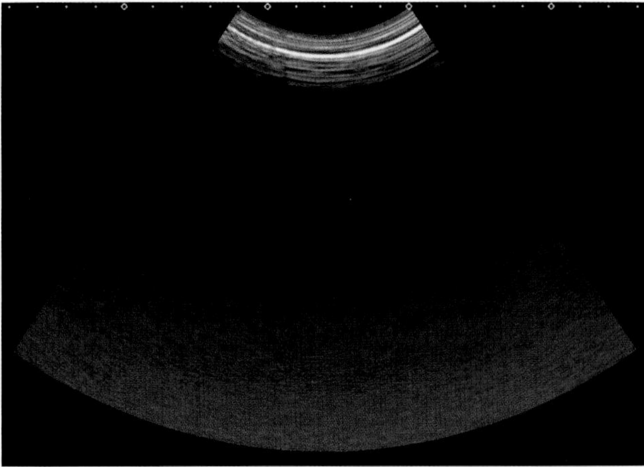

A

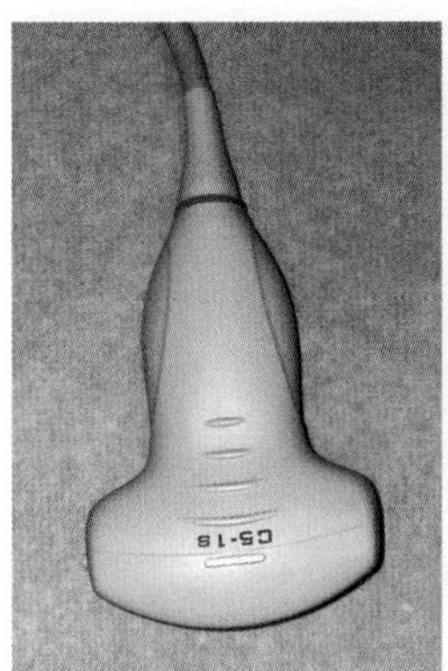

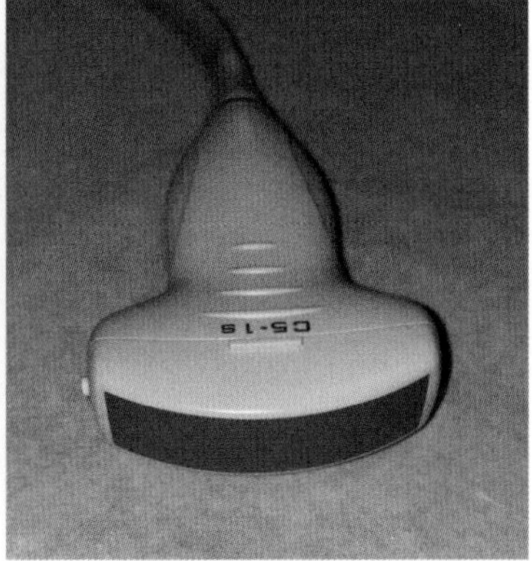

B

Figure 2-17 Curvilinear array transducer. **A.** The image shape of the curvilinear array transducer. **B.** Image of a curvilinear array transducer.

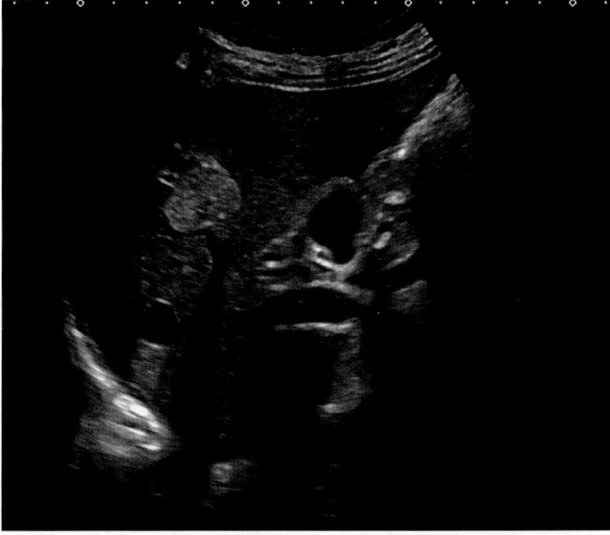

Figure 2-18 Image from curved sequenced array.

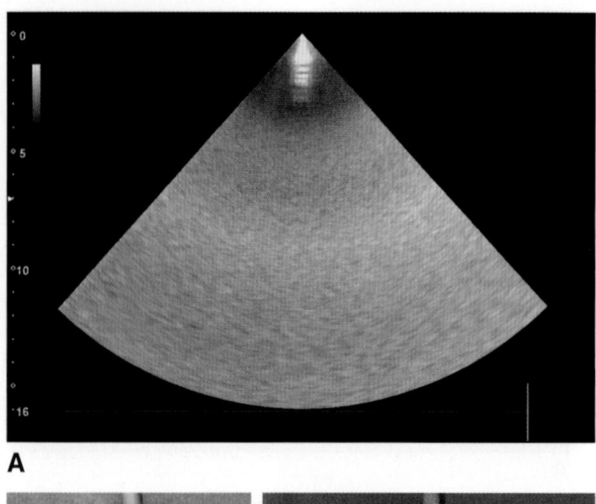

A

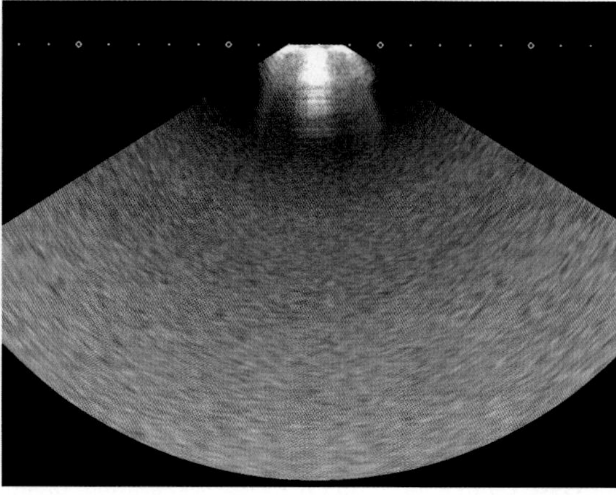

B

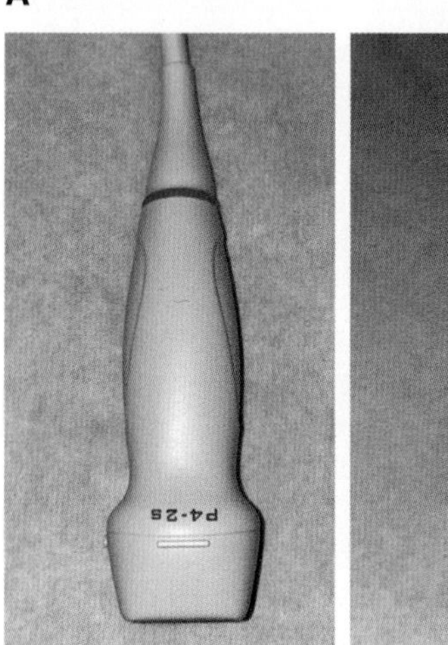

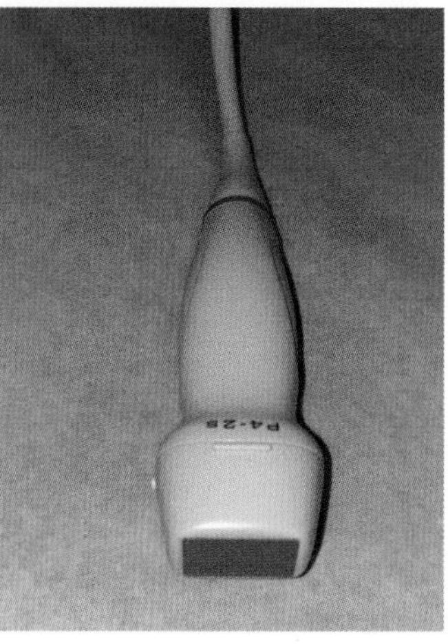

C

Figure 2-19 Phased array transducer. **(A)** Image from sector and **(B)** vector phased array transducers **(C)** Phased array transducer.

In order to create a sector image, electronic steering is needed for every scan line. Unlike the curved and linear sequenced arrays, where the shape of the transducer dictates the shape of the image, in the phased array, the shape of the face of the transducer does not resemble the shape of the image. This transducer can make either the sector, which yields a true "pie-shaped" image, or the vector image shape, which yields the flat-topped, trapezoidal image shape (Figure 2-21). With the sector phased array transducer, all of the scan lines originate from a common point of origin.

The phased array transducer uses **phasing** to steer and focus the beam (Table 2-10). Phasing is altering the

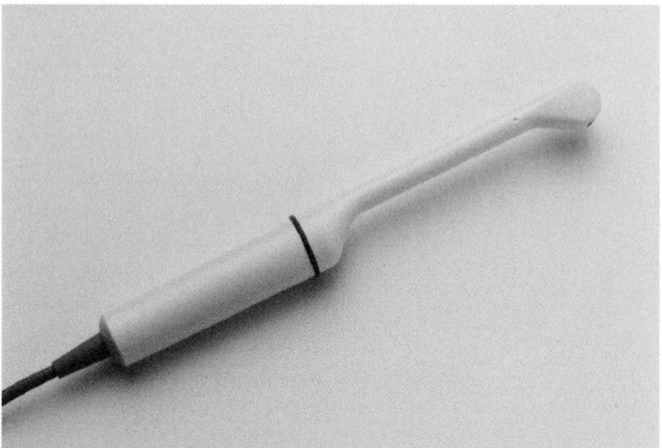

Figure 2-20 Endovaginal transducer. Endocavity transducers, including endovaginal and endorectal transducers, can be curved or phased arrays.

TABLE 2-9 Curved sequenced array

- Also referred to as a convex, curvilinear, or curved sequential array
- Curved-shaped image
- Elements shocked in sequence
- Electronically focused via phasing
- Used for abdominal, gynecology, and obstetrics imaging

TABLE 2-10 Phased array

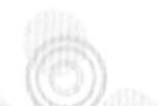

- Also referred to as sector or vector transducer
- Vector- or sector-shaped image
- Electronic phased steering and phased focusing
- Used for cardiac, abdominal, neonatal imaging, and endocavity transducers

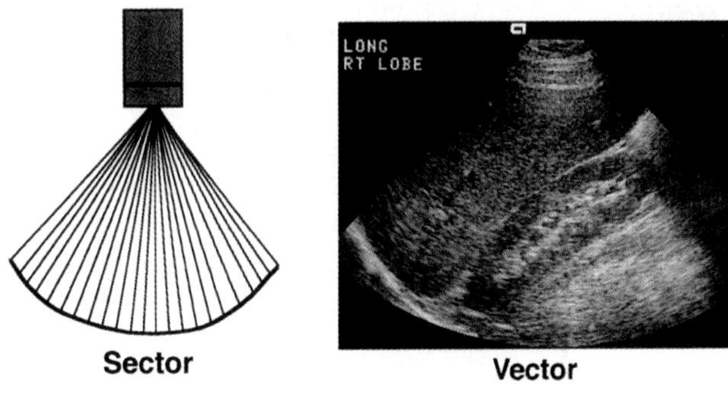

Figure 2-21 Phased array transducer and sector versus vector image shapes. **A.** A sector transducer produces a "piece of pie"-shaped image with a common point of origin on the transducer face. **B.** Vector transducers are sector transducers in which the scan lines do not have a common point of origin and the image is trapezoidal.

timing of the shocking of the elements in order to shape and steer the beam (Figure 2-22). All arrays, including sequenced arrays, are phased focused, that is, all of the array transducers mentioned in this section use phasing to control focusing in the scan plane. Phasing provides a sonographer with the ability to control the depth of the focal zone in the scan plane. The order in which the elements are shocked determines beam steering and focusing (Figures 2-23 to 2-25). Transducers can also focus when the beam returns to the patient,

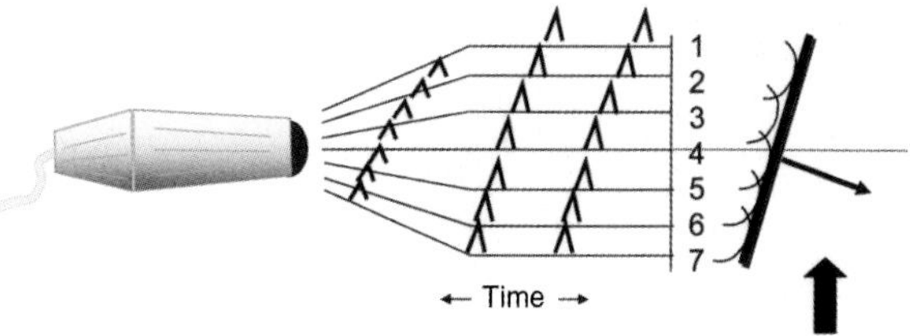

Figure 2-23 More about phasing and beam steering. Phased array technology permits steering of the ultrasound beam. By adjusting the timing of excitation of the individual piezoelectric crystals, the wavefront of ultrasound energy can be directed, as shown. Beam steering is a fundamental feature of how 2D images are created.

called a receive focusing or **dynamic focusing**. Refer to Figure 2-7 for an illustration of dynamic focusing in the transducer.

Three-Dimensional Transducers

Three-dimensional (3D) ultrasound images are traditionally made up of two-dimensional (2D) acquisitions placed next to each other (Figure 2-26). A 3D image allows the user to see a whole volume: width, height, and depth. Therefore, it may also be referred to as volume scanning. There are three different ways to create the 3D image: freehand, with a motorized 3D/4D transducer, or the newest method, with 2D array technology.

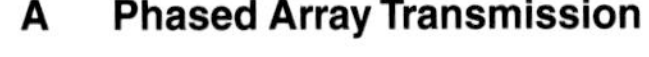

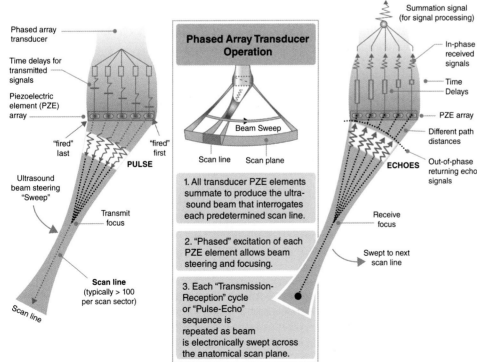

Figure 2-22 Phased array transducer operation. **A** and **B:** Simultaneous transmission and reception of ultrasound signals occur, although for simplicity, they are displayed separately. **A:** During phased array transmission, all transducer elements are excited and summate to form the ultrasound beam or scan line. **B:** During reception, the returning echoes (arising from that same scan line) are time-shifted, phase-adjusted, and summated.

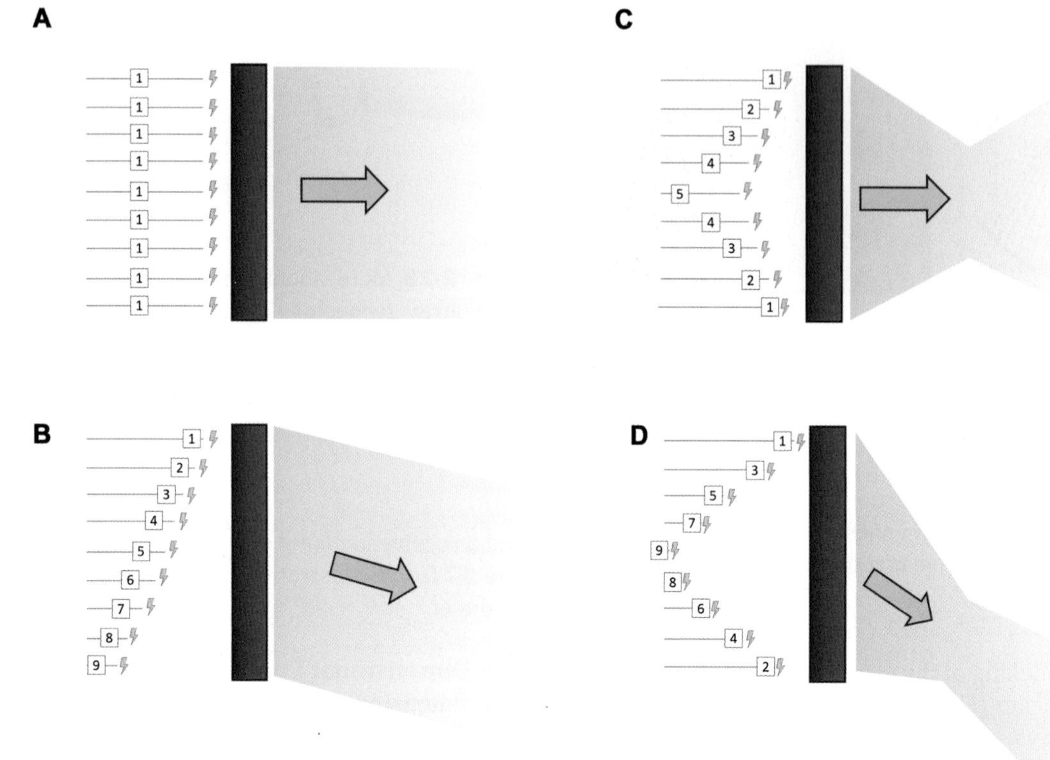

Figure 2-24 Phased steering and focusing of the beam. The steering and shape of the beam is determined by the pattern of electrical shocks sent to individual elements. **A.** All elements shocked at same time is a beam that is not steered. **B.** If the elements are shocked one at a time in a linear fashion, the beam is steered left or right. **C.** A curvature in the "shock pattern" implies that the beam is focused. If the two end elements are shocked at the same time, the beam is focused but not steered. **D.** If the shock pattern has a curvature but the end elements are shocked at different times, the beam is steered and focused.

In the freehand method, also referred to as manual, the sonographer is responsible for moving the transducer through a path to gather the 2D slices (Figure 2-27). This method is the most operator dependent, as it relies upon the steady hand of the sonographer

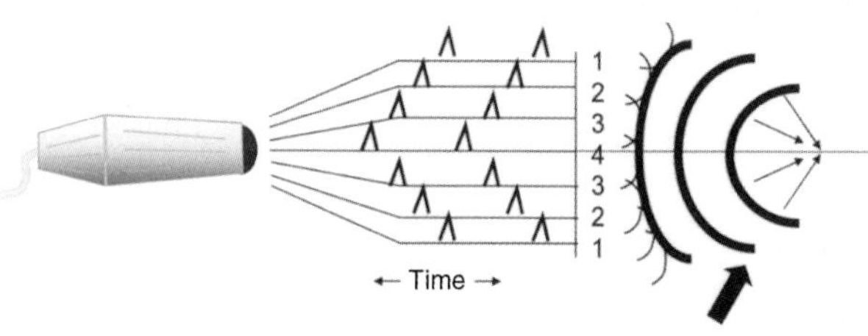

Figure 2-25 Phasing and focusing. By adjusting the timing of excitation of the individual crystals within a phased array transducer, the beam can be focused. In this example, the outer elements are fired first, followed sequentially by the more central elements. Because the speed of sound is fixed, this manipulation in the timing of excitation results in a wavefront that is curved and focused. This is called "transmit focusing." Changing the timing of when the elements are shocked focuses the beam.

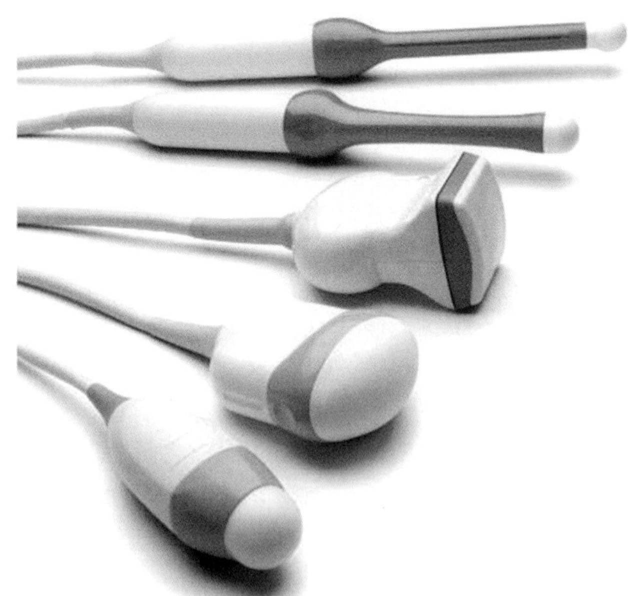

Figure 2-26 Motorized (mechanical) 3D/4D transducers contain a motor within the transducer housing that provides a consistent automated sweep. Endocavity linear, curved, and small-footprint 3D/4D transducers are available.

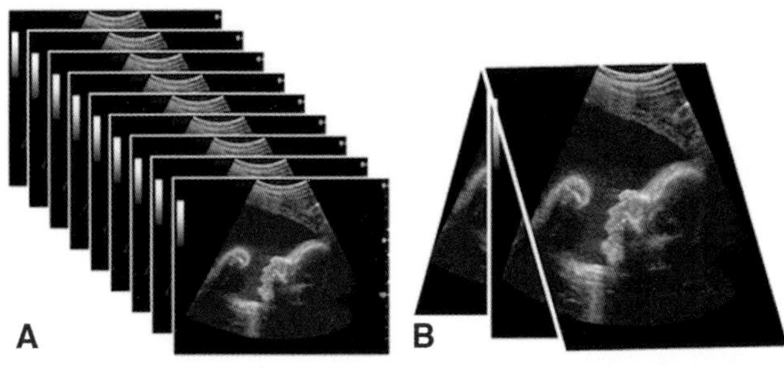

Figure 2-27 Freehand technique. **A.** Transducer is moved in a parallel fashion, and the 2D images are stacked together to form a 3D volume. **B.** Transducer is moved in a sweeping or fan motion. The 2D images are aligned together to form a 3D volume.

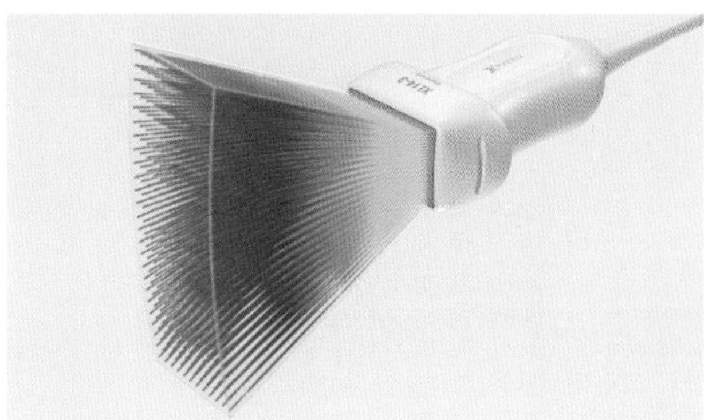

Figure 2-28 Linear 2D array transducer. (Courtesy of Philips Healthcare).

to move the transducer at the same speed over the tissue. Because of the potential variability in movement across the plane, measurements of the 3D image are not possible with the freehand 3D technique. The 2D slices, once converted to a 3D format, may then be sliced to view coronal, longitudinal, and axial planes and surface rendering of a structure (Figure 2-29).

SOUND OFF
There are three different ways to create the 3D image: freehand, with a mechanical transducer, or with a 2D array, which is the newest method.

With the motorized 3D/4D transducer, also referred to as the automated or mechanical 3D method, specialized transducers have been developed, which are linear or curved sequenced array transducers mounted onto a motor. These transducers permit the measurement on the screen of the 3D image as well as the use of real-time 3D ultrasound, also known as **four-dimensional (4D) ultrasound**. The **frame rate** of the 4D image is limited by the speed of the motor to which the transducer is attached. The newest technology for acquiring a 3D image is the 2D array or **matrix array transducer** (Figures 2-28 to 2-30). These transducers create scan lines in two planes (hence the term 2D array) and

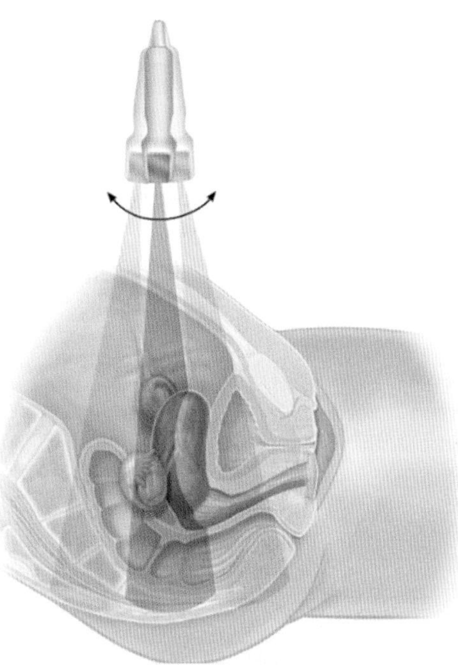

A

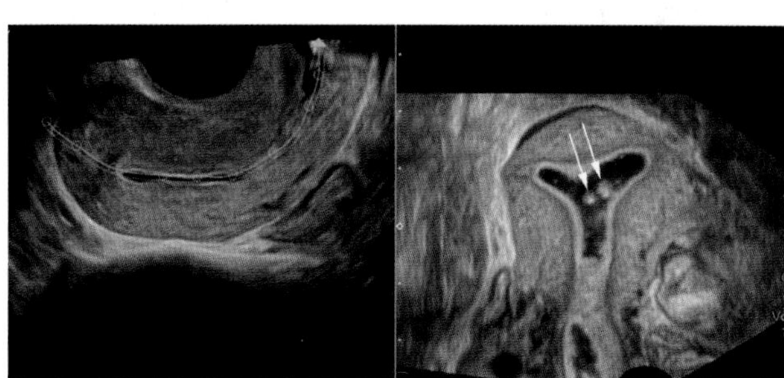

B

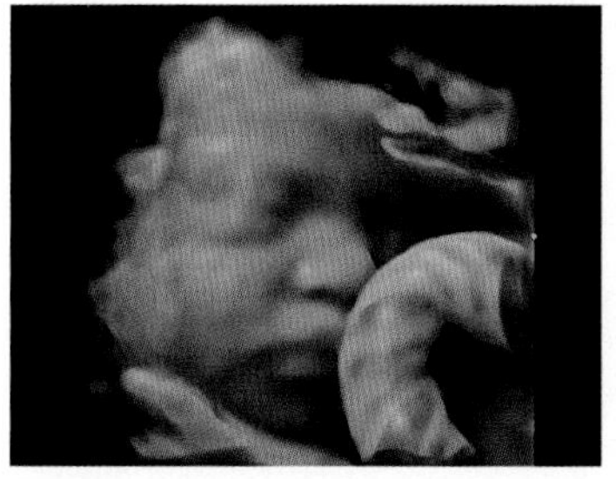

C

Figure 2-29 3D imaging. **A.** Freehand technique for obtaining 3D image (From Stephenson SR, Dmitrieva J. *Lippincott Connect for Obstetrics and Gynecology*. 5th ed. Wolters Kluwer Health; 2023). **B.** This machine has a package that allows the operator to scan through an organ and create a coronal image in post-processing (ie, after the image is frozen). This image is a reconstruction of the coronal uterus demonstrating polyps in the endometrial canal (*arrows*). **C.** Surface rendering image from mechanical curvilinear transducer. (Courtesy of Mindray North America).

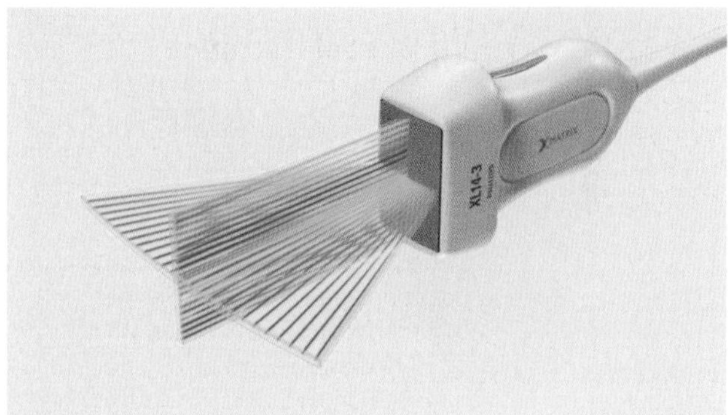

Figure 2-30 Image of a matrix or 2D array transducer. (Courtesy of Philips Healthcare).

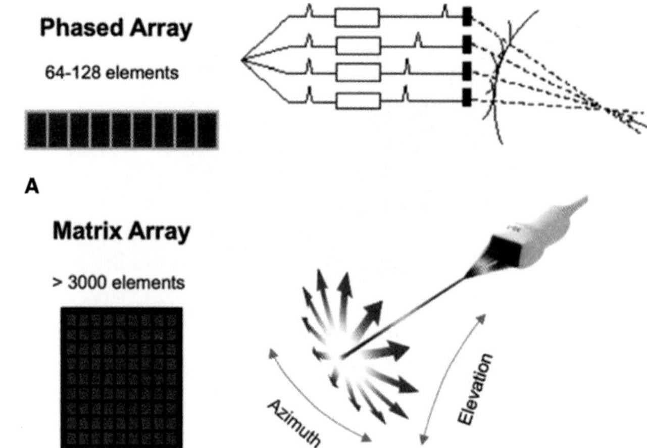

Figure 2-31 Comparison of phased (1D) array and matrix (2D) array. Schematic of the phased array **(A)** and the matrix array **(B)** transducer, with their respective steering capabilities. The phased array can only steer in one dimension, by firing elements in a specific sequence. In contrast, the checkerboard pattern of the 2D array allows phased firing of all the elements to offer a real-time 3D volume.

acquire real-time volumes using transducers with 3000 to over 90,000 elements compared with the 128 to 512 elements used in standard 1D array transducers (Figure 2-31). Figure 2-32 is an example of the ability of 2D arrays to produce a 3D volume in addition to imaging long and short axes simultaneously.

Continuous-Wave Transducers

CW transducers are utilized as part of Doppler studies. A dedicated CW transducer contains two piezoelectric elements: one to continuously transmit sound and one to continuously receive sound. No image is generated with these transducers because it is not possible to time how long it takes the echoes to return (Figure 2-33). Therefore, CW transducers have no **range resolution** (ie, they have depth ambiguity), and their only use is CW spectral Doppler. CW spectral Doppler can be performed either with a dedicated non-imaging probe (such as the Pedoff) or as part of a phased array transducer.

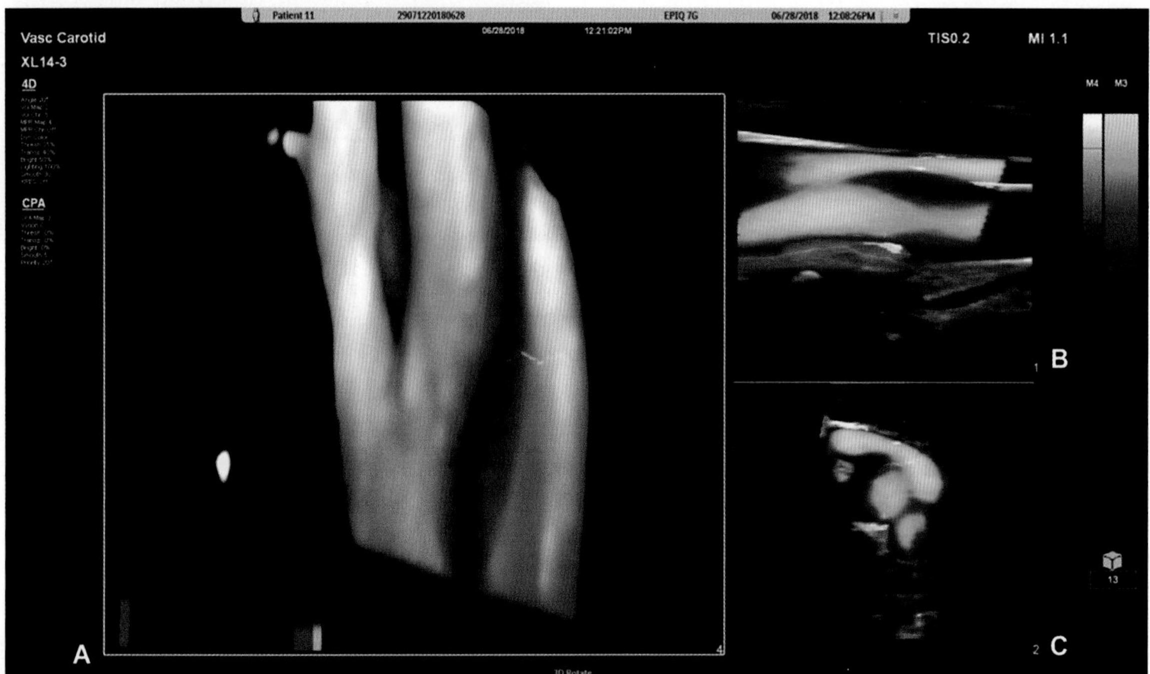

Figure 2-32 Images acquired by 2D array. **(A)** Surface rendering of extracranial blood vessels **(B)** Longitudinal and **(C)** Transverse images of the extracranial blood vessels. With a 2D array, long and short axis images can be acquired simultaneously in two dimensions and volumes can be acquired in real time. (Courtesy of Philips Healthcare).

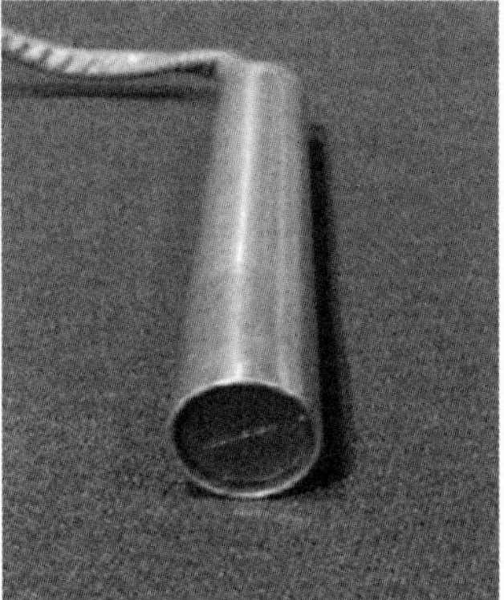

Figure 2-33 Dedicated CW transducer. A CW transducer uses two elements: one for producing sound and one for receiving sound. CW, continuous wave.

RESOLUTION

Spatial Resolution

Spatial resolution can be defined as the ability of a system to distinguish between closely spaced objects. Spatial (meaning space) resolution relates to the quality of the detail of an image. It can be divided into four components: **axial resolution**, **lateral resolution**, **elevational resolution**, and **contrast resolution** (Table 2-11 and Figure 2-34).

TABLE 2-11 Spatial resolution

Components of Spatial Resolution	Definition	Synonyms
Axial resolution	The minimum distance between two reflectors that are parallel to the beam and still appear on the screen as two dots	Longitudinal Axial Radial Range Depth
Lateral resolution	The ability to accurately identify reflectors that are arranged perpendicular to the ultrasound beam	Lateral Angular Transverse Azimuthal
Elevational resolution	The resolution in the third dimension of the beam: the slice-thickness plane	Slice- or section-thickness plane resolution
Contrast resolution	The ability to differentiate tissues with similar shades of gray	None

SOUND OFF
Remembering the word "LARRD" (*l*ongitudinal, *a*xial, *r*adial, *r*ange, *d*epth) can help one recall the different names for axial resolution.

Axial Resolution

Axial resolution is the minimum distance between two reflectors that are parallel to the beam and still appear on the screen as two separate dots, that is, if the transducer is aiming at two reflectors on the screen (parallel to the beam), then two dots should appear on the display (Figure 2-35). Axial resolution may also be referred to as longitudinal, axial, radial, range, and depth. Remembering the word "LARRD" (like the lard that goes in cookies and pies) can help one recall the different names for axial resolution.

SPL is determined when the transducer is built and is the wavelength (λ) multiplied by the number of cycles in a pulse (n). The SPL determines the system's axial resolution. Specifically, the shorter the pulse used, the better the axial resolution of the system. When a shorter pulse is desired, the manufacturer

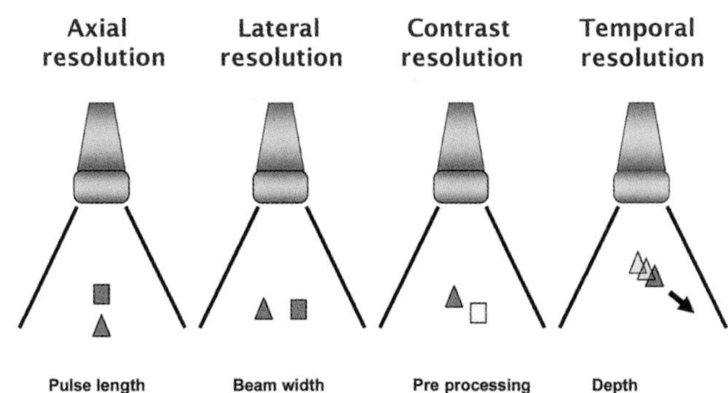

Figure 2-34 Primary determinants of axial, lateral, contrast, and temporal resolution.

Ultrasound Transducers

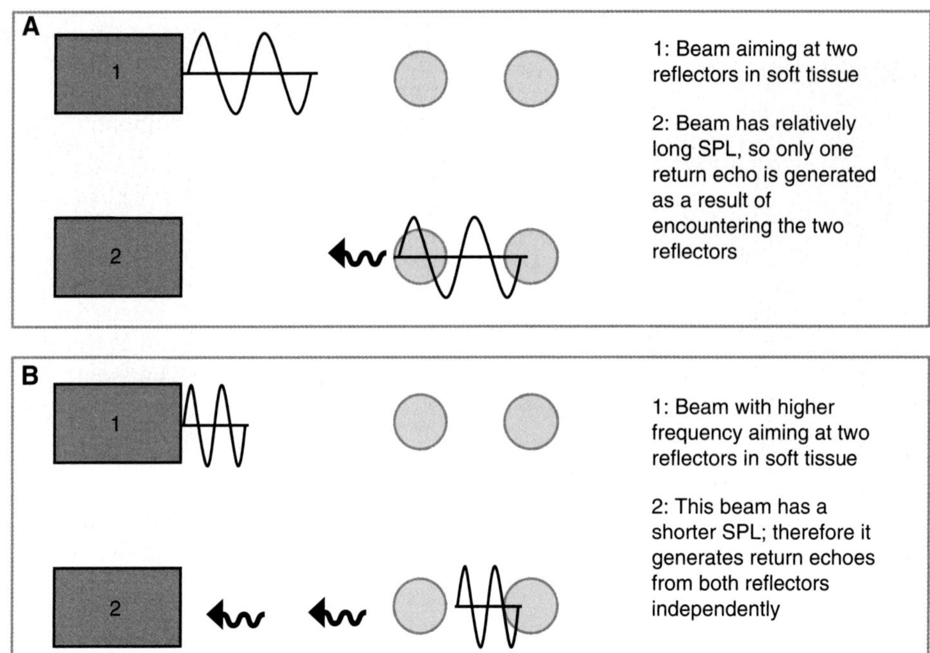
A
1
2
1: Beam aiming at two reflectors in soft tissue
2: Beam has relatively long SPL, so only one return echo is generated as a result of encountering the two reflectors
B
1
2
1: Beam with higher frequency aiming at two reflectors in soft tissue
2: This beam has a shorter SPL; therefore it generates return echoes from both reflectors independently

Figure 2-35 Axial resolution. Axial resolution is the minimum distance two reflectors can be, parallel to the beam, and still appear on the screen as two dots. **A.** A TD with a low-frequency beam is aiming at two reflectors in soft tissue. This beam has a relatively long SPL, so only one return echo is generated as a result of encountering the two reflectors. **B.** A TD with a higher frequency beam is aiming at the same two reflectors in soft tissue. This beam has relatively short SPL; therefore, it generates return echoes from both reflectors independently. TD, transducer; SPL, spatial pulse length.

of the transducer can decrease the length of the pulse by either decreasing the wavelength or decreasing the number of cycles per pulse (Table 2-12). The number of cycles can be decreased by adding more damping material. The wavelength can be decreased by increasing the frequency (Table 2-13). Therefore a higher frequency shortens the pulse, which is why higher frequency transducers offer better axial resolution than lower frequency transducers (Figure 2-36). Axial resolution is equal to one-half of the SPL (Table 2-14). It is important to note that if the SPL decreases, the numerical value for axial resolution decreases. Therefore, the lower the numerical value for axial resolution, the better the axial resolution of the transducer. In other words, an axial resolution of 0.2 mm is better than an axial resolution of 0.4 mm because two reflectors could be as close as 0.2 mm apart and still be resolved as two distinct echoes. Use caution when answering questions about axial resolution. Thus, in regard to these questions, you must ask yourself: "Are you provided with the SPL or the axial resolution?" If you are provided with the SPL, you will need to divide the number by 2 in order to obtain the axial resolution. Some examples of questions that may be asked about axial resolution are provided in Table 2-15.

> **SOUND OFF**
> The SPL determines the system's axial resolution. The shorter the pulse used, the better the axial resolution of the system.

> **SOUND OFF**
> Remembering the word "LATA" (*l*ateral, *a*ngular, *t*ransverse, *a*zimuthal) can help one recall the different names for lateral resolution.

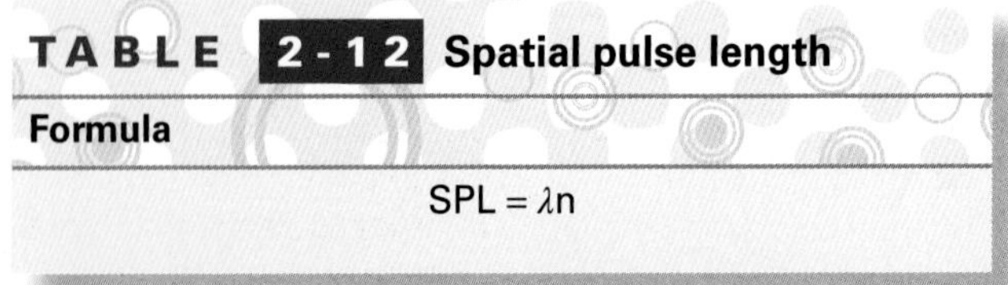

TABLE 2-12 Spatial pulse length

Formula
$SPL = \lambda n$

Spatial pulse length (SPL) is equal to the wavelength (λ) multiplied by the number of cycles (n) in the pulse.

TABLE 2-13 Wavelength

Formula
$\lambda = c/f$

Wavelength (λ) is equal to the propagation speed (c) divided by the frequency (f).

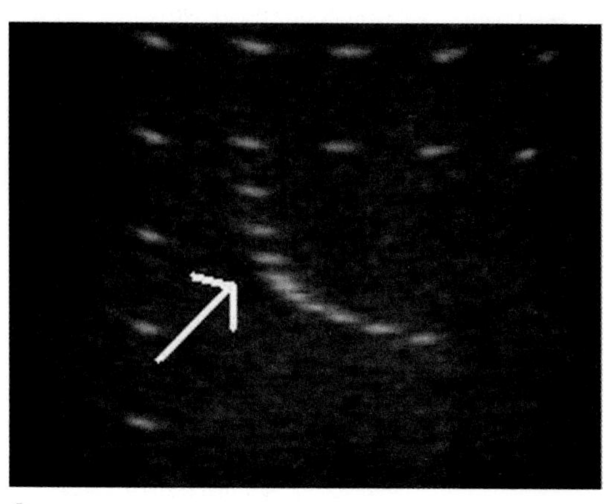

A

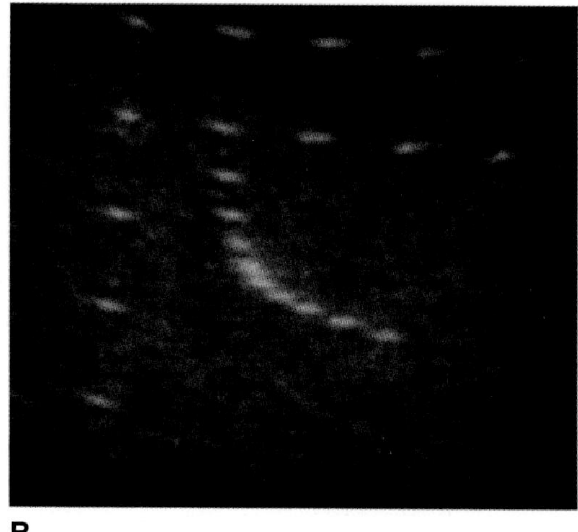

B

Figure 2-36 Frequency and axial resolution. The axial resolution of a high-frequency transducer **(A)** is much better at identifying separate pins (*arrow*) than the axial resolution of a lower-frequency transducer **(B)**, in which the pins merge and appear less distinct.

Lateral Resolution

Lateral relates to the width of the beam and the reflectors that lie perpendicular to it (Figure 2-37). Lateral resolution is the ability of a beam to pass between two reflectors that are perpendicular to the beam and not generate a return echo. Lateral resolution may also be referred to as lateral, angular, transverse, and azimuthal. Remembering the word "LATA" (like "latte," but LATA) can help with the different names for axial resolution (Table 2-11). Poor lateral resolution is apparent when reflectors appear to be wider than they are supposed to be (Figure 2-38).

The diameter of the beam is determined by the wavelength and the diameter of the element itself, also referred to as the **aperture**. In a conventional transducer, the beam takes on a shape in the appearance of an hourglass (Figure 2-39). As the beam leaves the transducer and travels into the patient, the diameter of the beam varies with distance. The beam begins to narrow immediately upon leaving the transducer. At its narrowest point, it is called the **focal point** or **focal zone**. The region from the transducer face to the focal point is called the **near zone** or **Fresnel zone**. Subsequently, the length of the near zone is referred to as the **near-zone length** (NZL). The depth of the focal point is called the **focal depth**. Distant to the focal depth, the beam starts to diverge, or spread. The region distal to the focal point is called the **far zone** or **Fraunhofer zone**. **Divergence**, or the spreading out of the beam, is detrimental to lateral resolution. Recall, a narrow beam width is desired in order to improve lateral resolution. Subsequently, the focal zone should be placed at or below the area of interest to obtain the best lateral resolution in that area.

TABLE 2-14 Axial resolution

Formula
Axial resolution = ½ SPL

The axial resolution is equal to one-half of the spatial pulse length (SPL).

SOUND OFF
The diameter of the beam is determined by both the frequency and the diameter of the element itself, also referred to as the aperture.

TABLE 2-15 Examples of questions relating to axial resolution

Question	Explanation
The axial resolution of the transducer is 0.2 mm. What is the smallest distance that two reflectors can be in order to appear as two echoes on the screen?	The answer is 0.2 mm. The two reflectors have to be the same as the axial resolution of the transducer or greater in order to be displayed as two distinct echoes.
The spatial pulse length of the transducer is 0.2 mm. What is the smallest distance two reflectors can be apart in order to appear as two echoes on the screen?	The answer is 0.1 mm. This time the SPL is given, not the axial resolution. The axial resolution of a transducer equals one-half of the SPL, so the SPL has to be halved in order to determine the axial resolution. In this case, ½ SPL = 0.1 mm.

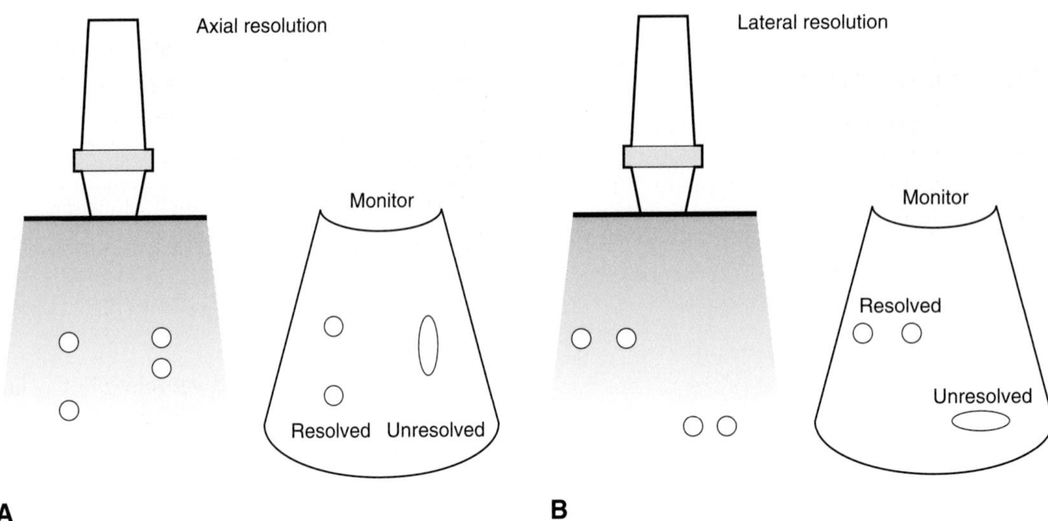

Figure 2-37 Difference between axial and lateral resolution **(A)**. Axial resolution is in line with the scanning plane **(B)**. Lateral resolution is perpendicular to the scanning plane.

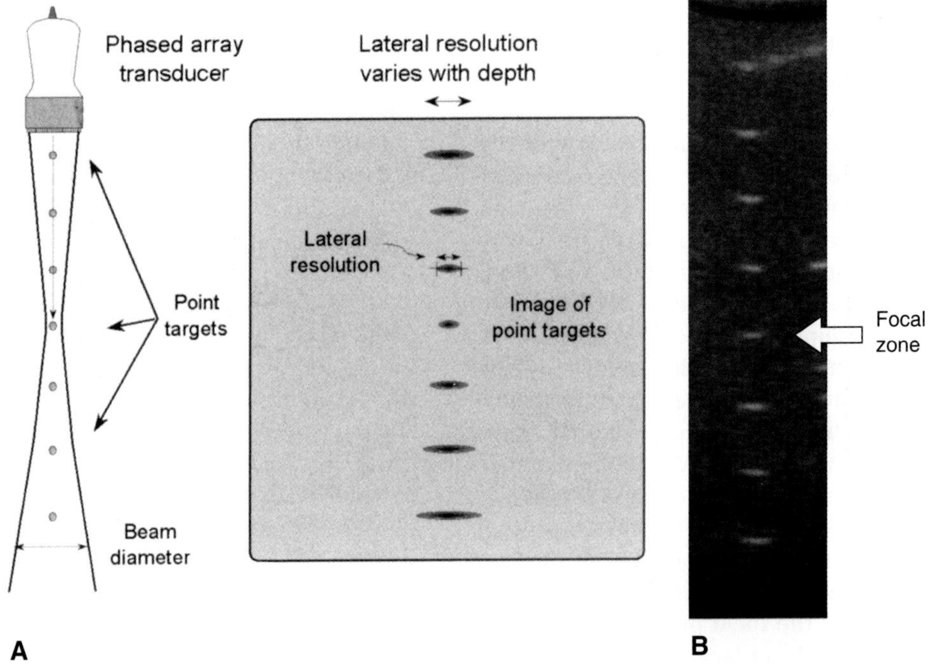

Figure 2-38 Lateral resolution. The beam changes shape as it travels deeper **(A)**. Depending on where the reflectors are located in the beam determines the lateral resolution. **B.** Notice how the reflectors appear to be wider where the beam diverges in this sonographic image of a tissue equivalent phantom showing lateral resolution.

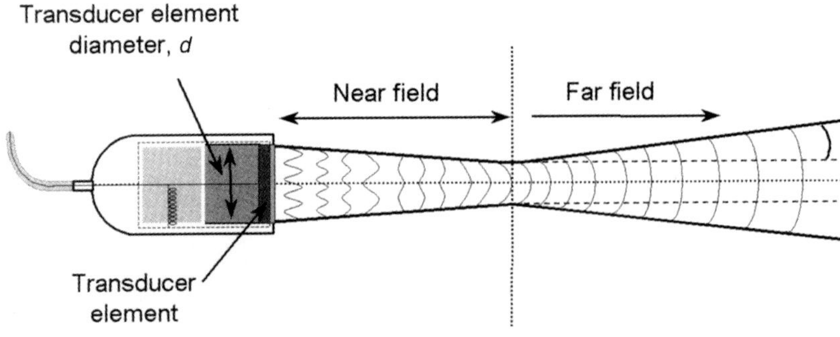

Figure 2-39 Hourglass-shaped ultrasound beam. Near field (zone) and far field (zone).

TABLE 2-16 Characteristics of an unfocused single-element transducer

- At the face of the transducer, the beam diameter is equal to the element diameter.
- At a distance of one near-zone length, the beam diameter is equal to one-half of the diameter of the element.
- At a distance of two near-zone lengths, the beam diameter again equals the element diameter.

TABLE 2-17 The relationship between frequency, aperture size, near-zone length (NZL), and divergence in the far field

Adjustment	Result
↑ Frequency	↑ NZL and ↓ divergence in far field
↑ Aperture	↑ NZL and ↓ divergence in far field

SOUND OFF
Like axial resolution, lateral resolution is best when the numerical value is smaller. Also, most transducers have better axial resolution than lateral resolution.

Discussions about lateral resolution usually use the example of a disk-shaped, single-element unfocused transducer to make the physics easier. However, even an unfocused transducer has a natural focal zone despite the absence of a lens. Assuming an unfocused beam from a single-element transducer, the beam diameter has several specific characteristics (Table 2-16 and Figure 2-40). As the beam propagates, its diameter changes. Therefore, lateral resolution does vary with depth. Both the actual diameter of the element and the frequency of the transducer have an effect on the NZL and the amount of divergence in the far field. A smaller aperture results in a shorter NZL and more divergence in the far field. If the transducer and the frequency do not change, but a larger aperture is utilized, a longer NZL will result, with less divergence in the far field. The same theory is true for identical aperture size, but different frequencies, that is, for a given aperture, the lower the frequency, the shorter the NZL, with an increase of divergence in the far field. Conversely, the higher the frequency, the longer the NZL, with less divergence in the far field (Table 2-17). Like axial resolution, lateral resolution is best when the numerical value is smaller. Therefore, a lateral resolution of 0.2 mm is better than a lateral resolution of 0.4 mm. It is important to note that most transducers have better axial resolution than lateral resolution. Table 2-18 reviews how to solve questions on lateral resolution.

Elevational Resolution and Contrast Resolution

A sonographic image is a 2D representation of 3D objects. The image seen on the ultrasound monitor is flat. However, in conventional ultrasound transducers, the beam is not razor thin but has definite thickness. The image on the ultrasound monitor is a compressed version of any object located within the ultrasound beam. Therefore, bogus echoes may be seen within a simple cyst because the beam is also slicing through the tissue next to the cyst. This third dimension of the beam

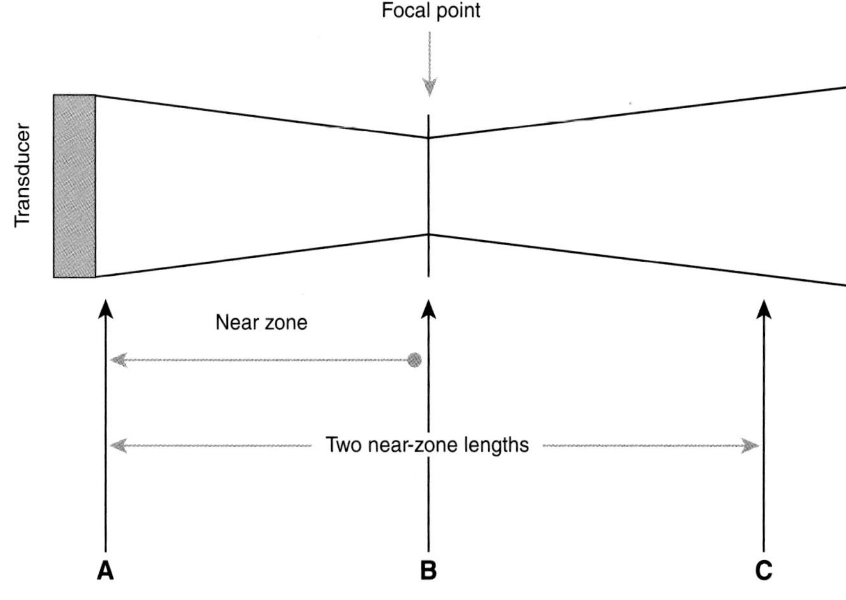

Figure 2-40 Single-element unfocused transducer. At the face of the transducer **(A)**, the beam width equals the element diameter. At a distance of one near-zone length **(B)**, the beam diameter is half the element diameter. At a distance of two near-zone lengths **(C)**, the beam diameter again equals the element diameter. Deep to this point, the beam continues to diverge.

Ultrasound Transducers

TABLE 2-18 Examples of questions on lateral resolution

1. You want to image a structure that is deeper than your current depth. In order to image deeper and have the area be in the near zone, what single-element transducer configuration do you want?
   - To increase the near-zone length, either increase the operating frequency or increase the element aperture. Of course, increasing the frequency limits penetration, so increasing the element diameter may be the best option.
2. What transducer configuration increases divergence in the far zone?
   - Beam divergence in the far zone is highest with transducers that are low frequency and/or have a small aperture.
3. Look at the image below and determine where the beam diameter will equal 20 mm deep to the transducer's face.

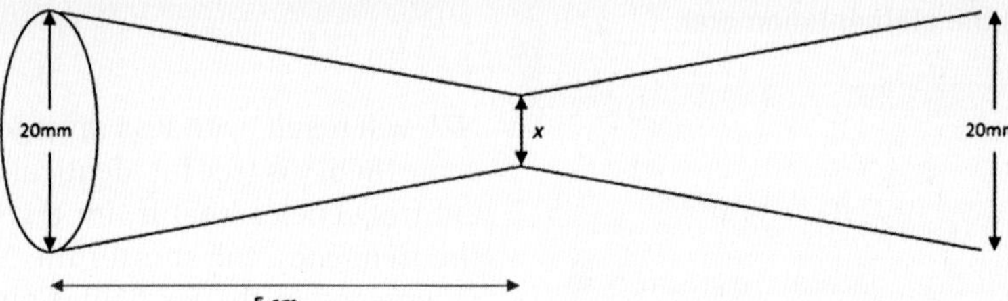

- The aperture is 20 mm. The beam diameter at the face of the transducer is 20 mm and 10 mm at the focal point (*x*). The beam diameter will again equal 20 mm at two near-zone lengths or 10 cm.

is called the **slice-thickness plane**. The slice-thickness plane may also be referred to as the **section-thickness plane** or the **elevational plane**. Elevational resolution is the resolution in the third dimension of the beam.

SOUND OFF
Elevational resolution is the resolution in the third dimension of the beam.

SOUND OFF
Contrast resolution is the ability to differentiate tissues with similar shades of gray.

To obtain the most diagnostic representation of the body, the thinnest plane possible should ideally be utilized. As with lateral resolution, the thinnest elevational plane is optimal. This is achieved by focusing. However, unlike electronic transducers with phased focusing, transducers are commonly focused with a lens in the slice-thickness plane. Because the slice-thickness plane is focused with a lens, the focus in this plane is fixed and does not change regardless of the depth (Figure 2-41).

Transducers with the ability to focus electronically in the elevational plane (Figure 2-42) are referred to as 1.5D transducers. These transducers allow for multiple focal zones in the elevational plane, yielding a narrower slice thickness.

Another type of spatial resolution is contrast resolution. **Contrast resolution** is the ability to differentiate tissues with similar shades of gray. It is related to dynamic range, which is discussed further in Chapter 3 of this book.

Temporal Resolution

As an introduction to this section, imagine your friend asks for help painting some walls for a project. You are going to paint one wall, and your friend is going to paint the other. You do not like painting, so you want to choose the easier job. Do you take the wall that is 8 feet long or 6 feet long? The 6-feet wall would take less time, right? Would you take the wall that is 5 feet high or 10 feet high? The shorter wall would take less time, right? Would you apply one coat? Or two coats? One coat would take less time, right? **Temporal resolution** represents the ability

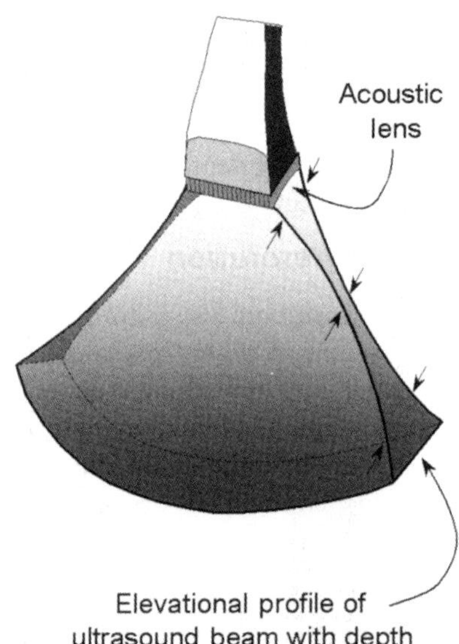

Figure 2-41 Elevational resolution. Elevational resolution is most commonly focused with a lens.

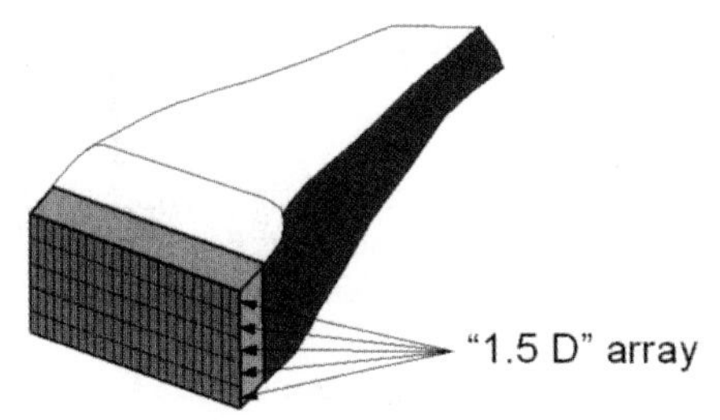

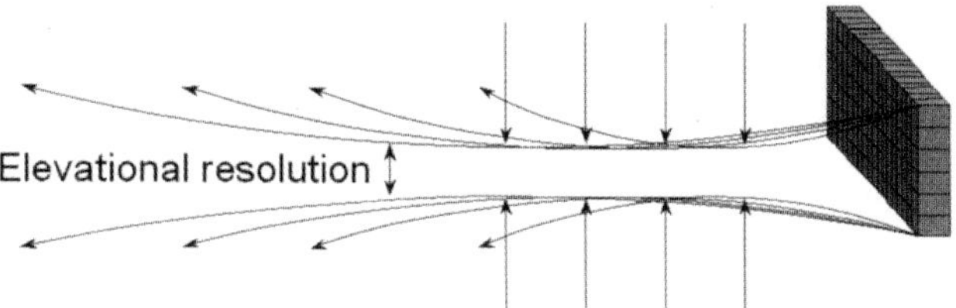

Figure 2-42 A 1.5D transducer. The 1.5D transducer is capable of electronically focusing the beam in the elevational plane.

to display structures in real time. Temporal (time) resolution relates to how quickly frames are generated. Another more commonly used term for temporal resolution is **frame rate**. A complete sonographic image, or frame, needs to be placed on the screen, scan line by line, before the next frame can begin to be placed. The longer it takes a frame to be displayed on the screen, the lower the frame rate and the worse the temporal resolution. The unit in which the frame rate can be expressed is hertz (Hz), which is equivalent to FPS.

SOUND OFF
Temporal resolution represents time or the ability to display structures in real time. It relates to how quickly frames are generated.

There are three adjustments that can be made to alter the frame rate in grayscale imaging: image depth (pulse repetition frequency (PRF)), the number of focal zones, and the number of scan lines per frame or line density (Figure 2-43). As the depth is increased, the pulse must travel farther or deeper into the body. A new pulse cannot be sent out until the previous pulse is received. Therefore, the machine has to wait before sending out the next pulse. The longer it takes to create one scan line, the longer it takes to display one frame. Therefore, PRF is directly related to the frame rate, that is, the higher the PRF, the shallower the image and the higher the frame rate. Recall that focal zones are created by phasing. However, there can only be one focal zone per scan line. If more than one focal zone is desired, it will take an extra pulse per scan line for each focal zone desired.

SOUND OFF
Line density, the spacing between the scan lines, also affects the frame rate. The higher the line density, the worse the temporal resolution.

Current ultrasound technology allows the width of the image to be increased or decreased. The more scan

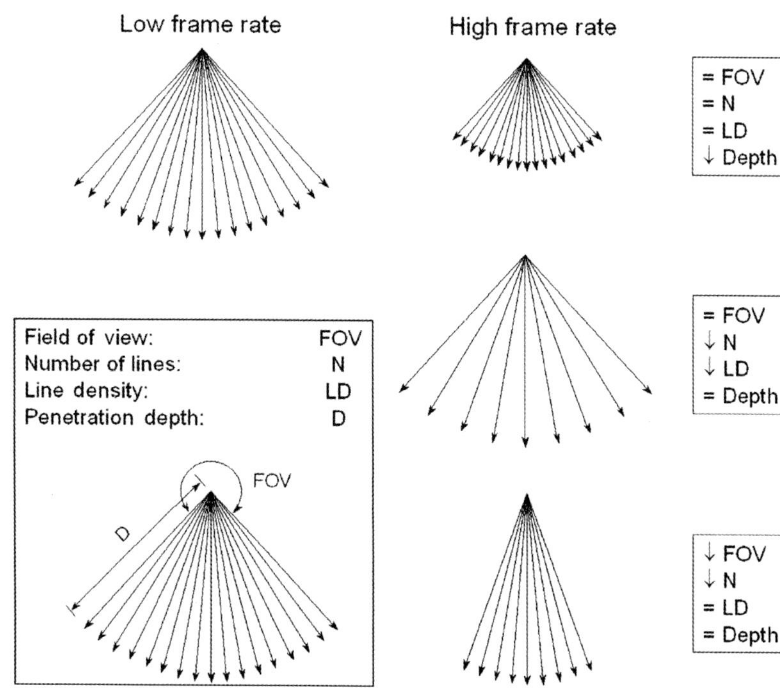

Figure 2-43 Temporal resolution and frame rate. Temporal resolution represents time, or the ability to display structures in real time. Ultrasound image quality depends on several factors, including the FOV, the number of scan lines per image (N), the line density (LD), and penetration depth (D) (**inset**), in addition to the image frame rate. Preserving the frame rate involves trade-offs. Changing any of the aforementioned parameters will affect the frame rate unless something else is changed to counter the effect. For example, if the depth is decreased, the frame rate will increase (**top right**). If the depth is then increased, in order to preserve the frame rate, either the line density or FOV must decrease (**middle and lower right**). FOV, field of view.

TABLE 2-19 Formula for frame rate

Formula
$$FR = \frac{PRF}{LPF}$$

The frame rate (FR) is equal to the pulse repetition frequency (PRF) divided by the lines per frame (LPF).

lines that need to be displayed, the longer it takes to create one frame, and therefore, the worse the temporal resolution. A wider image will usually require more scan lines than a narrower image. In the instance where the temporal resolution is inadequate, such as imaging a deep structure while using multiple focal zones, the frame rate can be improved by using a narrower image width, thereby decreasing the number of lines per frame. Line density, the spacing between the scan lines, also affects the frame rate. The higher the line density, the worse the temporal resolution. The frame rate is equal to the PRF divided by the number of lines per frame (Table 2-19). Figure 2-44 compares creating

TABLE 2-20 Examples of questions related to the frame rate

1. You decrease the depth but the frame rate stays the same. The number of focal zones did not change. What must have happened?
   - Decreasing the depth is the same as increasing the PRF. If the PRF increases, the FR should increase, but it did not. What must have happened is that the sector angle got wider, which would have lowered the frame rate, and canceling out the increase in the frame rate from decreasing the depth.
2. You double the number of focal zones to optimize lateral resolution in your image. What is effect on temporal resolution?
   - If you double the number of focal zones, the frame rate (temporal resolution) is halved.

scan lines with painting a wall, and the longer it takes to create a scan line, the longer it takes to create the image. Table 2-20 has sample problems on temporal resolution.

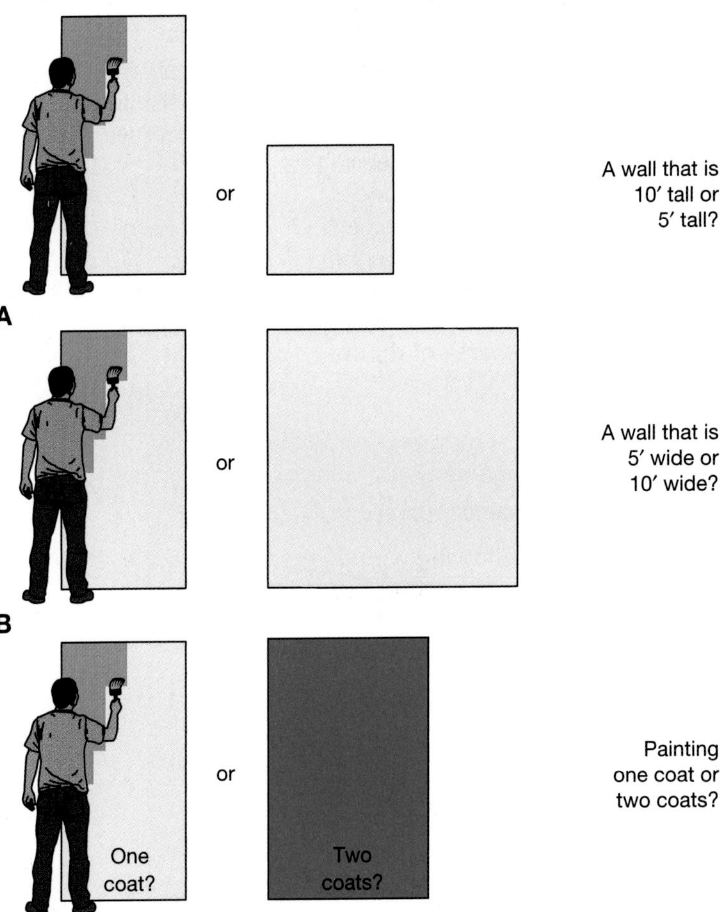
Which takes longer to paint?
or
A wall that is
10′ tall or
5′ tall?
A
or
A wall that is
5′ wide or
10′ wide?
B
One
coat?
or
Two
coats?
Painting
one coat or
two coats?
C

Figure 2-44 Temporal resolution (frame rate) is determined by PRF (depth), the number of focal zones, and the image width or number of lines per frame. This is analogous to painting a wall. **A.** Which takes longer? Painting a 10′ high wall or a 5′ high wall? The 10′ high wall will take longer because it is taller. This is analogous to image depth. **B.** Which takes longer? Painting a 10′ wide wall or a 5′ wide wall? The 10′ wide wall will take longer because it's wider. This is analogous to image width. **C.** Which takes longer? Painting a wall with one coat or with two? It takes more time to paint a wall twice. This is analogous to multiple focal zones. PRF, pulse repetition frequency.

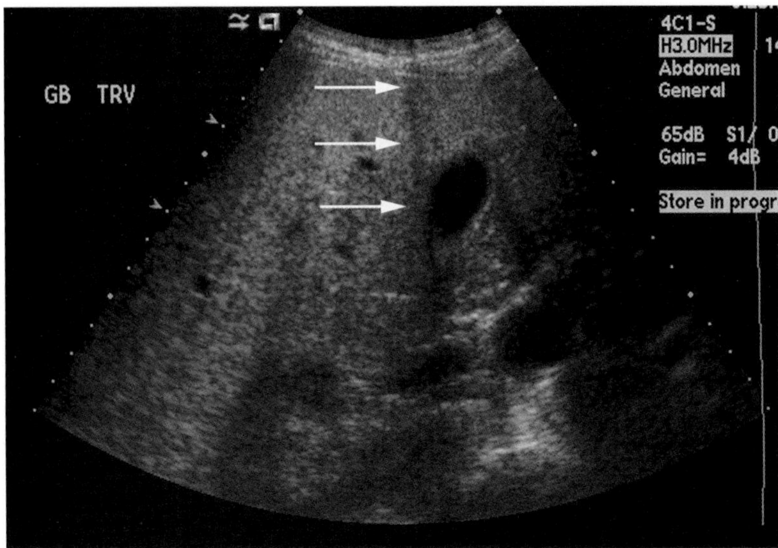

Figure 2-45 Transducer damage. An area of dropout (*arrows*) can be noted within this image.

TRANSDUCER CARE AND MAINTENANCE

Proper handling of the transducer is essential to prevent damage to the cord, housing, and piezoelectric elements. Transducers should be hung in the proper transducer holder on the equipment and never dangled over the handle of the machine. Hanging the transducer improperly places undue stress on the cord and may damage the wires inside. Likewise, dangling the transducer over the machine handle increases the risk of the transducer falling to the ground and potentially causing permanent and irreparable damage. Both the transducer and the power cords should be carefully placed so as to avoid rolling the machine over the cord as well. When the cord or probe is damaged, it may appear on the screen as an area of dropout (Figure 2-45). Any damage to the transducer or the cord should be immediately resolved.

The American Institute of Ultrasound in Medicine (AIUM) has an official statement on transducer testing and repair. They state:

> The quality of an ultrasound image is strongly dependent on the quality of the ultrasound transducer used to acquire it. Defective as well as poorly remanufactured transducers can lead to a wrong or missed diagnosis. Regular assessment of transducer operation and quality control of repaired transducers are critical for optimal patient care.

Further discussion concerning transducer care including disinfection related to infection control is provided in Chapter 6 of this book.

REVIEW QUESTIONS

1. Which of the following would be considered the narrowest part of a sound beam?
   a. Far zone
   b. Near zone
   c. Fresnel zone
   d. Focal zone

2. Which of the following is the part of the transducer that shortens the vibration of the element?
   a. Matching layer
   b. Housing
   c. Damping material
   d. Insulator

3. Along with image depth which of the following also determines the frame rate?
   a. Axial resolution
   b. Damping
   c. Number of lines per frame
   d. Lateral resolution

4. Which type of resolution is necessary for providing an accurate representation of moving structures?
   a. Lateral resolution
   b. Azimuthal resolution
   c. Spatial resolution
   d. Temporal resolution

5. If the depth is increased and the frame rate is unchanged, what else must have decreased?
   a. The pulse repetition period
   b. The number of lines per frame
   c. The pulse duration
   d. The output power

6. Which of the following transducers can be described as having the scan lines originate from a common point of origin?
   a. Sector phased array
   b. Vector phased array
   c. Curvilinear array
   d. Linear sequenced array

7. You are using a 6-MHz broadband transducer that offers the lowest frequency at 4.5 MHz and the highest frequency at 7.5 MHz. What is the bandwidth of this transducer?
   a. 1.5 MHz
   b. 3 MHz
   c. 4.5 MHz
   d. 6 MHz

8. Along with crystal diameter (aperture), the divergence in the far field is also determined by which of the following?
   a. Spatial pulse length
   b. Frequency
   c. Propagation speed
   d. Line density

9. Which of the following would cause a decrease in temporal resolution?
   a. Increased line density
   b. Decreased sector size
   c. Single transmit focal zone
   d. Increased PRF

10. Which of the following would cause an increase in the frame rate?
    a. Multifocusing
    b. Increased line density
    c. Increased imaging depth
    d. Increased PRF

11. Which of the following is true of the diameter of the sound beam in the Fresnel zone?
    a. It increases with distance from the transducer
    b. It decreases with distance from the transducer
    c. It does not change with distance from the transducer
    d. It is unpredictable

12. Which resolution typically has the lowest numerical value in clinical imaging?
    a. Longitudinal
    b. Lateral
    c. Transverse
    d. Azimuthal

13. Which of the following would most likely increase the near-zone length?
    a. Large crystal diameter, low frequency
    b. Small crystal diameter, low frequency
    c. Large crystal diameter, high frequency
    d. Small crystal diameter, high frequency

14. Which of the following would most likely decrease beam divergence in the far field?
    a. Large crystal diameter, low frequency
    b. Small crystal diameter, low frequency
    c. Large crystal diameter, high frequency
    d. Small crystal diameter, high frequency

15. Imaging transducers typically have:
    a. Low-quality factors, wide bandwidths
    b. High-quality factors, narrow bandwidths
    c. Low-quality factors, narrow bandwidths
    d. High-quality factors, wide bandwidths

16. Damping material produces all of the following except:
    a. Decreased sensitivity
    b. Increased SPL
    c. Wide bandwidths
    d. Low-quality factors

17. Which of the following electrical patterns produces electronic focusing of the ultrasound beam?
    a. Curved
    b. Sloped
    c. Spiral
    d. Circular

18. In an unfocused, single-element transducer, the width at the focal point of the sound beam measures how much compared to the beam width at the face of the transducer?
    a. One-fourth
    b. One-third
    c. One-half
    d. Equal

19. Which of the following facilitates the transmission of sound from the element into the patient's skin?
    a. Damping material
    b. Matching layer
    c. Tungsten covering
    d. Focusing material

20. Which of the following describes the range of frequencies present within the beam?
    a. Matching layer
    b. Bandwidth
    c. Array
    d. Wavefront

21. Which type of interference results in a higher amplitude sound wave?
    a. Constructive interference
    b. Destructive interference
    c. True interference
    d. False interference

22. Which of the following will NOT affect temporal resolution?
    a. Line density
    b. Image depth
    c. Spatial pulse length
    d. Number of focal zones

23. Which of the following best describes the components of the damping material?
    a. Epoxy resin loaded with tungsten
    b. Resin made with lead zirconate titanate
    c. Polyvinylidene fluoride
    d. Tungsten impregnated with lead

24. Which of the following is NOT true of the linear sequenced array transducer?
    a. Rectangular shape image
    b. Firing is sequential
    c. Electronically focused
    d. The elements are arranged in a ring

25. Which of the following is a true statement?
    a. Lateral resolution varies with depth
    b. A larger aperture results in a shorter near-zone length
    c. A larger aperture produces more divergence in the far field
    d. Lateral resolution may also be referred to as range resolution

26. Which of the following is true of damping?
    a. Damping increases the number of cycles in a pulse
    b. Damping increases spatial pulse length
    c. Damping improves axial resolution
    d. Damping increases the sensitivity of the transducer

27. The transducer that has a trapezoidal image shape and is from a phased array transducer is a:
    a. Sector
    b. Vector
    c. Linear
    d. Curved

28. Temporal resolution relates to which of the following?
    a. Lateral resolution
    b. Frame rate
    c. Range ambiguity
    d. Element diameter

29. Which of the following may also be referred to as the far zone?
    a. Frame zone
    b. Fresnel zone
    c. Fraunhofer zone
    d. Azimuthal zone

30. What states that waves are the result of the interference of many wavelets produced at the face of the transducer?
    a. Curie's principle
    b. Snell's law
    c. Bernoulli's law
    d. Huygen's principle

31. Which of the following is the resolution in the third dimension of the beam?
    a. Lateral resolution
    b. Elevational resolution
    c. Contrast resolution
    d. Longitudinal resolution

32. Which of the following is true concerning the frequency and the near-zone length, assuming a single-element, unfocused transducer?
    a. The higher the frequency, the longer the near-zone length
    b. The lower the frequency, the longer the near-zone length
    c. Frequency and near-zone length are not related
    d. Increasing the frequency causes increased divergence in the near field

33. Which of the following is defined as shocking the piezoelectric elements one at a time or more than one at a time with very small time differences in between in order to shape and steer the beam?
    a. Angulation
    b. Focusing
    c. Phasing
    d. Bundling

34. Which of the following is NOT a component of spatial resolution?
    a. Temporal resolution
    b. Contrast resolution
    c. Axial resolution
    d. Elevational resolution

35. Which transducer has no range resolution?
    a. Continuous-wave transducers
    b. Curved sequenced array transducers
    c. Linear sequenced array transducers
    d. Phased array transducers

36. Which of the following transducers is NOT used for imaging?
    a. Continuous-wave transducers
    b. Curved sequenced array transducers
    c. Linear sequenced array transducers
    d. Phased array transducers

37. Which of the following transducers is also referred to as a sector or vector transducer?
    a. Linear sequential array
    b. Phased array
    c. Continuous-wave transducer
    d. Curved sequential array transducer

38. Which of the following shortens the length of the pulse by decreasing the number of cycles in the pulse?
    a. Matching material
    b. Piezoelectric element
    c. Backing material
    d. PZT

39. Which of the following produces a pie-shaped image?
    a. Linear sequenced array
    b. Phased array
    c. Curved sequenced array
    d. Convex transducer

40. The portion of the transducer that is closest to the patient is the:
    a. Backing material
    b. Matching layer
    c. Wire
    d. Damping material

41. What does heat sterilization do to an ultrasound transducer?
    a. Gives it better axial resolution
    b. Improves the lateral resolution of the transducer
    c. Kills all the bacteria and viruses
    d. Kills pathogens and destroys the transducer

42. Which of the following is defined as the minimum distance two reflectors can be, parallel to the beam, and still appear on the screen as two dots?
    a. Range resolution
    b. Angular resolution
    c. Contrast resolution
    d. Transverse resolution

43. Which of the following describes the result of destructive interference?
    a. The resulting wave is much larger than the original wave
    b. The resulting wave is a little larger than the original wave
    c. The resulting wave is smaller than the original wave
    d. Destructive interference does not occur with diagnostic imaging

44. To produce a transducer with a higher frequency one should:
    a. Use a thinner piezoelectric element
    b. Use a thicker piezoelectric element
    c. Use more damping
    d. Use less damping

45. A transducer is being used to image two reflectors parallel to the beam that are 0.2 mm apart. The spatial pulse length of the transducer is 0.3 mm. What is seen on the display, one reflector or two?

46. Which of the following would be best utilized for imaging of deep structures in the abdomen?
    a. Endocavity transducer
    b. Linear sequenced array transducer
    c. Curved sequenced array transducer
    d. Continuous-wave transducer

47. Which of the following 3D/4D methods mounts a transducer on a motor?
    a. 1.5D array technology
    b. 2D array technology
    c. Freehand technique
    d. Mechanical transducer

48. Which of the following best describes the frame rate?
    a. The frame rate is equal to the pulse repetition frequency multiplied by the lines per frame
    b. The frame rate is equal to the pulse repetition frequency divided by the lines per frame
    c. The frame rate is equal to the pulse repetition period divided by the lines per frame
    d. The frame rate is equal to the pulse repetition period multiplied by the lines per frame

49. Which of the following is represented as time, or the ability to display structures in real time?
    a. Temporal resolution
    b. Axial resolution
    c. Longitudinal resolution
    d. Contrast resolution

50. When high-level disinfection is needed, how are ultrasound transducers commonly disinfected?
    a. Heating transducers to the Curie point
    b. With cold-disinfection methods
    c. Autoclaving
    d. Alcohol immersion

SUGGESTED READINGS

AIUM. Transducer testing and repair. Accessed September 10, 2023. https://www.aium.org/resources/official-statements/view/transducer-testing-and-repair, 2019.

Brant W. *The Core Curriculum: Ultrasound.* Wolters Kluwer; 2001.

Bushberg JT, Seibert JA, Leidholdt EM Jr, Boone JM. *The Essential Physics of Medical Imaging.* 4th ed. Wolters Kluwer; 2020.

Cosby K, Kendall J. *Practical Guide to Emergency Ultrasound.* Wolters Kluwer; 2007.

Edelman SK. *Understanding Ultrasound Physics.* 4th ed. ESP Inc.; 2012.

Kremkau FW. *Diagnostic Ultrasound: Principles and Instruments.* 10th ed. Saunders; 2020.

Miele F. *Ultrasound Physics and Instrumentation.* 6th ed. Miele Enterprises; 2022.

Nanosonics. The Nanosonics Story. Available at: http://www.nanosonics.com.au.

Penny SM. *Introduction to Sonography and Patient Care.* 2nd ed. Wolters Kluwer; 2020.

Sanders RC, Hall-Terracciano B. *Clinical Sonography: A Practical Guide.* 5th ed. Wolters Kluwer; 2016.

Szabo TL. *Diagnostic Ultrasound Imaging: Inside Out.* Elsevier; 2014.

Tai A, Gelly JF, Easterbrook S. Xdclear transducer technology. White paper. http://landing1.gehealthcare.com/rs/005-SHS-767/images/DOC1231110-Global%20LOGIQ%20E9%20with%20Xdclear%20Technology%20Whitepaper.pdf, 2012.

3

Imaging Principles and Instrumentation

Outline

Introduction

This chapter discusses how sound is produced and what happens when the return echo is received by a transducer. In addition, a description of the imaging artifacts that may occur as a result of sound transmission through soft tissue is offered.

Key Terms

13 μs rule—the rule that states that it takes 13 μs for a sound to propagate to a depth of 1 cm in soft tissue and return to the transducer

acoustic speckle—the interference pattern caused by scatterers that produces the granular appearance of what is called "parenchyma" on a sonographic image

ALARA—as low as reasonably achievable; the principle that states one should always use the lowest power and shortest scanning time possible to reduce the potential for bioeffects

A-mode—amplitude mode; ophthalmology-specific mode in which the height of the spike on the image is related to the strength (amplitude) of the echo generated by a reflector

amplification—the part of the receiver that increases or decreases the received echoes equally, regardless of depth

amplitude—the maximum (positive or negative) deviation of an acoustic variable from the average value of that variable; the strength of the reflector

amplitude mode—*see* the key term "A-mode"

analog-to-digital (A-to-D) converter—the part of the digital scan converter that converts the analog signals from the receiver to binary signals for processing by the computer

anechoic—without echoes or black

apodization—the technique that changes the amplitude of the voltage to the individual elements to reduce grating lobes

artifacts—echoes on the screen that are not representative of actual anatomy, or reflectors in the body that are not displayed on the screen

B-flow imaging—a non-Doppler technology that offers real-time imaging of blood flow while scanning in grayscale

binary system—the digital language of zeros and ones

bistable—purely black-and-white image

bit—the smallest unit of memory in a digital device

B-mode—brightness mode; the brightness of the dots is proportional to the strength of the echo generated by the reflector

brightness mode—*see* the key term "B-mode"

byte—8 bits of memory

cathode ray tube (CRT)—obsolete display that uses an electron gun to produce a stream of electrons toward a phosphor-coated screen

channel—part of the transducer containing a pulse delay and its corresponding piezoelectric element

coded excitation—a way of processing the pulse to improve contrast resolution and reduce acoustic speckle

comet tail—a small reverberation artifact caused by small reflectors (eg, surgical clips)

compensation—the function of the receiver that changes the brightness of the echo amplitudes to compensate for attenuation that occurs with depth

compression—the function of the receiver that decreases the range of signal amplitudes present within the machine's receiver; opposite of the dynamic range

contrast resolution—the ability to differentiate tissues with similar shades of gray or differences in echogenicities in tissue

demodulation—the function of the receiver that makes the signal easier to process by performing the functions rectification and smoothing; also called detection

digital-to-analog (D-to-A) converter—part of the digital scan converter that converts the binary signals from computer memory to analog for display and storage

digitizer—*see* the key term "analog-to-digital converter"

dynamic range—the range of echo amplitudes present within the signal, which corresponds to the shades of gray available

echogenic—a medium that has the ability to produce return echoes

echogenicity—a measure of relative brightness compared to adjacent structures

echotexture—measure of the relative "smoothness" of a structure imaged on B-mode ultrasound

edge shadowing—refraction artifact caused by the curved surface of the reflector

electrical interference—arc-like bands that occur when the machine is too close to an unshielded electrical device

enhancement—an artifact of increased brightness in the tissue deep to a structure caused by sound passing through an area of lower attenuation

fill-in interpolation—places grayscale pixels in between scan lines, where there is no signal information; also referred to as pixel interpolation

frame—one complete ultrasound image

frame rate—the number of frames per second (in FPS or Hz)

frequency compounding—averages the frequencies across the image to improve contrast resolution and reduce acoustic speckle

fundamental frequency—the operating or resonating frequency emitted by a transducer

grating lobes—an artifact caused by the extraneous sound that is not located along the primary beam path; occurs with arrays; reduced or eliminated by apodization, subdicing, and tissue harmonics

harmonics—the harmonic signal produced by the patient's tissue and that is a multiple of the fundamental frequency

hyperechoic—displayed echoes that are relatively brighter than the surrounding tissue

hypoechoic—displayed echoes that are relatively darker than the surrounding tissue

isoechoic—echogenicity that is identical to the surrounding tissue

liquid crystal display (LCD)—display that uses the twisting and untwisting of liquid crystals in front of a light source; also called a flat panel

master synchronizer—the timing component of an ultrasound machine that notes how long it takes for signals to return from reflectors

mirror-image artifact—an artifact caused by sound bouncing off a specular reflector and causing a structure to appear on both sides of the reflector

M-mode—motion mode; used to display the motion of the reflectors

motion mode—*see* the key term "M-mode"

multipath—an artifact caused by the beam reflecting off several reflectors before returning to the transducer

noise—low-level echoes on the display that do not contribute to useful diagnostic information

output—output power; strength of voltage pulse and therefore the strength of the sound wave transmitted into the patient

overall gain—the receiver function that increases or decreases all echo amplitudes equally

persistence—averaging of frame information to reduce image noise

picture archiving and communication system (PACS)—a type of display and storage device commonly used in sonography and other imaging modalities

pixel (picture element)—the smallest component of a two-dimensional (2D) digital image

pixel interpolation—*see* the key term "fill-in interpolation"

postprocessing—changes that can be made on a frozen image because the scan information has been stored in memory

preprocessing—changes made before the scan information has been stored in memory (ie, while the image is live)

propagation speed errors—artifact that occurs because the actual propagation speed of the tissue is greater than or less than 1540 m/s, the machine places the reflector at the wrong location on the display

pulse inversion technology—harmonic imaging technology in which the fundamental frequency is flipped 180°, which cancels out the fundamental frequency via destructive interference, leaving only the harmonic signal for processing

pulser—part of the beamformer that controls the amount of energy in the pulse (ie, the amplitude of the signal)

range equation—the equation used to calculate the distance to the reflector; in soft tissue, $d = 0.77t$, where "d" is the depth of the reflector and "t" represents the round-trip time of the pulse

read zoom—the type of magnification performed in the postprocessing that magnifies the image by enlarging the pixels and can be used on a frozen image

receiver—the component of the machine that processes the signals coming back from the patient

rectification—the part of the receiver that inverts the negative voltages to positive voltages

rejection—the function of the receiver that is used to reduce image noise; sets a threshold below which the signal will not be displayed

reverberation—an artifact caused by the beam bouncing between two strong reflectors

ring-down artifact—an artifact caused by the vibration of air bubbles

scan converter—the part of the ultrasound machine that processes the signals from the receiver

scan line—created when one or more pulses of sound return from the tissue containing information related to the depth and amplitude of the reflectors

shadowing—an artifact caused by the failure of sound to pass through a medium with increased attenuation

side lobes—an artifact caused by extraneous sound that is not found along the primary beam path; occurs with single-element transducers

signal processor—*see* key term "receiver"

slice-thickness artifact—artifact that occurs as a result of the elevational plane not being razor-thin; thus, unintended echoes may appear in the image as the beam slices through structures adjacent to intended reflectors; also known as the elevational plane artifact or partial volume thickness artifact

smoothing—part of the demodulation component of the receiver; an "envelope" is wrapped around the signal to eliminate the "humps" or "ripples"

spatial compounding—a technique that eliminates edge shadowing and reduces acoustic speckle because the object is imaged from different angles

speckle reduction—the algorithm used in signal processing to reduce the amount of acoustic speckle and to make the image appear smoother

specular reflectors—large, flat, smooth boundaries that cause strong reflections

subdicing—dividing the piezoelectric elements into very small pieces to reduce grating lobes

summer—creates the scan line on the receive end by adding together the received signals

time-gain compensation—time-gain compensation; *see* the key term "compensation"

transmitter—*see* the key term "pulser"

transmit/receive switch—ensures the electrical signals travel in the correct direction

voxel (volume element)—the smallest component of a three-dimensional (3D) image

write zoom—the type of magnification performed in the preprocessing that magnifies the image by redrawing it before it is stored in memory

***x*-axis**—the plane that is perpendicular to the beam path (ie, horizontal)

***y*-axis**—the plane that is parallel to the beam path (ie, vertical)

***z*-axis**—the brightness, or amplitude, of the dots on a B-mode display

DISPLAY MODES

There are different modes used in ultrasound imaging for displaying the return echo information on the display (Table 3-1).

A-Mode

One of the original methods of displaying the return echo information utilizes a display similar to an oscilloscope, where the depth is represented along the ***x*-axis** and the strength of the reflector is represented

TABLE 3-1 Imaging modes

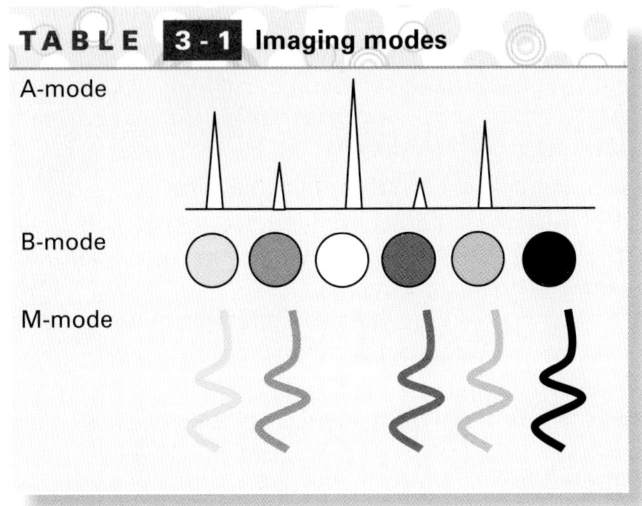

as a "spike" along the ***y*-axis**. This display method is called the **amplitude mode** or **A-mode**, and it may still utilized in dedicated ophthalmology sonography units. A pulse of sound is sent out to create one **scan line** of information, which contains the depth and **amplitude** of the reflectors. No image is generated, but only a set of spikes representing the amplitude of reflectors and their depth is generated (Figure 3-1).

> **SOUND OFF**
> With A-mode, a pulse of sound is sent out to create one scan line of information, which contains the depth and amplitude of the reflectors.

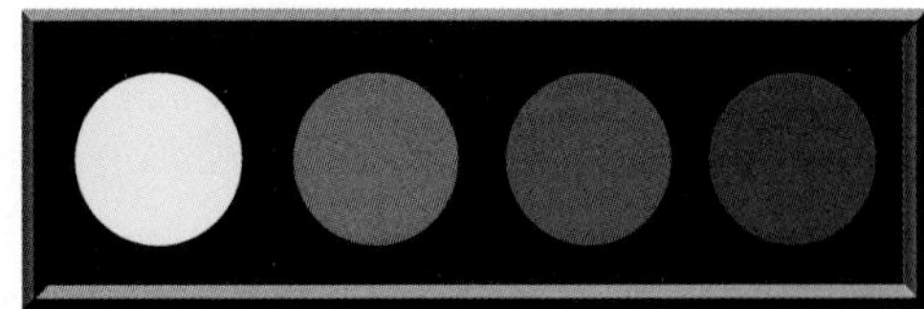

Figure 3-2 The different shades of gray. The brighter the dot, the stronger the returning echo.

> **SOUND OFF**
> With B-mode, stronger the return echo, the brighter the dot.

B-Mode

Brightness mode, or **B-mode** imaging (Figure 3-2), displays the returning echoes as dots of varying brightness. The brightness of the dot represents the strength of the return echo (Figure 3-3). Modern equipment uses a white dot on a black background. The stronger the return echo, the brighter the dot. Stronger reflectors will be brighter shades of white, weaker reflectors will be darker shades of gray. Ultrasound images on B-mode are often characterized by echotexture and echogenicity. **Echotexture** is subjective and is a measure of the relative "smoothness" of a tissue. Tissue, such as the liver, may be described, as "coarse" or "smooth." **Echogenicity** is a measure of relative brightness. If a structure is brighter than the surrounding tissue, it is described as **hyperechoic**. A structure that is darker than the surrounding tissue is described as **hypoechoic.** The absence of return echoes is called

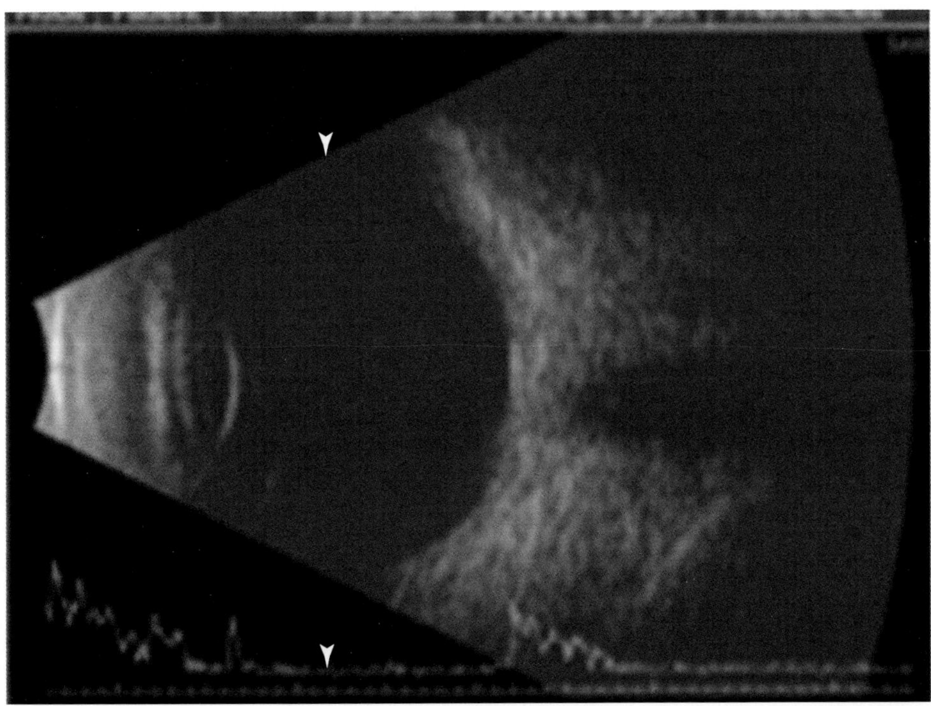

Figure 3-1 A-mode display superimposed over a B-mode image. Note that the amplitude (height) of the A-mode signal is proportional to the shade of gray on the B-mode image. Where the image is black, the corresponding amplitude is very low (*arrows*).

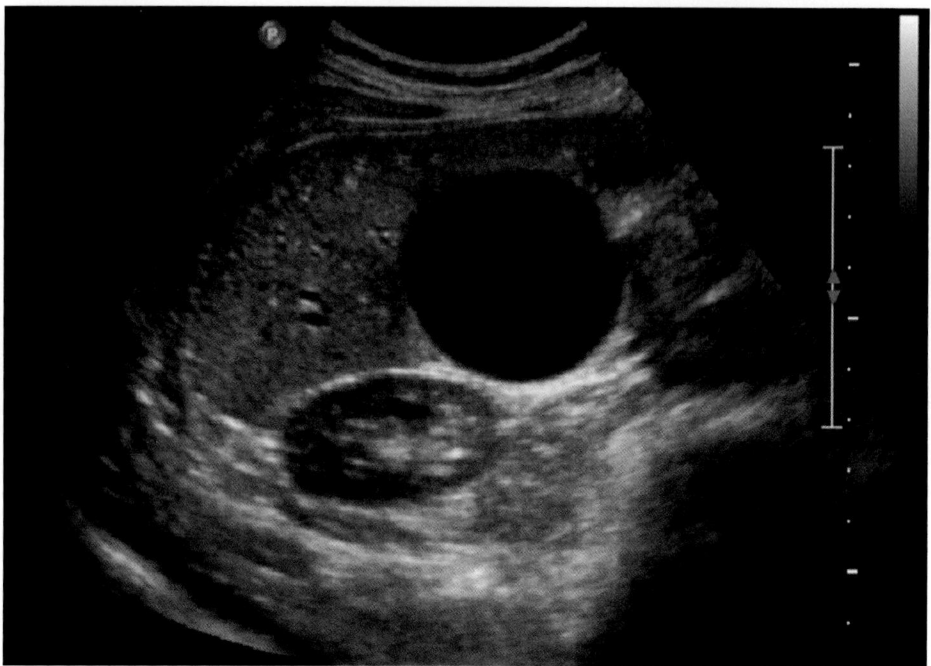

Figure 3-3 B-mode image of a solid organ, in this case, the liver, the anechoic circle in the middle is the gallbladder.

anechoic, which appears black on ultrasound. Fluids, such as water or urine, are commonly anechoic as there are no reflectors to reflect the sound wave, so unless there are particulates in the fluid to reflect sound, no dot is "painted" on the display. In echogenicity, tissue that is identical to its background is called **isoechoic**. Structures that are capable of producing echoes are called **echogenic**. In most literature and in the clinical lexicon, echogenic has long been a synonym for "hyperechoic." According the American Institute of Ultrasound in Medicine's (AIUM's) manual on *Recommended Ultrasound Terminology*, 4th ed. (AIUM, 2019), the term echogenic should be used to mean "capable of producing echoes," and it is not necessarily a synonym for "hyperechoic."

The brightness of the dot, representing the amplitude of the return echo, corresponds to the height of the spike on the A-mode display. On B-mode, it is the same as the spike, but along the ***z*-axis** of the image (ie, coming out of the display). Therefore, the amplitude of the B-mode image is displayed along the *z*-axis. The B-mode image is made up of many scan lines placed next to each other. Each scan line is made up of one or more pulses of sound. For the machine to know where to place the dots on the screen, it must know where the return echoes came from. To determine where the echo came from, the time it takes for the sound to reach the reflector and return must be known. This is summed up by the **range equation**, which states that the distance to the reflector (d, in mm) is equal to the propagation speed (c, in mm/µs) multiplied by the round-trip time (t, in µs), or time to the reflector and back, divided by 2 (Table 3-2). To simplify the range equation formula, it is important to understand that the ultrasound machine is programmed to always assume that the beam is traveling through soft tissue, and thus the propagation speed of 1.54 mm/µs can be used to reveal an equation that assumes soft tissue: $d = 0.77t$, where t is always the round-trip time of the echo. When answering questions about the depth of the reflector, verify that the information that is provided in the question is the round-trip time and not the one-way time. For example, if the time given is only *to the reflector*, you must double it to make it the round-trip time. It is useful to know the **13 µs rule**: It takes 13 µs for sound to travel to a depth of 1 cm and return (Table 3-3). In other words, it takes 6.5 µs to get to the reflector and 6.5 µs to return to the transducer, assuming soft tissue is the medium. Learners are often

TABLE 3-2 Range equation

Range Equation Formula
$d = c \times t/2$
Remember that t is always the round-trip time

TABLE 3-3 Summary of the range equation

The Range Equation
In soft tissue:
$d = 0.77t$
Remember that t is always the round-trip time It takes 13 µs to travel 1 cm (10 mm) in soft tissue (round-trip time)

Imaging Principles and Instrumentation

confused about when to multiply or divide when practicing range equation sample questions. A helpful shortcut is as follows: When solving for *depth*, and you are given a one-way time, multiply your result by 2. When solving for *time*, and you are only asked to solve for a one-way time, divide your result by 2.

> **SOUND OFF**
> "When do I double the time, and when do I halve the time?" The short way to remember is:
>
> - If solving for *depth*, and you have a one-way time, *double* the time.
> - If solving for *time*, and you only need the one-way time, *halve* the time.
> - If solving for *depth*, and you have a round-trip time, *do nothing.*
> - If solving for *time*, and you need a round-trip time, *do nothing.*
> - When do I double or halve depth? *Never.* Leave depth alone.

The machine is programmed with only one propagation speed, the speed of soft tissue; however, different tissues of the body do have different propagation speeds. Therefore, reflectors may be displayed in a wrong location when sound travels through tissue at a speed that is either greater than or less than 1540 m/s. This will be explained in greater detail in the "Imaging Artifacts" section of this chapter.

> **EXAMPLE 1:** A sound wave travels for 13 μs and impinges on a reflector. How far away is the reflector?
>
> Note that in this example, the round-trip time is not given, but only the one-way time to the reflector is provided. Therefore, the time given (13 μs) must be doubled, and 26 μs should be plugged into the equation as follows: $d = 0.77(26\ \mu s) = 20$ mm. The distance from the transducer to the reflector is thus 20 mm.

> **EXAMPLE 2:** A reflector is 25 mm away from the transducer. How long does it take sound to get to the reflector and return back to the transducer?
>
> In this example, we are given the distance to the transducer and seeking the round-trip time. Rearrange the equation so that $t = d/0.77$.
>
> $$t = 25\ \text{mm}/0.77 = 32.46\ \mu s.$$
>
> **REMEMBER:** *t* is the round-trip time. If the question is asked, "how long does it take for a pulse of sound to get to the reflector," and if no mention is made of the sound getting back to the transducer, then the number provided should be divided by 2.

> **SOUND OFF**
> The M-mode tracing is one scan line spread out over time, with depth along the *y*-axis and time along the *x*-axis.

M-Mode

With B-mode imaging, we are interested in the anatomy represented in the whole image (Figure 3-4). However, there are times when we are more concerned with the movement of the reflectors and not the anatomy. **M-mode**, or **motion mode**, is used in the instances when the documentation of the movement of a reflector is needed, such as looking at the motion of a heart valve or myocardial wall thickness during systole and diastole. Newer applications for M-mode at the time of this writing include evaluating lungs for pneumothorax, respiratory distress, and infection. M-mode is often used in adult and pediatric echocardiography and in obstetrics to demonstrate fetal heart motion and perform fetal echocardiography (Figure 3-5).

B-Mode (Grayscale) Image Display Options

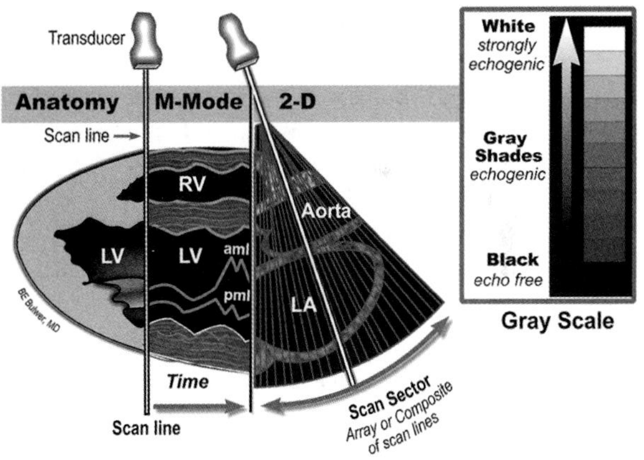

Parasternal Long-Axis Views

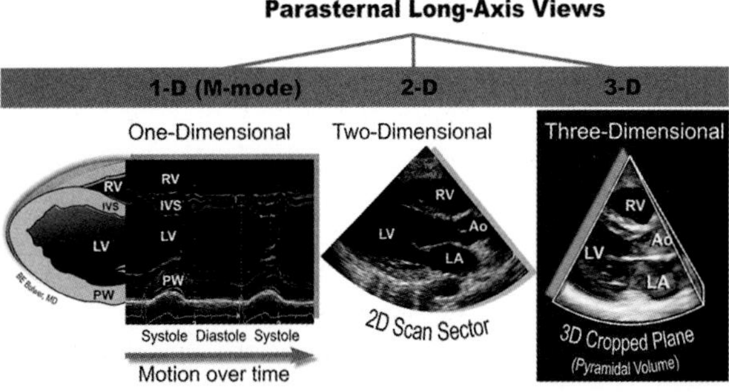

Figure 3-4 B-mode or grayscale display options. **Upper panel, from left to right:** Imaging of cardiac anatomy can be optionally displayed as M-mode or as a 2D image. Both M-mode and 2D are image display options that are based on grayscale or brightness modulation (B-mode). **Lower panel, from left to right:** The amplitudes of the received echoes can be processed into B-mode data that can be displayed using M-mode, 2D (cross-sectional anatomy), or 3D formats.

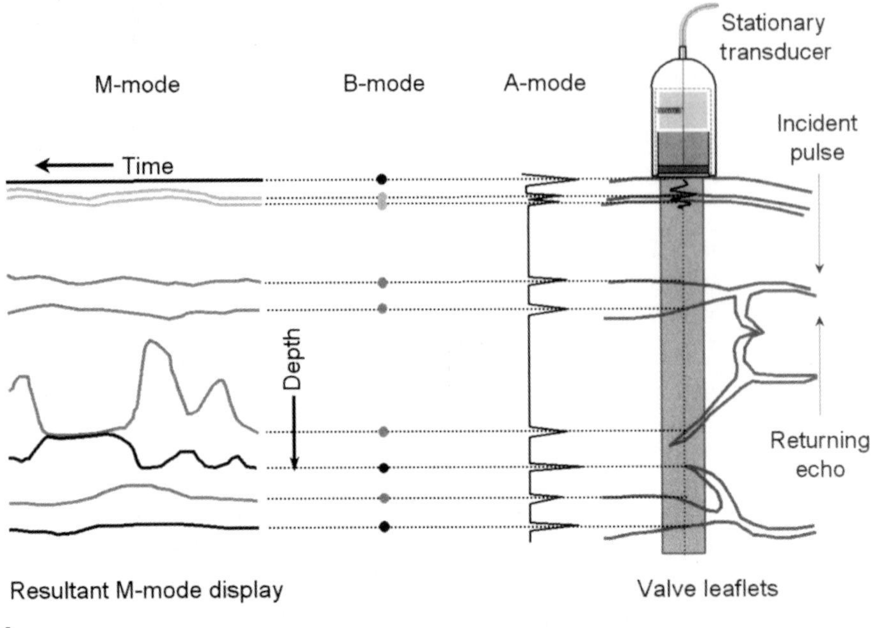

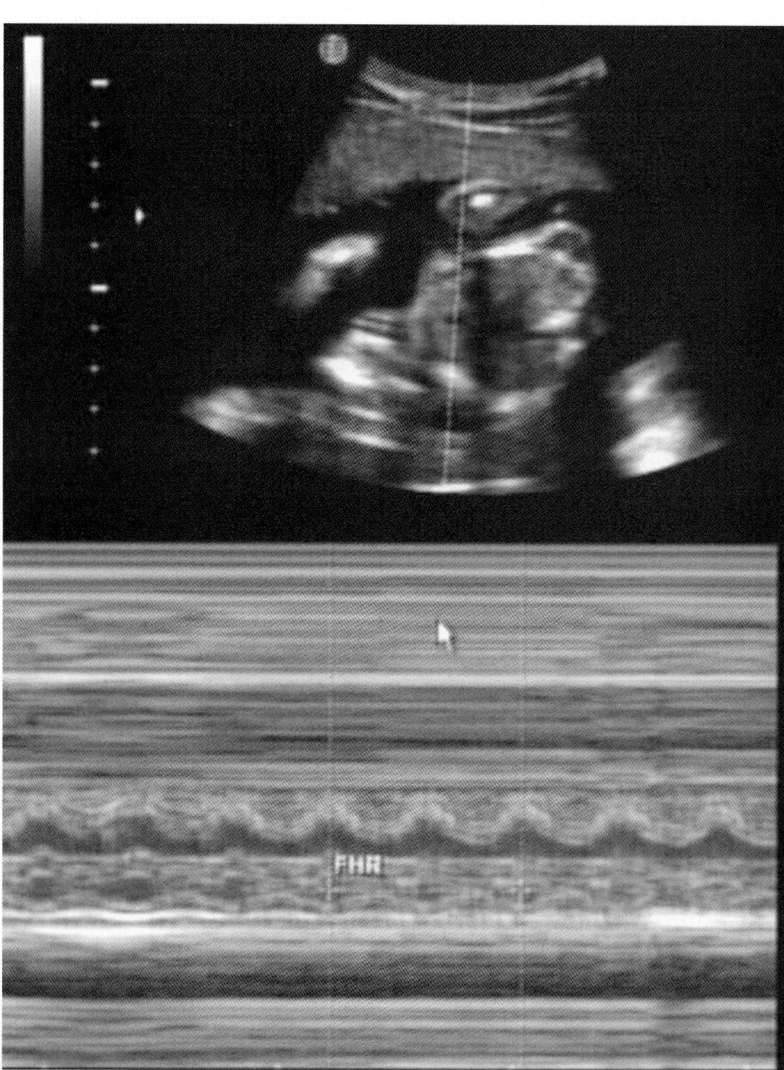

Figure 3-5 M-mode. **A.** M-mode display of valve leaflets and corresponding appearance on B-mode and A-mode. **B.** In this image, the M-mode tracing depicts the motion of the fetal heart. The vertical white line is the cursor that lets the operator select which scan line to use for tracing the motion of the reflectors.

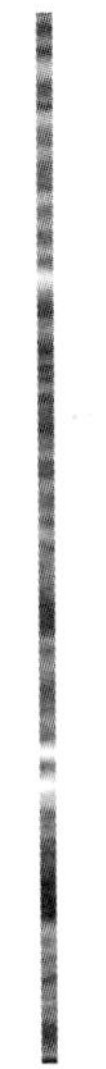

Figure 3-6 One scan line.

With M-mode imaging, the motion of the reflectors along a single scan line is analyzed. The M-mode tracing is one scan line represented over time, with depth along the *y*-axis and time along the *x*-axis. The M-mode image is one B-mode scan line represented over time (Figure 3-6).

TRANSMISSION OF ULTRASOUND

The ultrasound system is a complex piece of diagnostic equipment (Figure 3-7). Table A-1 summarizes the components of an ultrasound machine.

> **SOUND OFF**
> The beamformer works to decrease the risk of grating lobes through a process called apodization.

Beamformer

The beamformer has transmit and receive components. The **transmit beamformer** controls the timing of signals sent to individual elements in an array transducer for the steering and focusing of the beam. It is the job of the beamformer to determine the sequence of voltage pulses sent to the individual elements in the array transducer. These minute differences in timing steer and focus the beam (see Chapter 2). The beamformer also controls **apodization**, which is used to decrease the risk of **grating lobes** that are artifacts caused by extraneous sound that lies outside of the primary beam path. Apodization works by decreasing the strength of the voltage pulse sent to the outermost elements (Figure 3-8). Grating lobes are described on page 80. Other parts of the beamformer (aka transmit beamformer), described in the subsequent sections, include the master synchronizer, the pulser, pulse delays, and the transmit/receive switch.

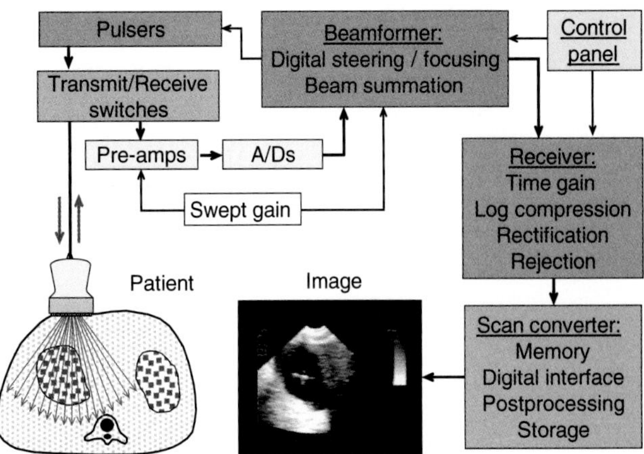

Figure 3-7 Schematic of an ultrasound machine showing the components that produce sound waves and interpret the returning signal. Components of the ultrasound imager. This schematic depicts the design of a digital acquisition/digital beamformer system, where each of the transducer elements in the array has transmit and receive channels (eg, for a 128-element phased array, there are 128 transmit channels and 128 receive channels). The transmit/receive switch ensures that signals go to the transmit or receive channel, whichever is appropriate. From the transducer the return signal goes to the receiver, then the scan converter, and then image output and display, as needed. Thick lines indicate the path of ultrasound data through the system. ADC, analog-to-digital converter.

Master Synchronizer

The **master synchronizer** is the part of the beamformer and is responsible for controlling the timing of the pulse. It ensures that a new pulse is not sent out until the previous echoes have returned.

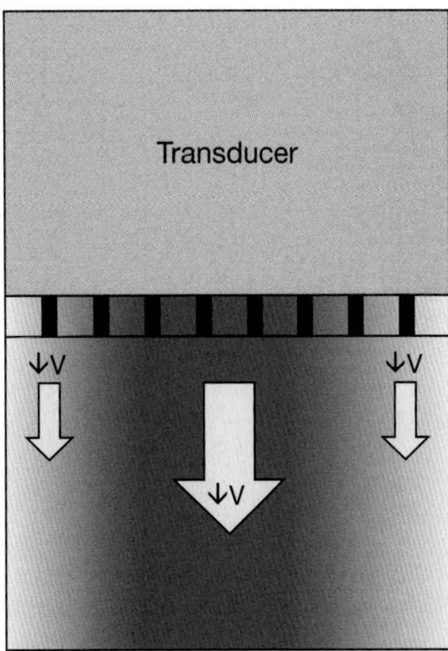

Figure 3-8 Apodization is used to help reduce the appearance of grating lobes. The center elements receive stronger voltages, whereas the edge elements receive weaker voltages.

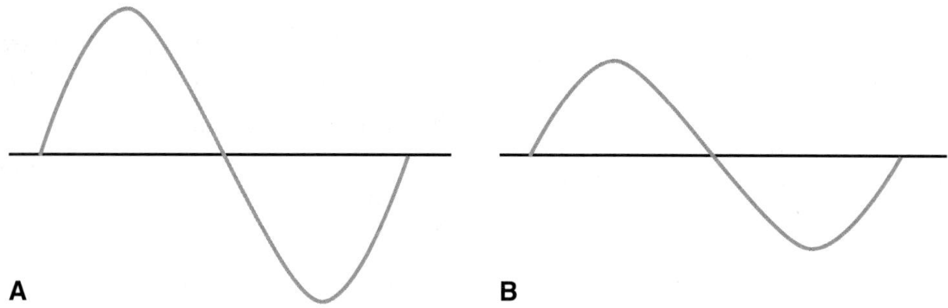

Figure 3-9 Diagram showing the direct relationship between amplitude voltage and pulse strength. High-amplitude voltage pulse equals high-amplitude pulse **(A)**, whereas low-amplitude voltage pulse equals low-amplitude pulse **(B)**.

Pulser

The **pulser**, or **transmitter**, controls the strength, or amplitude, of the electricity striking the elements, as well as the pulse repetition frequency and pulse repetition period. The strength of a sound wave entering a medium is directly proportional to the strength of the signal (voltage) impinging upon the elements. The stronger the output power, the stronger the beam (ie, higher the amplitude) of the sound entering the medium, and therefore the proportionally stronger the signal that returns from the reflectors in the medium (Figure 3-9). It is also important to note that frequency and amplitude are not related. Increasing or decreasing the strength of the pulse sent out of the transducer does not change the operating frequency of the transducer; it only changes the amplitude (strength) of the pulse (Figure 3-10). The pulser is connected to multiple channels. A **channel** is part of a transducer that consists of one pulse delay and its piezoelectric element. A typical 2D imaging transducer may have hundreds of channels.

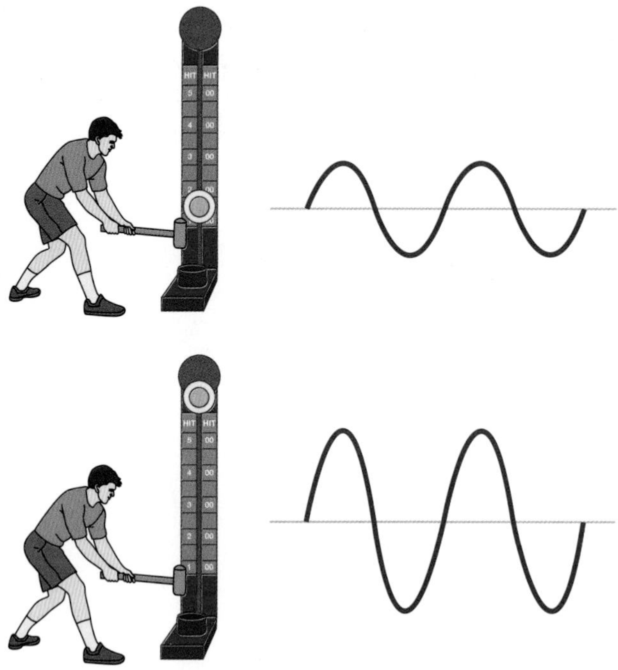

Figure 3-10 This illustration of a carnival game demonstrates how the amplitude (strength) of the voltage pulse corresponds to the amplitude of the pulse. In the top image, a weaker effort (ie, a weaker voltage pulse) results in a weaker pulse of sound. In the bottom image, a stronger effort results in a stronger pulse of sound.

SOUND OFF
The strength of a sound wave entering a medium is directly proportional to the strength of the signal (voltage) impinging upon the elements. Altering the amplitude does not affect the frequency because the frequency is primarily determined by the thickness of the element. They are not related to each other.

Power is known by several names (**output**, output gain, output power, acoustic power, etc). Only the pulser controls the amount of power entering the patient. If the word "output" or "power" is used in a term (ie, output gain), consider that this is a pulser function. Keep in mind that the higher the output power, the stronger the return echo. Increased output power has a few advantages: (1) higher amplitude return echoes for a better signal-to-noise ratio (ie, less image noise) and (2) improved depth penetration (Table 3-4). Increased output power is not without disadvantages. Increasing the output power increases the exposure to the patient and therefore creates an increased risk of potential bioeffects. Therefore, the lowest power should always

TABLE 3-4 Benefits and risks of increasing output power

Benefits of Increasing Output Power	Risks of Increasing Output Power
Higher amplitude return echoes result in a higher signal-to-noise ratio	Increases patient exposure (opposes the ALARA concept)
Improves depth penetration	

be used, following the principle of **ALARA** (as low as reasonably achievable), which states that the lowest power and shortest scanning time should be used to reduce the potential risk of bioeffects. A sonographer can adjust the output power by adjusting the control that may be labeled "output," "power," or "transmit." However, if the image is too dark, the receiver gain should always be increased before the output power.

SOUND OFF
If the word "output" or "power" is used in a term (ie, output gain or acoustic power), consider that this is a pulser function.

SOUND OFF
Coded excitation allows for multiple focal zones, improved penetration, speckle reduction, B-flow imaging, and improved contrast resolution.

SOUND OFF
If the image is too dark, the receiver gain should always be increased before the output power.

Coded excitation is a more complicated way of driving the energy pulse. This technique sends a series of encoded pulses to form one scan line instead of the one-pulse-per-scan-line method. This technique allows for multiple focal zones, improved penetration, **speckle reduction**, **B-flow imaging**, and improved **contrast resolution**.

As discussed in Chapter 2, one side effect of damping is that pulsed-wave transducers have many frequencies in the beam (ie, wide bandwidth). With **frequency compounding**, soft tissue is imaged at various frequencies and averaged. The displayed image is the result of all of the frequencies, and there is another way to produce an image with improved contrast resolution and reduction in **noise** and **acoustic speckle**.

TABLE 3-5 Important points to remember concerning tissue harmonic imaging

Tissue Harmonic Imaging
• Is possible because of the nonlinear propagation of sound
• Harmonic signals are produced by the patient, not the transducer
• Is a narrow beam that improves lateral resolution
• Images using the second harmonic that is twice as much as the transmitted (fundamental) frequency
• Elimination of near-field artifacts (eg, noise and reverberation)
• Elimination of grating lobes
• Harmonic beam is weaker (lower amplitude than the fundamental) but travels only one way—from the patient to the transducer

Tissue Harmonic Imaging

As stated in previous chapters, sound is a traveling pressure wave. As a pressure wave travels through tissue, beyond a few centimeters from the surface, its shape is deformed so that the high-pressure peak of the wave starts traveling faster than its low-pressure trough. The deeper the wave travels, the more deformed it becomes. Because of the deformed wave, sound waves are generated by vibrations of the patient's own tissue, called **harmonics** (Table 3-5). At the surface, no harmonics are generated; they are only generated as the beam travels deeper. The original transmitted frequency, called the **fundamental frequency** (f_0), is filtered out of the received beam, and only the harmonic signal is processed. These harmonic signals are multiples of the fundamental frequency. It is the second harmonic ($2f_0$), or two times the fundamental frequency, that is most often used. Therefore, if a 2 MHz beam is passed through a patient, a 4 MHz harmonic signal, which is generated by the patient's own tissue, is displayed. This harmonic signal is very narrow, thereby offering improved lateral resolution (Figure 3-11).

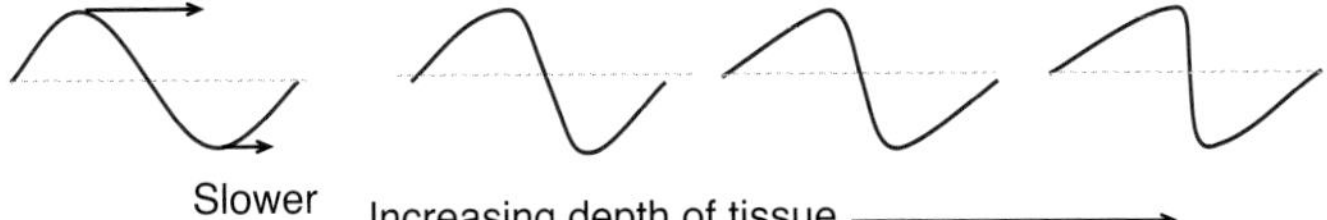

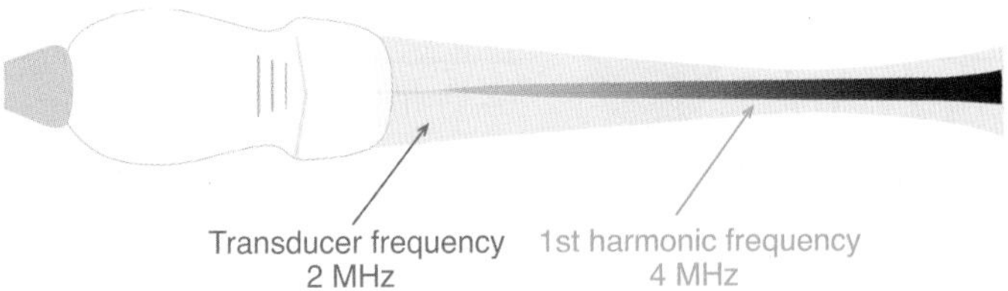

Figure 3-11 With depth, the sound wave distorts, producing the vibration in the tissue that causes the harmonic signals to form. The harmonic signal (black) is more narrow than the fundamental signal (light blue), producing better lateral resolution.

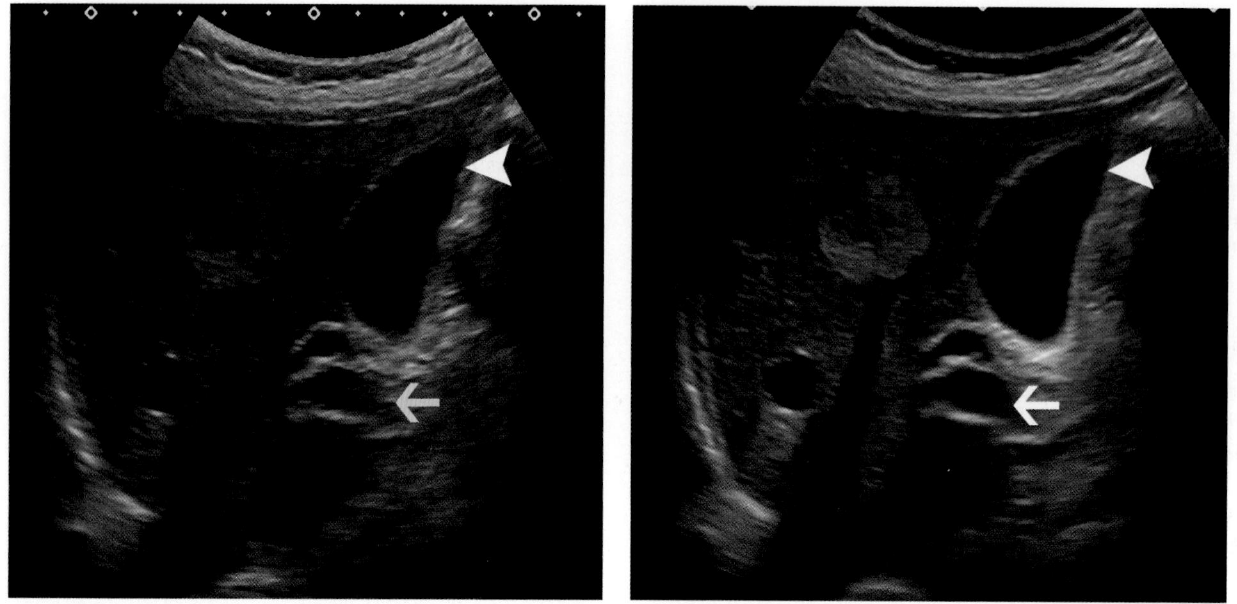

Figure 3-12 Images produced with fundamental and tissue harmonic imaging. **A.** Ultrasound of the liver with fundamental imaging. The arrow points to echoes within the main portal vein. The arrowhead points to an area of reverberation. **B.** Correlative images with tissue harmonic imaging enabled.

As a result of harmonic signals being generated deep to the surface, most superficial **artifacts**, such as **reverberation**, are reduced or possibly eliminated (Figure 3-12). The fundamental frequency may be eliminated using various technologies, including **pulse inversion** and others. With pulse inversion, the fundamental frequency is flipped 180° and transmitted, which cancels out the fundamental frequency via destructive interference, leaving only the harmonic signal (Figure 3-13).

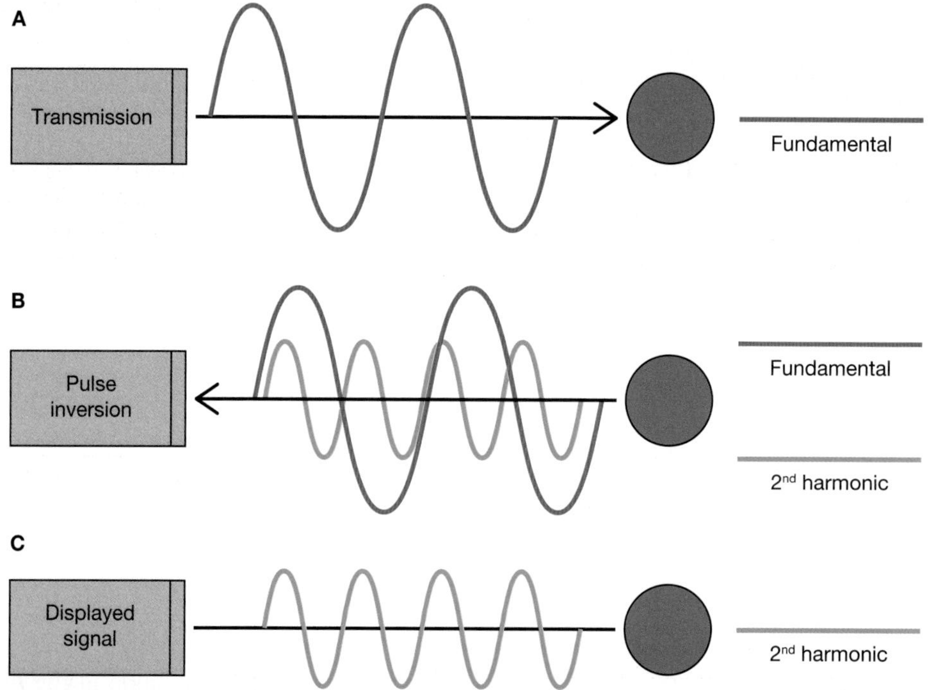

Figure 3-13 Tissue harmonic imaging. **A.** Sound propagates into the tissue at the fundamental frequency. **B.** The fundamental frequency and the harmonic signal return to the transducer. **C.** Technology such as pulse inversion is used to eliminate the fundamental frequency so that only the harmonic signal is displayed.

RECEPTION OF ULTRASOUND

Receiver

Sound returns to the transducer and strikes the piezoelectric element(s). Remember that sound is a pressure wave, so there is a mechanical force hitting the element, which causes electricity to be produced. The signal then enters the **receiver**. The return signal goes through the receiver of the beamformer and then undergoes amplification, which is needed to increase the relatively weak signal coming from the patient. The amplitude of the signal must be increased to allow for signal processing. The receiver has several functions, including **amplification**, **compensation**, **compression**, **demodulation**, and **rejection**. Altering the following receiver functions does not change the amount of energy entering the patient, because these functions are all happening to the sound coming back from the patient:

- **Amplification**, or **overall gain**, increases or decreases the strength of all of the returning echoes equally (Figure 3-14).
- Compensation, also referred to as **time-gain compensation** (TGC), adjusts the strength of echoes in a different way than amplification. As the beam propagates, the signal strength decreases because of attenuation. Therefore, echoes farther away from the transducer will be weaker than those that are closer. Compensation provides adjustment (ie, compensates) for the fact that attenuation occurs, and the more distant echoes are increased in brightness to achieve a uniform level of brightness on the image The TGC slide pot controls, also called pods or sliders, are adjusted to achieve a more uniform level of brightness across the entire image. This physical control has now become an electronic adjustment in some machines or has disappeared because of "auto-optimize" settings (Figures 3-15 and 3-16).
- Compression is needed to decrease the difference between the largest and smallest amplitudes within the signal, referred to as the **dynamic range**. The dynamic range is the series of echo amplitudes present within the signal (Figure 3-17). Compression is inversely related to the dynamic range. As the compression of the signal increases, the dynamic range decreases (Figure 3-18).
- Demodulation processes the signal to make it easier for the machine to handle. The two components of demodulation are **rectification** and **smoothing**. Rectification turns negative voltages into positive

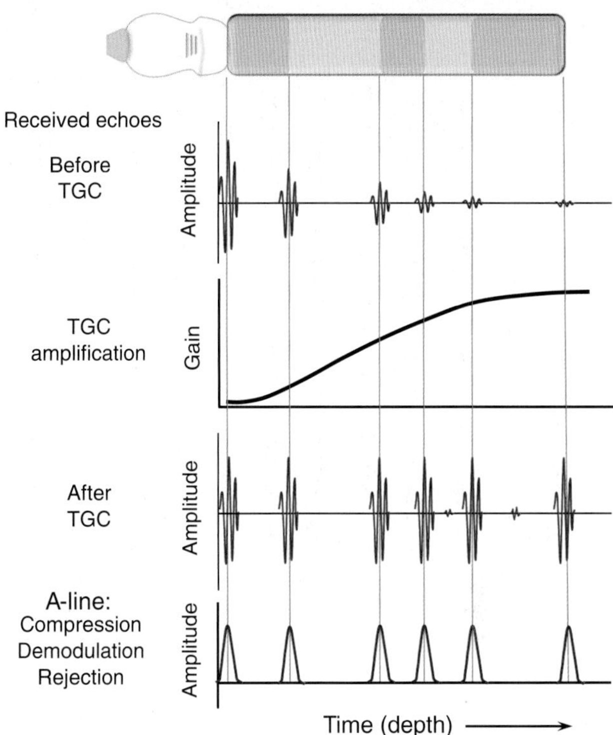

Figure 3-15 Time-gain compensation. Diagram showing how the returning echoes farther away from the transducer are increased in amplitude to account for attenuation.

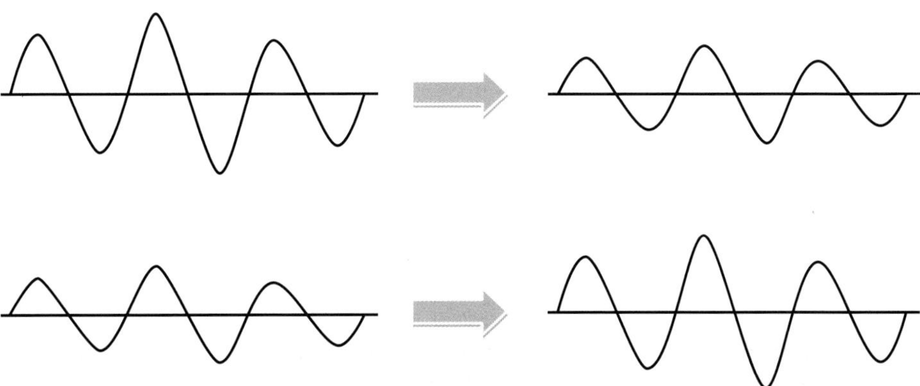

Figure 3-14 Amplification. All echo amplitudes increased or decreased equally, regardless of depth.

Imaging Principles and Instrumentation

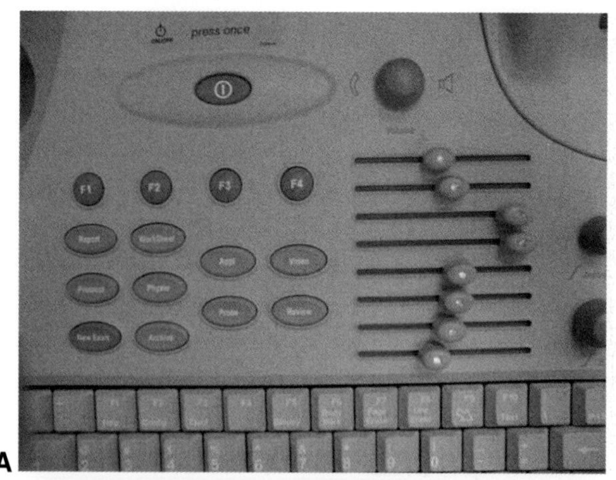

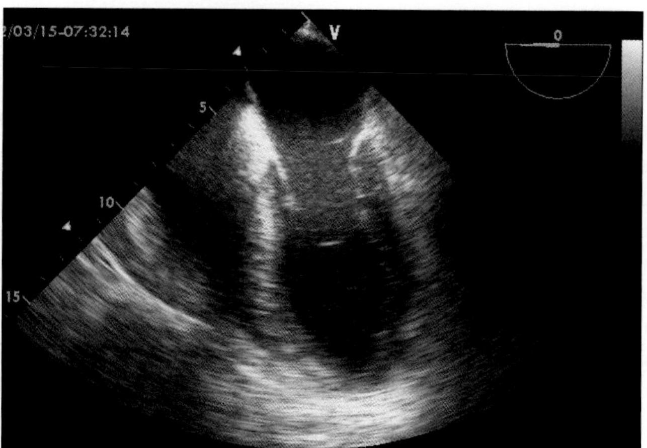

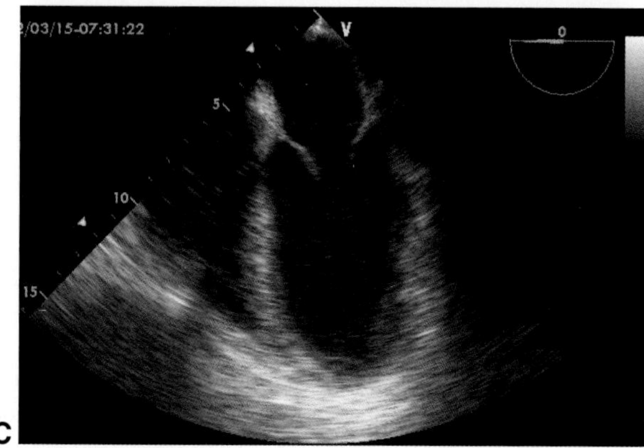

Figure 3-16 Influence of TGC adjustment on an image. **A.** The TGC is typically controlled by a series of slide pots. The upper controls affect the near field and the lower controls the far field. Note the high settings of the third and fourth controls and their effects on the midfield in B. **B.** In this image, the upper-middle part of the image is obscured by specular noise. **C.** The TGC controls were subsequently reduced, thus revealing the mitral valve more clearly. TGC, time-gain compensation.

voltages, whereas smoothing wraps an envelope around the signal to make it less "bumpy" or removes the "humps" (Figure 3-19).

- Rejection discards signal amplitudes below a certain threshold to reduce image noise (Figure 3-20).

SOUND OFF

The transmit/receive switch makes sure that pulser voltages pass through the transducer and received voltages from the transducer pass through the amplifier.

Transmit/Receive Switch

The **transmit/receive (T/R) switch** ensures that the electrical signals travel in the correct direction. Relatively high voltages (10 to 500 V) coming from the pulser would damage the circuitry in the receiver because the receiver is accustomed to receiving low voltages, about 2 μV to 1 V. The T/R switch ensures that the pulser voltages go through the transducer, and the received voltages from the transducer go through the amplifier. Figure 3-21 portrays the T/R switch as a traffic officer controlling the flow of traffic. The T/R switch ensures the correct flow of the signal to the transmit or receive channel as appropriate.

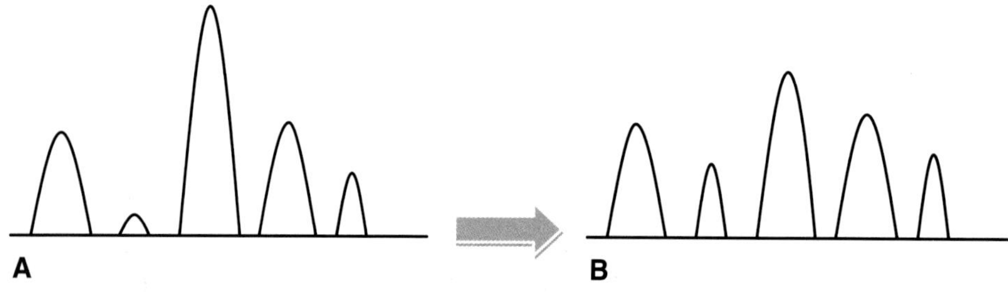

Figure 3-17 Compression. Compression is needed to decrease the difference between the largest and smallest amplitudes within the signal (the dynamic range). **A.** Signal before compression is applied. Notice the large difference between the largest and the smallest signal amplitudes. **B.** Signal after compression is applied. Compression decreases the differences between the largest and smallest amplitudes.

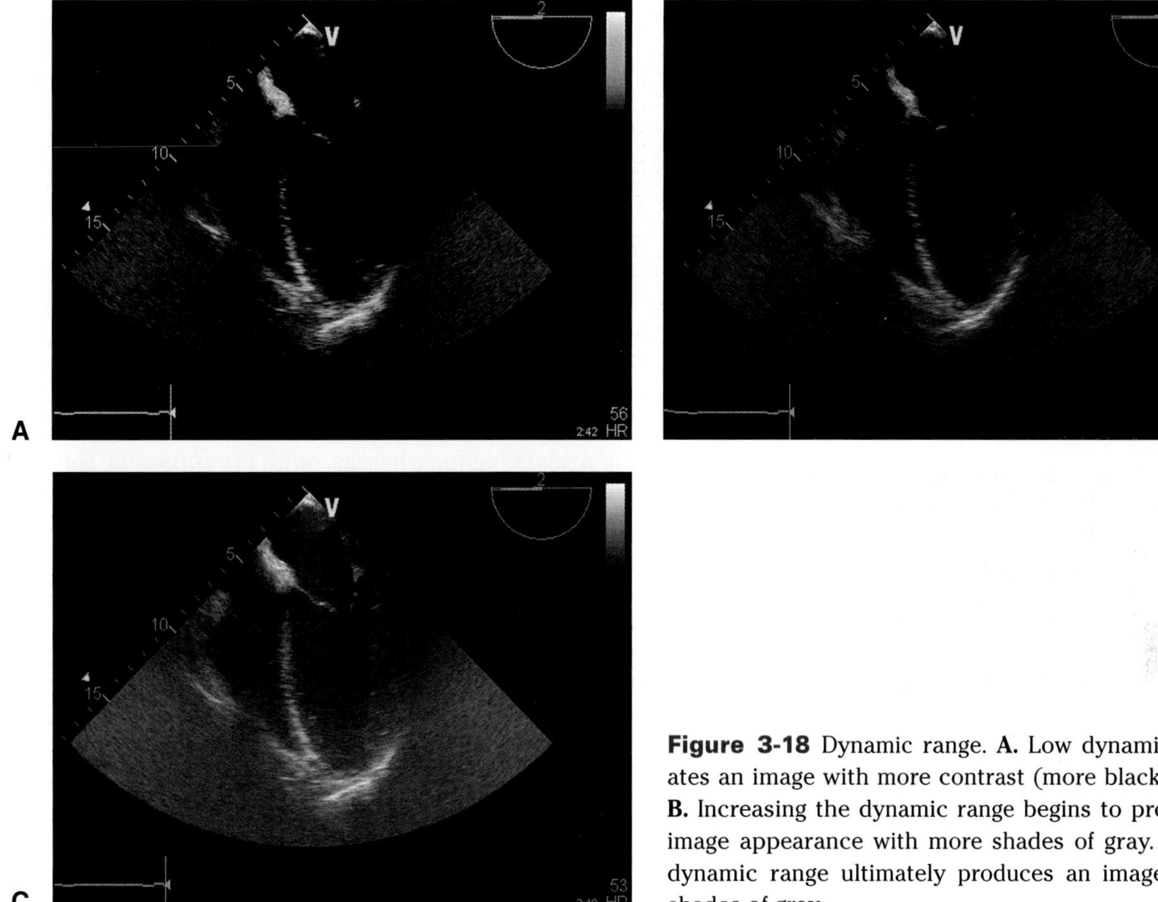

Figure 3-18 Dynamic range. **A.** Low dynamic range creates an image with more contrast (more black and white). **B.** Increasing the dynamic range begins to produce softer image appearance with more shades of gray. **C.** A higher dynamic range ultimately produces an image with more shades of gray.

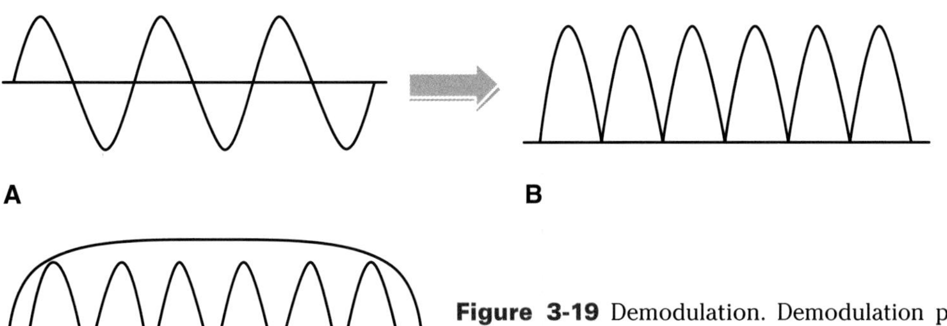

Figure 3-19 Demodulation. Demodulation processes the signal to make it easier for the machine to handle. Two components: **(A)** rectification turns negative voltages into positive voltages **(B)** and smoothing **(C)** wraps an envelope around the signal to make it less "bumpy."

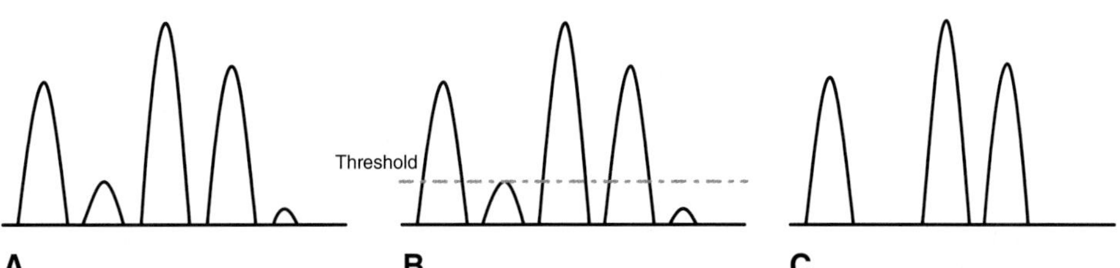

Figure 3-20 Rejection. Rejection discards signal amplitudes below a certain threshold to reduce image noise. **A.** Signal before rejection is applied. **B.** The threshold eliminates "noise" by removing signals below a certain set point. **C.** Signal result.

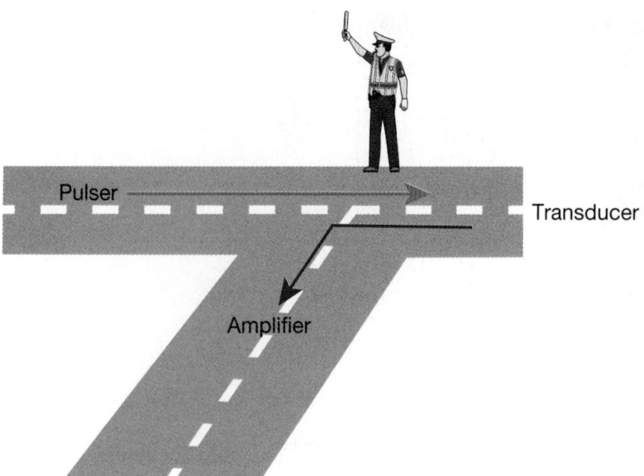

Figure 3-21 T/R switch. The T/R switch operates in the similar manner as a police officer directing traffic. The T/R switch ensures sound from the transducer's pulser only goes to the transducer elements, and sound returning from the patient only goes to the amplifier. T/R, transmit/receive.

SOUND OFF
Present-day scan converters are digital devices.

Scan Converter

The **scan converter** is the part of the machine that makes grayscale imaging possible and is responsible for the storage of the image data. The original scan converters were analog. Analog means infinite, and these scan converters could store a large range of signal amplitudes, thus allowing for many shades of gray. An often-used example of an analog device is the dimmer switch. Present-day scan converters are digital devices. Digital means finite in that there are far fewer choices available. For example, whereas a dimmer switch lets you adjust an infinitely variable light setting, the on–off switch is a "digital" device that offers discrete, finite choices (on or off, with nothing in between). Digital devices such as computers use the **binary** system that utilizes only zeroes and ones instead of the numbers zero through nine. Computers only communicate and process signals in binary, so any signal coming into the computer has to be converted into zeroes and ones. In ultrasound machines, signals are represented by black-and-white dots, or echoes; zero (0) represents "off" or a black echo, whereas one (1) represents "on" or a white echo. Before scan converters made grayscale imaging possible, images were purely black and white or **bistable**.

Signals travel from the receiver to the **analog-to-digital (A-to-D) converter**, to the scan converter/image memory, and then to the **digital-to-analog (D-to-A) converter**. **Preprocessing** occurs before the scan converter. Preprocessing is where incoming signals are assigned shades of gray based on their amplitudes. At this point, the image is still "live." Any changes to the image that need to be made while the image is live (ie, not frozen) occur in the preprocessing phase.

There are occasions where gaps exist between the scan lines, such as the diverging scan lines of sector scans. In these cases, the machine guesses what pixel should be placed there based on the surrounding shades of gray, a process called **pixel interpolation** or **fill-in interpolation** (Figure 3-22). After the signal is converted to a digital form, it can be processed by the computer. The image is stored in a computer where it can be displayed.

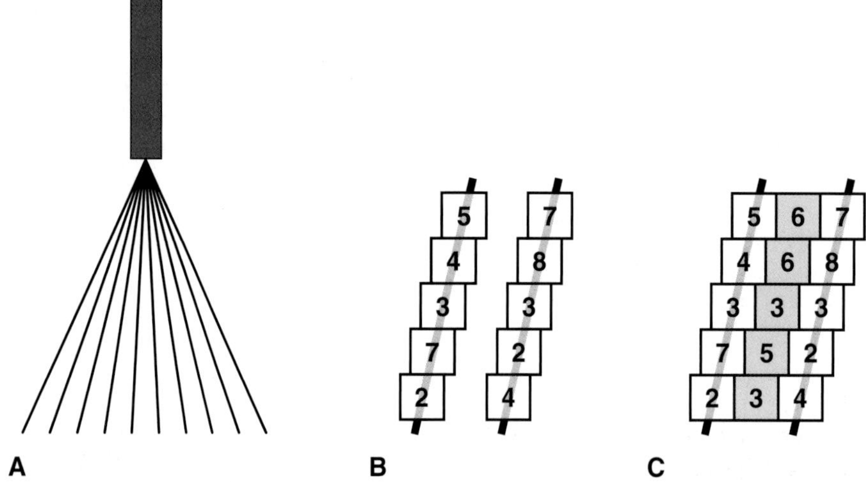

Figure 3-22 Divergence and fill-in interpolation. Divergence causes gaps between the scan lines **(A)**. Pixels along the scan lines are assigned a shade of gray **(B)**. Phantom pixels are added in between the scan lines where there is no signal information. The machine guesses what shade of gray to put in this space, a process called fill-in interpolation **(C)**.

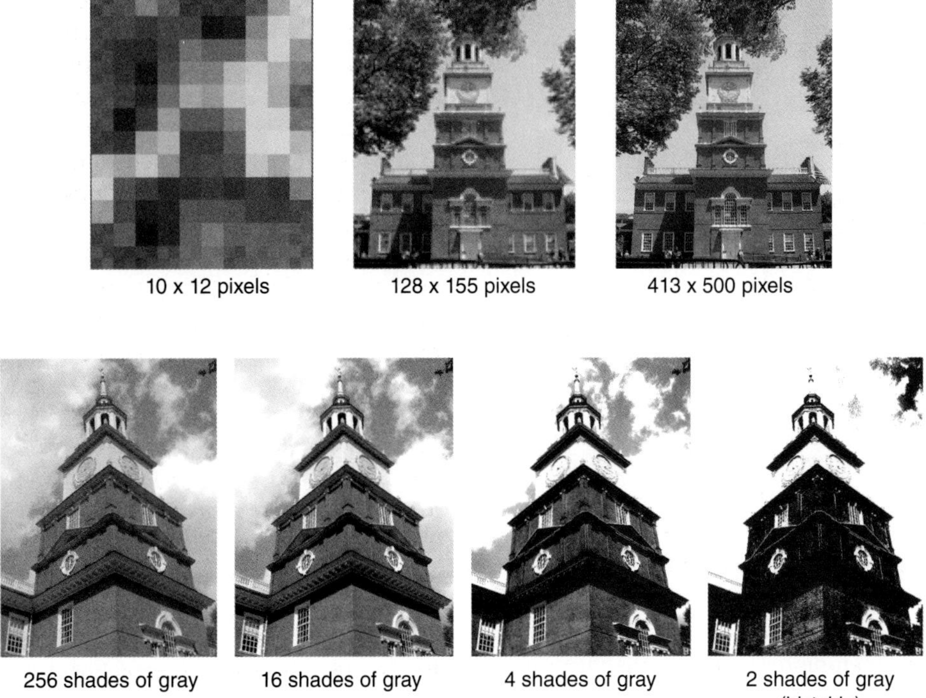

Figure 3-23 Pixels. In general, it is better to have more pixels than to have more shades of gray. The more pixels on a display, the better the spatial resolution of that display.

Sometimes it is desirable to "stack" frames (images) on top of each other instead of a new frame replacing the previous frame. The frames are averaged, and the resultant frame has reduced noise. This averaging of the frames is called **persistence** and is built into some manufacturer's presets and may be labeled on the machine under a trademarked name.

> **SOUND OFF**
> Preprocessing is where incoming signals are assigned shades of gray based on their amplitudes.

Recall that computers use the binary system, where the image information consists of zeroes and ones (Table A-2). A **bit** is the smallest amount of computer memory possible. Eight bits = 1 **byte**. The number of bits in memory determines the number of possible shades of gray. With only one bit there are only two shades available: black and white (known as "bistable"). The formula to determine the number of shades of gray is 2^n, where n is the number of bits. Two bits of memory = 4 (2^2) shades of gray, from the shade of gray 0 to the shade of gray 3. Eight bits of memory = 256 (2^8) shades of gray. Most ultrasound machines use 8 bits of memory, which equates to 256 available shades of gray, from the shade of gray 0 to the shade of gray 255.

The image is divided into rows and columns, called an image matrix. The ultrasound machine's image memory has a storage location corresponding to every **pixel** of the display. A pixel is short for the picture element, the smallest part of any digital image. A pixel is created at the intersection of the rows and columns in the image matrix. The more pixels on a display, the better the spatial resolution of the display. Therefore, an image matrix of 512 × 512 pixels is better than 256 × 256 pixels. In general, it is better to have more pixels per inch (ie, a higher pixel density) than to have more shades of gray (Figure 3-23). For 3D imaging, the term used is **voxel**, which is short for the volume element. Table 3-6 sums up computer terminologies.

TABLE 3-6 Computer terminology and description

Binary	Computer language of zeroes and ones
Bit	Binary digit. The smallest amount of computer memory
Byte	Eight bits of memory
Pixel	A picture element. The smallest unit of a 2D image
Voxel	A volume element. The smallest unit of a 3D image
Image matrix	Storage in memory corresponding to each pixel on the display

Imaging Principles and Instrumentation

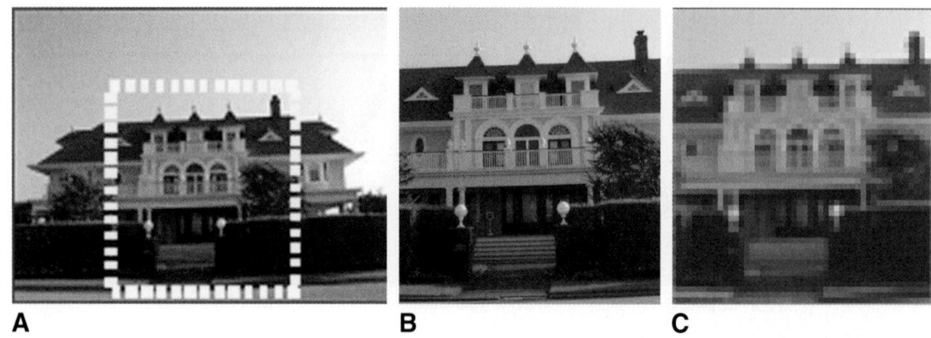

Figure 3-24 Write zoom versus read zoom. The original image **(A)** in this figure is being analyzed. Write zoom is a preprocessing function that enlarges the image by redrawing it **(B)**. This offers a high-quality zoomed image. Read zoom, a postprocessing function, enlarges the image by making the pixels bigger **(C)**. This type of zoom offers a coarser, less optimal type of zoom.

SOUND OFF
Most modern machines offer postprocessing image settings that can be changed once the image is frozen, including TGC, overall gain, and some Doppler settings.

Once the signal is stored in memory, it may be sent to the D-to-A converter. In the D-to-A converter, the signal is converted back to the analog form so that it can be displayed. The image information may also be sent to a **picture archiving and communication system** (PACS), hard drive, DVD, or thermal paper. Although it varies by manufacturer, modern ultrasound machines offer **postprocessing** image settings that can be changed after the image is frozen, including gain and some Doppler settings. There are two ways of magnifying the ultrasound image: **write zoom** and **read zoom** (Figure 3-24). Write zoom, a preprocessing function, enlarges the image by redrawing it. Because the image has not been stored in memory yet, it is possible to enlarge the image while maintaining the pixel density. This offers a high-quality zoomed image. Write zoom is a preprocessing function, and therefore the image must be live. Read zoom, a postprocessing function, enlarges the image by magnifying the pixels. The image has already been stored in memory, so it is not possible to maintain the pixel density in this case. Read zoom offers a coarser, less optimal type of zoom. With read zoom, the image may be a frozen or live image. To recall which is which, remember: Write zoom is the "write" way to do it (Table 3-7).

Display

Today's modern ultrasound equipment utilizes a **liquid crystal display (LCD)**. The older technology used for display was the **cathode ray tube (CRT)** (Figure 3-25). The CRT was like a vintage television, and it is no longer used in clinical practice. The LCD, also called a flat-panel display, works with a light source, either fluorescent or light emitting diode (LED), positioned behind two polarized filters with liquid crystals sandwiched between them. The twisting or untwisting of the crystals determines whether light shines through to the face of the display.

Recording and Storage Devices

PACS is the most recent display and storage medium (Figures 3-26 and 3-27). Other storage devices, most of which have fallen out of favor, include the following: film; video recording, such as VHS that uses a magnetic tape; CDs/DVDs that are optical storage devices; and magneto-optical (MO) storage. Images can also be sent to a piece of paper or thermal printers. PACS systems use a redundant array of independent disks (RAID array) to store large quantities of data and back up the PACS.

Imaging computers use a standardized format called digital imaging in communications and medicine (DICOM) to communicate with each other and exchange data. DICOM is used in sonography, CT, MRI, and other medical imaging systems.

TABLE 3-7 Write and read zoom comparison

Write Zoom	Read Zoom
Preprocessing function	Postprocessing function
Image must be live	Image may be frozen or live
Higher quality zoom	Lower quality zoom
Memory tip: Write zoom is the "write" way to do it!	

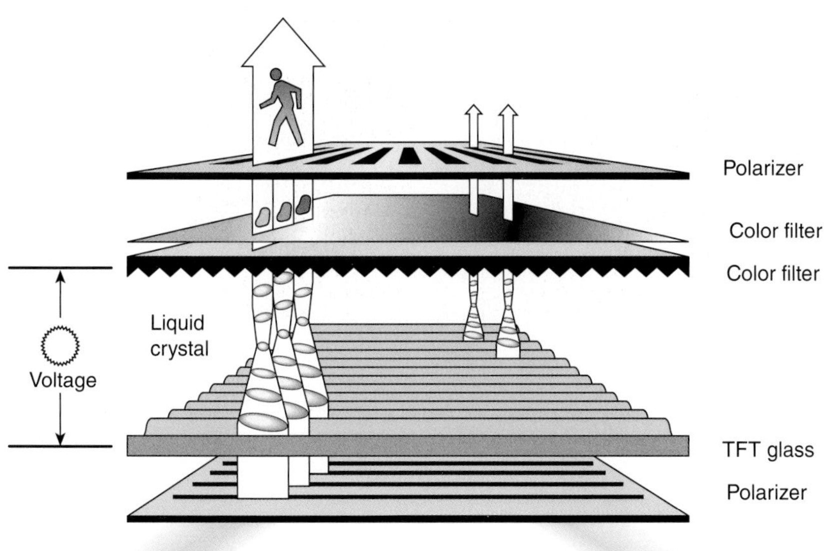

Figure 3-25 Diagram of a liquid crystal display.

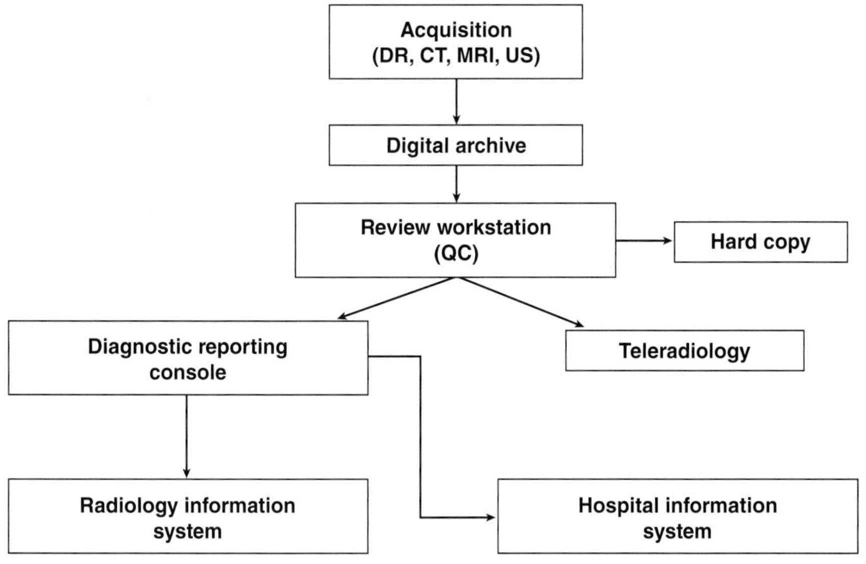

Figure 3-26 Diagram of a picture archiving and communication system.

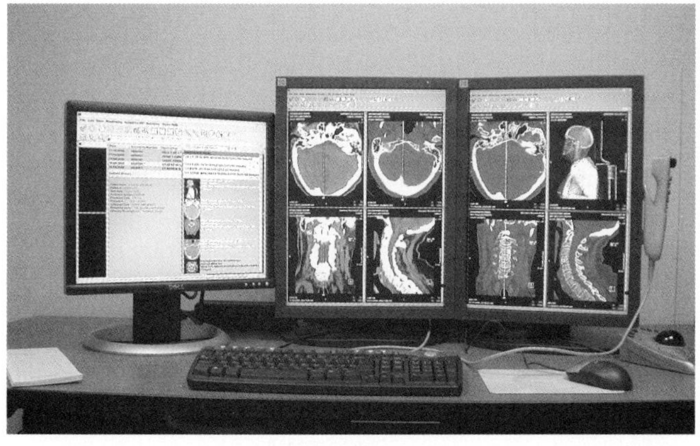

Figure 3-27 Photograph of a picture archiving and communication system workstation.

IMAGING ARTIFACTS

Artifacts are echoes on the screen that are not representative of actual anatomic features or occur when there are anatomic structures in the body that are not displayed on the screen (Table 3-8). Artifacts may also occur as a result of electrical interference or a problem with the ultrasound machine.

Artifacts result from assumptions that the ultrasound machine makes. These include:

- Sound beams travel in a straight line and go directly to the reflector and back to the transducer.
- The only propagation speed in the body is 1540 m/s (ie, the 13 μs rule).
- Any reflection that comes back to the transducer is from a reflector along the path of the beam.
- The slice-thickness plane is razor-thin.

A common artifact is **reverberation** that is described as multiple reflections, and it occurs when the sound bounces back and forth between two closely spaced strong **specular reflectors** (Figures 3-28 and 3-29). This produces the appearance of parallel echoes that are equally spaced and decrease in brightness (amplitude) with depth. One subtype of reverberation is the **comet tail** that is caused by small structures such as

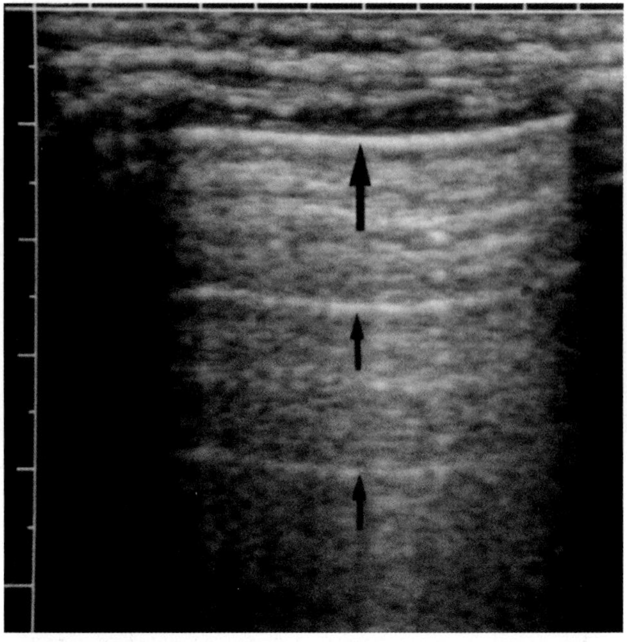

Figure 3-28 Reverberation artifact. Intercostal linear array image of the normal lung surface shows intense reflections at the soft tissue–air interface (*large arrow*) that reflects back and forth between the transducer surface and the interface to produce a series of reverberation bands (*small arrows*) deeper in the image.

TABLE 3-8 Imaging artifacts

Imaging Artifacts	Description
Reverberation	Closely spaced parallel echoes of decreasing brightness deep to two parallel specular reflectors
Mirror image	Artifact caused by sound reflecting off a strong specular reflector and displaying an object on both sides of the reflector
Multipath	Beam reflects off objects in the body and makes two or more changes in the direction before returning to the transducer
Edge shadowing	Refraction artifact caused by sound refracting off the curved surface. Eliminated/reduced by spatial compounding
Side/grating lobes	Extraneous energy not along the path of main beam causes erroneous reflections
Propagation speed errors (aka boundary displacement)	If the actual propagation speed of the tissue is greater than or less than 1540 m/s, the machine places the reflector at the wrong location on the display Remember: The machine is using $d = (c \times t)/2$, but assumes $c = 1540$ m/s
Shadowing	Potentially useful artifact occurs when sound traverses a highly attenuating structure. May help to identify stones
Enhancement	Potentially useful artifact that occurs when sound travels through a weakly attenuating structure. Appears as an area of increased brightness distal to weakly attenuating reflectors
Slice-thickness artifact (also known as partial-volume artifact)	Artifact that occurs as a result of the elevational plane of the beam not being razor-thin. Unintended echoes may appear in the image as the beam slices through structures adjacent to intended reflectors
Electric interference	Disturbance on display that appears as "arc-like" moving bands caused by the ultrasound machine being placed too close to unshielded electrical equipment

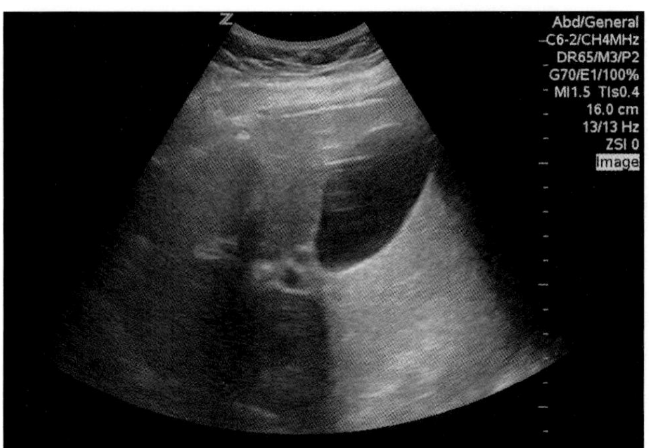

Figure 3-29 Reverberation in the gallbladder. Reverberation produces a "stepladder" appearance within the anterior aspect of the gallbladder.

surgical clips or adenomyomatosis within the gallbladder wall (Figure 3-30). The **ring-down artifact** appears like a comet tail but with long streamers/streaks or a curtain of echoes; it is caused by the interaction of sound with small air bubbles, making the bubbles vibrate (Figure 3-31). This artifact is potentially useful because it indicates the presence of air and therefore might demonstrate pneumobilia or abscess. The ring-down artifact may also occur from nonair structures, such as needles or foreign bodies.

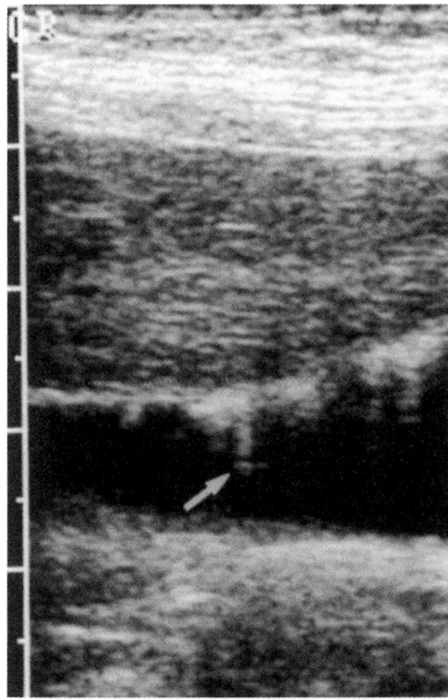

Figure 3-30 Comet-tail artifact. Image of the gallbladder shows a series of bright tapering echoes (*arrow*) extending from its walls. This is a sonographic finding that is commonly associated with cholesterol crystal accumulation within the gallbladder wall, a condition known as adenomyomatosis.

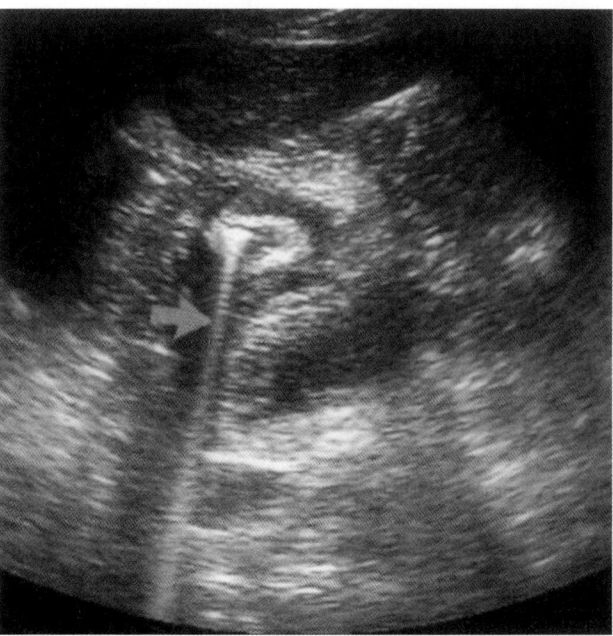

Figure 3-31 Ring-down artifact. Longitudinal image of the gastric antrum shows a prominent ring-down artifact (*arrow*) caused by air bubbles in the stomach.

SOUND OFF

The ring-down artifact appears like a comet tail, but it is caused by the interaction of sound with small air bubbles, making the bubbles vibrate.

SOUND OFF

The mirror-image artifact occurs when the sound is aimed toward a large specular reflector that acts like a mirror and directs some of the sound in a direction other than back to the transducer.

SOUND OFF

Spatial compounding eliminates edge shadowing and improves margin delineation. It also reduces the speckle artifact and reverberation, resulting in a smoother image with improved contrast.

SOUND OFF

Side lobes occur with all transducers, and grating lobes occur with linear arrays.

The **mirror-image artifact** occurs when the sound is aimed toward a large specular reflector that acts like a mirror and directs some of the sound in a direction other than back to the transducer. This causes the reflector

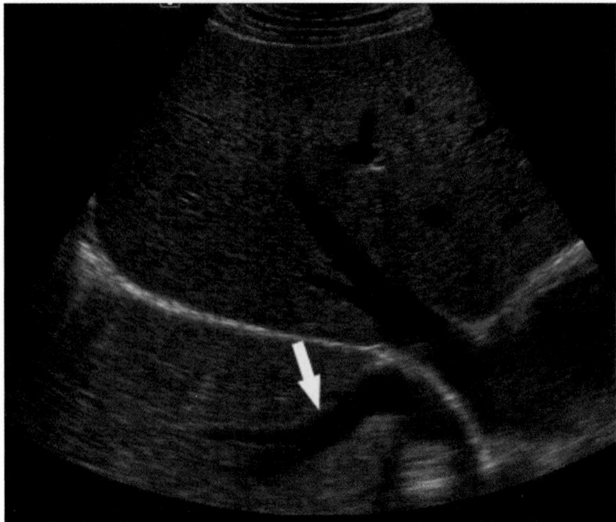

Figure 3-32 Mirror-image artifact. In this transverse image of the liver, a duplicate hepatic vein (*arrow*) is noted deeper than the actual structure in this image.

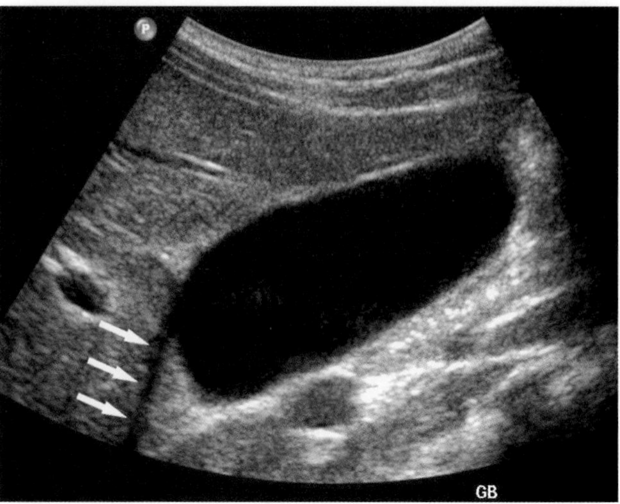

Figure 3-33 Edge shadow. Edge shadow (*arrows*) arising from the edge of the gallbladder.

to appear equally spaced apart from either side of the strong reflector. This artifact is commonly seen near the diaphragm and pleura. Note that the duplicate object always appears deeper than the actual structure being duplicated (Figure 3-32).

Refraction causes artifacts as the beam is directed away from the path in which it was originally intended to go. One refraction artifact is **edge shadowing** that is seen when sound strikes a curved reflector like the transverse gallbladder or carotid artery (Figure 3-33). **Spatial compounding** eliminates edge shadowing because the object is imaged from different angles. Thus, spatial compounding improves margin delineation. It also reduces the speckle artifact and reverberation, resulting in a smoother image with improved contrast (Figure 3-34). Different manufacturers have different names for spatial compounding (eg, Crossbeam, Aplipure, SonoCT, etc).

One of the assumptions made by the machine is that sound energy travels along the main axis of the beam. If there is extraneous sound energy not along the main axis (Figure 3-35), the possibility exists that this sound will cause reflections back to the transducer. As the machine assumes that all reflectors lie along the path of the beam, the artifacts produced are called **side lobes** or grating lobes (Figure 3-36). Side lobes occur with

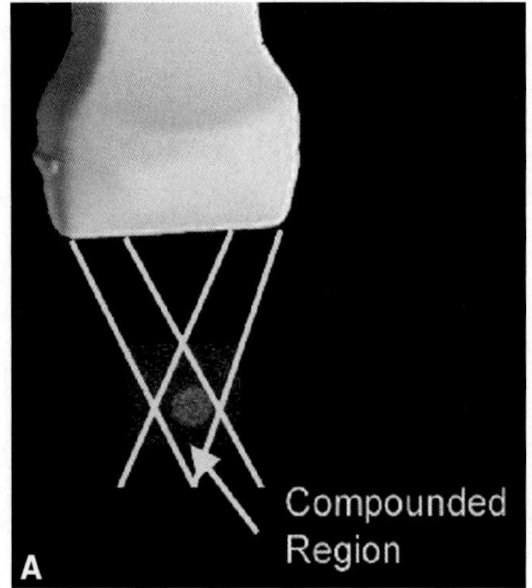

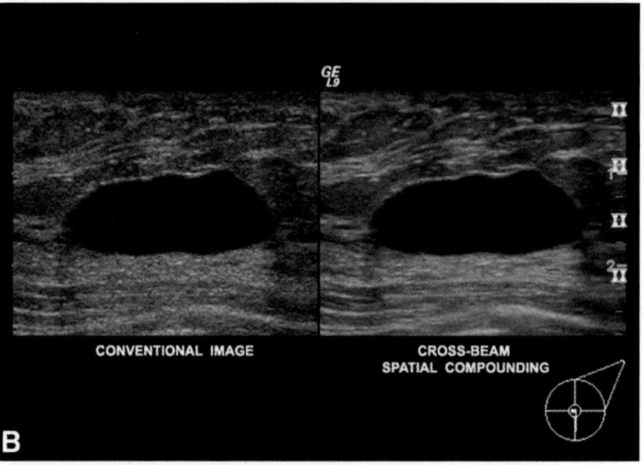

Figure 3-34 Benefits of spatial compounding. **A.** Spatial compound technique utilizing varying transmit angles. The area of compounding occurs in the region where transmit beams overlap. **B.** The image on the left of a breast cyst was produced with conventional imaging, whereas the image on the right employed spatial compounding. Note that the image with spatial compounding improves the margin delineation of the cyst. It also reduces the speckle artifact and reverberation, resulting in a smoother image with improved contrast.

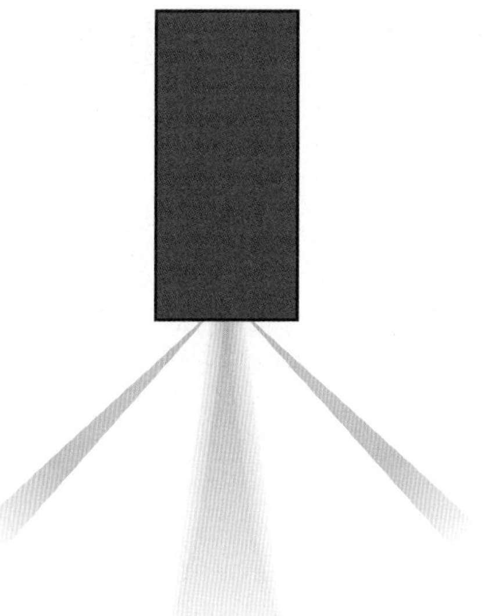

Figure 3-35 Illustration depicting the grating lobe artifact, with sound beams directed outward and are not part of the primary beam. These grating lobes add additional echoes to the image.

single-element transducers, and grating lobes occur with array transducers. Tissue harmonic imaging, apodization, and **subdicing**, the techniques used to slice the crystals into much smaller sections, are used to reduce or eliminate grating lobes.

Propagation speed errors can take place as well. Recall that although the ultrasound machine is programmed to assume that sound travels through all tissues at 1540 m/s, this does not actually occur, because the body consists of many different types of tissue with many different propagation speeds. Nonetheless, the machine is programmed to assume 1540 m/s regardless of which type of tissue, or group of tissues, the beam encounters. If the actual propagation speed through which the sound is traveling is less than 1540 m/s, reflectors will be displayed on the screen too far away. Likewise, if the actual propagation speed of the tissue is greater than 1540 m/s, reflectors will be displayed too close. Propagation speed errors may also be called boundary or speed displacement because they can make boundaries, such as the diaphragm, appear displaced because of the propagation speed error.

SOUND OFF
Shadowing and enhancement are both potentially useful artifacts because they help in the differentiation of some benign and malignant processes.

Two potentially useful artifacts are **shadowing** and **enhancement**. Shadowing occurs when the sound travels through an area of higher attenuation, such as a rib or other calcified or bony structure (Figure 3-37). The shadow artifact occurs because there is insufficient ultrasound energy deep to the highly attenuating reflector, and no echoes return to the transducer. This artifact is potentially useful, like when it helps with the identification of kidney stones or gallstones, but

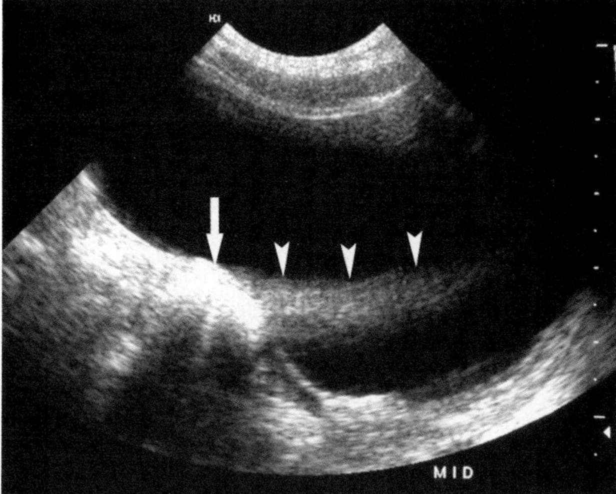

Figure 3-36 Grating lobe artifact. Longitudinal view of the urinary bladder showing the grating lobe artifact (*arrowheads*) arising from bowel gas (*arrow*) extending well into the bladder.

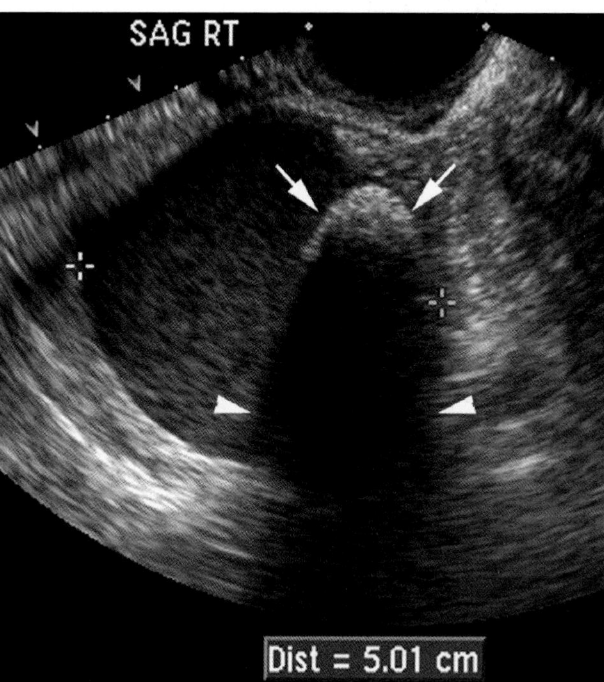

Figure 3-37 Shadowing. This ovarian dermoid tumor (between *calipers*) has a solid component (between *arrows*) that produces a prominent acoustic shadow (between *arrowheads*).

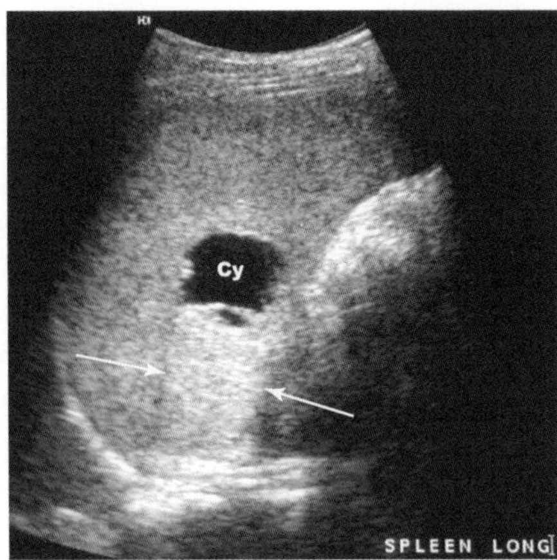

Figure 3-38 Enhancement. Longitudinal view of the spleen showing acoustic enhancement (between *arrows*) posterior to a splenic cyst (*Cy*).

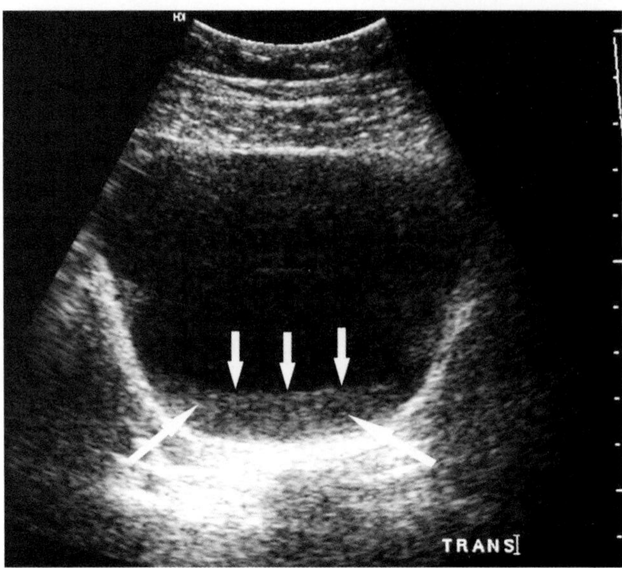

Figure 3-39 Slice-thickness artifact. False echoes created by adjacent bowel gas simulate layering debris (*arrows*) within this urinary bladder.

shadowing is potentially detrimental when the shadow obscures part of the anatomy. Acoustic enhancement occurs when the sound beam travels through areas of decreased attenuation compared to the surrounding tissue, such as fluid (Figure 3-38). Because less sound is attenuated when traveling through this region (eg, a cyst), there is more signal strength distal to the object. This makes the tissue deep to the weak attenuator appear brighter. Note that solid masses may enhance depending on their internal makeup and vascularity.

With ultrasound technology using conventional beamforming, the ultrasound beam is not razor-thin; it has a definite thickness called the slice thickness or elevational plane. Any reflectors appearing in this plane will appear in the image. An often-seen example of this is scanning through an ovarian cyst and seeing what appears to be echoes within it or scanning through a narrow blood vessel and echoes appear that resemble thrombus. After the transducer is turned 90°, the echoes disappear, indicating that they are not really within the cyst. The **slice-thickness artifact** occurs because the beam is scanned through both the cyst and soft tissue adjacent to the cyst, causing both to appear on the image (Figure 3-39). The solution to the slice-thickness artifact is utilizing a 1.5D transducer, which allows for a narrower elevational plane (see Chapter 2).

The presence of electrical equipment near the ultrasound machine (eg, unshielded ventilators) may cause an artifact related to **electrical interference**. This causes arc-like bands that move across the screen as long as the machine is in proximity to the unshielded equipment (Figure 3-40).

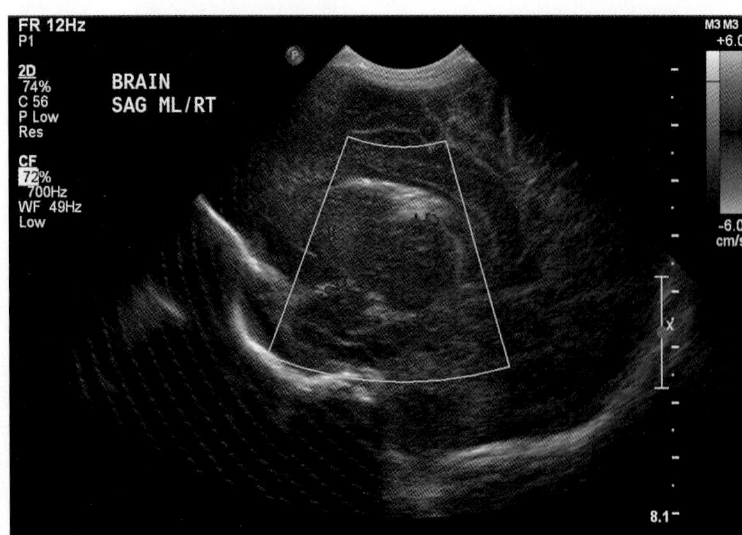

Figure 3-40 Electronic noise. The arc-like bands seen on an image in proximity to electronic noise degrade the image quality. Try to keep the machine from sources of unshielded electronic equipment when possible.

REVIEW QUESTIONS

1. The output of the pulser determines the _______ of the acoustic pulse.
   a. Frequency
   b. Intensity
   c. Duration
   d. Pulse repetition period

2. What is the function of the receiver that changes the brightness of the echo amplitudes to adjust for attenuation with depth?
   a. Compression
   b. Condensation
   c. Confirmation
   d. Compensation

3. Which of the following tasks is incorporated in the process of demodulation?
   a. Rejection
   b. Amplification
   c. Rectification
   d. Receiving

4. What is the smallest element in a digital picture called?
   a. The bit
   b. The pixel
   c. The byte
   d. The fractal

5. The part of the transducer called a "transmit channel" consists of a transducer element and a __________
   a. Pulse delay
   b. Reciprocator
   c. Pulser
   d. Synchronizer

6. The part of the machine that ensures that the signal from the pulser goes to the transducer and the signal from the patient goes to the amplifier is:
   a. Amplifier
   b. T/R switch
   c. RAID array
   d. A-to-D converter

7. A video display that is limited to only black and white with no other shades of gray is called ______.
   a. Bistable
   b. Monochrome
   c. Binary
   d. Unichrome

8. What type of display uses a backlight with two polarized filters to produce an image?
   a. LCD
   b. Plasma
   c. CRT
   d. OLED

9. In tissue harmonic imaging, what frequency is used to produce the image?
   a. The fundamental frequency
   b. Half of the fundamental frequency
   c. Double the fundamental frequency
   d. Three times the fundamental frequency

10. What backup system is used to protect the stored data on a PACS?
    a. Optical drive
    b. RAID array
    c. Tape backup
    d. Flash drive

11. With 6 bits, what is the largest number of different shades of gray that can be stored?
    a. 16
    b. 8
    c. 256
    d. 64

12. In B-mode imaging, the stronger the return echo,
    a. The darker the dot on the display
    b. The brighter the dot on the display
    c. The worse the temporal resolution
    d. The weaker the transmit power

13. What happens to a digital image when the pixel density is increased?
    a. There is more spatial detail
    b. There is less spatial detail
    c. The temporal resolution increases
    d. There are more shades of gray

14. You are using a transducer that produces a beam with a very wide elevational plane. Which of the following problems are you most likely to encounter as a result?
    a. Slice-thickness artifact
    b. Increased reverberation
    c. Increased side lobes
    d. Increased electrical interference

15. The potentially useful artifact that one might see behind a weakly attenuating structure is:
    a. Shadowing
    b. Reflection
    c. Enhancement
    d. Refraction

16. When you adjust the output power control, you affect the following system component:
    a. Pulser
    b. Memory
    c. Scan converter
    d. Receiver

17. The part of the receiver that reduces low-level system noise is:
    a. Demodulation
    b. Compensation
    c. Amplification
    d. Rejection

18. What receiver function is responsible for decreasing the difference between the largest and smallest received signal amplitudes?
    a. Amplification
    b. Compensation
    c. Compression
    d. Rejection

19. Sound bouncing off a strong reflector and producing an image on the opposite site of the strong reflector is:
    a. Range ambiguity
    b. Mirror image artifact
    c. Slice-thickness artifact
    d. Enhancement

20. What must be known to calculate the distance from a transducer to a reflector?
    a. Attenuation, propagation speed, tissue density
    b. Attenuation, impedance
    c. Tissue density, propagation speed
    d. Round trip time, propagation speed

21. Contrast resolution is:
    a. The ability to see differences in shades of gray
    b. The ability to display moving structures in real time
    c. The ability to identify two reflectors parallel to the beam
    d. The ability to identify two reflectors perpendicular to the beam

22. Which of the following occurs after the image has been stored in memory?
    a. Preprocessing
    b. Postprocessing
    c. Conversion to binary
    d. Write zoom

23. In which mode is the strength of the reflector represented by the brightness of the dot?
    a. A-mode
    b. B-mode
    c. 3D mode
    d. Z-mode

24. Which mode displays the movement of the reflectors along a single scan line?
    a. A-mode
    b. B-mode
    c. M-mode
    d. C-mode

25. In M-mode imaging, what is represented by the *x*-axis?
    a. Depth
    b. Amplitude
    c. Intensity
    d. Time

26. The harmonic signal
    a. Is produced by the transducer's elements
    b. Is produced by the patient's tissue
    c. Is of a stronger amplitude than the fundamental
    d. Has worse lateral resolution than the fundamental

27. When imaging in tissue harmonic imaging:
    a. The fundamental frequency is filtered out
    b. The fundamental beam's frequency is increased
    c. The harmonic signal is filtered out
    d. There are more artifacts

28. A sound wave travels 26 μs to a reflector. How far away is the reflector, assuming the medium is soft tissue?
    a. 0.5 cm
    b. 1.0 cm
    c. 2.0 cm
    d. 4.0 cm

29. A reflector is 20 mm away from the transducer. How long does it take for sound to travel to the reflector and back to the transducer?
    a. 13 μs
    b. 20 μs
    c. 26 μs
    d. 39 μs

30. Which of the following is a technique used to reduce the presence of grating lobes?
    a. Output power adjustment
    b. Apodization
    c. Wall filter adjustment
    d. Rejection

31. The strength of the voltages sent to each element is determined by the:
    a. Beamformer
    b. Receiver
    c. Scan converter
    d. Display

32. An advantage of coded excitation is improved:
    a. Azimuthal resolution
    b. Temporal resolution
    c. Signal-to-noise ratio
    d. Lateral resolution

33. If the far field of the image is too dark, the preferred technique is to:
    a. Apply less pressure to the patient
    b. Optimize the TGC
    c. Increase the output power
    d. Raise the focal zone

34. Read zoom is a _________ function
    a. PACS
    b. Postprocessing
    c. Preprocessing
    d. Pulser

35. Which type of zoom offers a high-quality zoom but must be selected while the image is live?
    a. Postprocessing zoom
    b. Read zoom
    c. Write zoom
    d. Compensated zoom

36. As the sound beam propagates deeper, the strength of the beam is attenuated. This explains the need to have which receiver function?
    a. Compression
    b. Demodulation
    c. Amplification
    d. Compensation

37. The smallest component of a 3D image is the:
    a. Bit
    b. Byte
    c. Voxel
    d. Pixel

38. The technique that uses made-up pixel information to replace areas between the scan lines where there is no actual signal information is:
    a. Compression
    b. Fill-in interpolation
    c. Tissue harmonics
    d. Frequency compounding

39. Which of the following is the standard for data exchange among imaging systems?
    a. RAID
    b. PACS
    c. RIS
    d. DICOM

40. An artifact that occurs when a sound beam bounces back and forth between two strong reflectors, creating a series of repeating lines is:
    a. Reverberation
    b. Side lobes
    c. Multipath
    d. Edge shadowing

41. Additional reflectors on the screen (with an array transducer) that are from extraneous sound waves off the primary axis of the beam are:
    a. Ring-down artifacts
    b. Edge shadows
    c. Harmonics
    d. Grating lobes

42. Sound travels through a large quantity of muscle tissue. The reflector will be displayed:
    a. Too close to the transducer
    b. Too far away from the transducer
    c. In the correct location
    d. Sound does not travel through muscle tissue.

43. A shadow occurs when sound:
    a. Propagates through an area of decreased attenuation
    b. Propagates through an area of increased attenuation
    c. Reflects off a weak attenuator
    d. Travels through a cystic structure

44. The digital echo information is taken from the memory and sent to the __________ so that it can be shown on an analog display.
    a. Beamformer
    b. Receiver
    c. A-to-D converter
    d. D-to-A converter

45. Which older mode may still be used today in ophthalmology?
    a. A-mode
    b. B-mode
    c. M-mode
    d. C-mode

46. Which part of the US machine does not affect the amount of energy entering the patient?
    a. Receiver
    b. Pulser
    c. Transmitter
    d. Transmit beamformer

47. An image with 1 bit of memory can display _____ shades of gray.
    a. None
    b. One
    c. Two
    d. Four

48. Sound that strikes air and creates a streak-like artifact is called:
    a. Ring-down
    b. Comet-tail
    c. Reverberation
    d. Ghost image

49. A technique that averages out the frequencies present within the beam to improve contrast resolution and reduce speckle is:
    a. Spatial compounding
    b. Frequency compounding
    c. Coded excitation
    d. Tissue harmonics

50. Artifacts related to propagation speed occur because:
    a. The machine can measure the propagation speed of the tissue
    b. The beam bounces off strong reflectors
    c. The beam travels in a straight line
    d. The machine assumes 1540 m/s for all tissue

SUGGESTED READINGS

AIUM.org. *Recommended Ultrasound Terminology*. 4th ed. Accessed October 1, 2023. https://www.aium.org/docs/default-source/aium-publications/rut.pdf

Bushberg JT, Seibert JA, Leidholdt EM Jr., Boone, JM. *The Essential Physics of Medical Imaging*. 4th ed. Wolters Kluwer; 2020.

Digital Imaging and Communications in Medicine (DICOM). Accessed May 5, 2024. http://dicom.nema.org

Edelman SK. *Understanding Ultrasound Physics*. 4th ed. ESP Ultrasound; 2012.

Feldman MK, Katyal S, Blackwood MS. US artifacts. *Radiographics*. 2009;29(4):1179–1189.

Hedrick WR. *Technology for Diagnostic Sonography*. Elsevier Health Sciences; 2012.

Hedrick WR, Hykes DL, Starchman DE. *Ultrasound Physics and Instrumentation*. 4th ed. Elsevier Mosby; 2005.

Hughes S. *Sonography Principles and Instrumentation*. Society of Diagnostic Medical Sonographers; 2009.

Kremkau FW. *Diagnostic Ultrasound: Principles and Instruments*. 10th ed. Saunders; 2020.

Miele F. *Ultrasound Physics and Instrumentation*. 6th ed. Miele Enterprises; 2022.

Sanders RC, Hall-Terracciano B. *Clinical Sonography: A Practical Guide*. 5th ed. Wolters Kluwer; 2016.

Szabo TL. *Diagnostic Ultrasound Imaging: Inside Out*. Elsevier; 2014.

Tranquart F, Grenier N, Eder V, Pourcelot L. Clinical use of ultrasound tissue harmonic imaging. *Ultrasound Med Biol*. 1999;25(6):889–894.

4

Hemodynamics and Doppler

Outline

Introduction

This chapter is divided into two parts. The first part will cover hemodynamics—the science of how and why blood flows through the blood vessels of the body. Normal arterial and venous flow will be examined, along with what happens when there is a stenosis. The second part of the chapter will discuss Doppler; review the Doppler equation; and will discuss spectral, color, and power Doppler, as well as the artifacts that are associated with Doppler examinations.

Key Terms

aliasing—the wraparound of the spectral or color Doppler display that occurs when the frequency shift exceeds the Nyquist limit; occurs only with PW Doppler

angle-correction—the Doppler tool used to inform the machine what the angle to flow is so that velocities can be accurately calculated

autocorrelation—the color Doppler processing technique that assesses pixels as stationary or in motion

BART—the acronym used to describe color Doppler scale: "blue away, red toward"

baseline—the operator-adjustable dividing line between positive frequency shifts and negative frequency shifts on spectral and color Doppler (also called the *zero-flow baseline*)

Bernoulli's principle—the principle that describes the inverse relationship between velocity and pressure

boundary layer—the stationary (or near-stationary) layer of blood cells immediately adjacent to the vessel wall

brightness—the term describing the intensity or luminance of the color Doppler display

calf muscle pump—the muscles in the calf that, upon contraction, propel venous blood toward the heart

capacitance—the ability of veins to store blood

clutter—acoustic noise in the color and/or spectral Doppler signal

collateral blood vessels—accessory vessels that dilate to permit blood flow in the presence of an obstruction in the main blood vessel

color Doppler imaging—Doppler shift information presented as a color (hue) superimposed over the grayscale image

color priority—the setting for color Doppler that allows the operator to select the frequency shift threshold; it determines whether color pixels should be displayed preferentially over grayscale pixels

continuity equation—the equation that describes the change in velocity as the area changes in order to maintain the volumetric flow rate

continuous-wave Doppler—non-imaging Doppler device that consists of two elements: one element is used by the system to constantly transmit sound and the other is used to constantly receive sound

critical stenosis—the point at which a stenosis is hemodynamically significant with a drop in pressure or volume flow distal to the stenosis

depth ambiguity—the inability to determine the depth of the reflector if the pulses are sent out too fast for them to be timed (also called *range ambiguity*)

diastole—the relaxation of the cardiac ventricles following contraction

Doppler effect—the change in the frequency of the received signal related to the motion of a reflector

Doppler equation—the equation that explains the relationship of the Doppler frequency shift (F_D) with the frequency of the transducer (f), the velocity of the blood (v), the angle of blood flow ($\cos\theta$ (in °)), and the propagation speed (c)

duplex—real-time two-dimensional imaging combined with the spectral Doppler display

effective resistance—the sum of the individual resistances when multiple vessels are connected in series

ensemble length—the number of pulses per scan line in color Doppler; also referred to as packet size

extrinsic pressure—pressure applied from the outside of an object

fast Fourier transform—a mathematical process used for analyzing and processing the Doppler signal to produce the spectral waveform

flash artifact—a motion artifact caused by the movement of tissue when using power Doppler

frequency shift—the difference between the transmitted and received frequencies

friction—a form of resistance, caused by two materials rubbing against each other, thereby converting energy to heat

hemodynamically significant stenosis—*see* the key term "critical stenosis"

hemodynamics—the study of blood flow through the blood vessels of the body

hue—a term used to describe displayed colors (eg, red, blue, and green)

hydrostatic pressure—describes the relationship between gravity, density of the blood, and the distance between an arbitrary reference point

inertia—Newton's first law of motion stating that an object at rest stays at rest and an object in motion stays in motion, unless acted on by an outside force

innervated—supplied with nerves

kinetic energy—the energy form of flowing blood

laminar flow—the flow profile represented by blood that travels in nonmixing layers of different velocities, with the fastest flow in the center and the slowest flow near the vessel walls

law of conservation of energy—the total amount of energy in a system never changes, although it might be in a different form from which it started

luminance—the brightness of the color Doppler image

mm Hg—millimeters of mercury; unit of pressure

noise—low-level echoes on the display that do not contribute to useful diagnostic information

nondirectional Doppler—a Doppler device that cannot differentiate between positive and negative frequency shifts

nonhemodynamically significant stenosis—a stenosis that has not reached a critical threshold for volume flow or pressure distal to the stenosis.

Nyquist limit—the maximum frequency shift sampled without aliasing; equal to one-half of the pulse repetition frequency

Ohm's law—a law used in electronics in which flow (current, I) is equal to the pressure difference (Volts, V) divided by resistance (R)

oscillator—the component of a continuous-wave Doppler device that produces the voltage that drives the piezoelectric elements

packet size—the number of pulses per scan line; also called ensemble length

persistence—the averaging of color frames in order to display blood flow with a low signal-to-noise ratio

phase quadrature—the component of the Doppler device that determines positive opposed to negative frequency shifts and, therefore, the direction of blood flow

phasicity—in arteries, the phasicity describes the shape of the waveform based on the resistiveness of the distal bed (eg, multiphasic and monophasic); in veins, phasicity describes the flow pattern that results from respiratory variation (eg, respiratory phasicity or respirophasicity)

plug flow—the flow profile represented by blood flowing at the same velocity

Poiseuille's law—the law that describes the relationship between the resistance, pressure, and flow

potential energy—pressure energy created by the beating heart

power Doppler—a Doppler mode in which the signal is determined by the amplitude (strength) of the shift, not the shift itself; amplitude is directly proportional to the number of red blood cells; also referred to as amplitude Doppler

pressure difference—the difference between pressures at two points of a blood vessel

pulsatility—blood that flows in a pattern representative of the beating heart, with increases and decreases in pressure and blood flow velocity

pulsatility index—Doppler measurement used to determine how pulsatile a vessel is over time

pulse repetition frequency—the number of pulses of sound produced in 1 s

pulsed-wave Doppler—the Doppler technique that uses pulses of sound to obtain Doppler signals from a user-specified depth

RABT—color scale set so that red is away from the transducer (negative Doppler shift) and blue is toward the transducer (positive Doppler shift)

range gate—the gate placed by the operator in the region where Doppler sampling is desired; used with pulsed-wave Doppler

range resolution—the ability to determine the depth of echoes by timing how long it takes for the echoes to go from the transducer to the reflector and back; utilized by pulsed-wave devices

Rayleigh scatterers—very small reflectors, like red blood cells

resistance—the downstream impedance to flow determined by vessel length, vessel radius, and viscosity of blood

resistive index—Doppler measurement used to quantitate the resistiveness of the distal bed

respirophasic flow—the characteristic waveform of peripheral veins; flow is determined by respiratory variations as a result of intrathoracic pressure changes (also called *respiratory phasicity*)

Reynolds number—the formula used to quantitate the presence of turbulence; Reynolds numbers greater than 2000 typically indicate turbulence

sample volume—the area within the range gate where the Doppler signals are obtained

saturation—the amount of white added to a hue; the more white is there, the less saturated the color

scale—the spectral Doppler and color Doppler tool that controls the number of pulses transmitted per second to obtain the Doppler information; also known as pulse repetition frequency in spectral Doppler and color Doppler

speckle tracking—the method used to obtain the strain information

spectral broadening—the filling of the spectral window

spectral window—the area underneath the envelope on the spectral display

stenosis—pathologic narrowing of a blood vessel

strain—the changing of the shape of the muscle as it lengthens and contracts

sweep speed—the operator-adjustable spectral Doppler control that increases or decreases the number of heartbeats visualized on the spectral display

systole—the time period of the cardiac cycle when the ventricles of the heart are contracting

tardus parvus—an arterial waveform shape with a delayed peak systolic upstroke that indicates proximal obstruction (also called *parvus et tardus* and, more recently, *dampened*)

thrombus—combination of platelets, red blood cells, and fibrin that make up a blood clot

tissue Doppler imaging—the color Doppler imaging technique using a low-pass filter to document wall motion and eliminate the signal from flowing blood

transmural pressure—the difference in pressure inside a vessel compared with the pressure outside of the vessel

triplex—the ability to visualize real-time grayscale, color Doppler, and spectral Doppler simultaneously

tunica adventitia—the outer layer of a blood vessel

tunica intima—the inner layer of a blood vessel that is closest to the flowing blood

tunica media—the middle, muscular layer of a blood vessel

turbulent flow—chaotic, disorderly flow of blood cells in which they may move in any direction.

variance mode—the color Doppler scale with mean velocities displayed vertically on the scale in shades of red or blue, and turbulence displayed horizontally in green

vasa vasorum—a network of small blood vessels that supply blood to the walls of arteries and veins

vasoconstriction—the narrowing of a blood vessel caused by the contraction of the vessel wall

vasodilatation—the widening of a blood vessel caused by the relaxation of the vessel wall

velocity mode—the color Doppler scale with mean velocities displayed vertically

viscous energy—the energy loss caused by friction

volume flow—the volume of blood per unit time; typically measured in liter per minute or milliliter per second; represented by the symbol Q

wall filter—the operator control that eliminates low-frequency, high-amplitude signals caused by wall or valve motion; also called the high-pass filter

***z*-axis**—the brightness, or amplitude, of the dots on a B-mode display; the brighter the dots of the spectral waveform, the more red blood cells that make up the signal

zero-flow baseline—*see* the key term "baseline"

HEMODYNAMICS

Pressure Energy

> **SOUND OFF**
> A pressure difference (ΔP, or $P_1 - P_2$) is needed for flow to move through a blood vessel. Without a pressure difference, there is no flow.

Hemodynamics is the study of blood flow through the blood vessels of the body.

It is because of a difference in fluid energy that there is flow through a blood vessel. This difference in fluid energy is called a **pressure difference** (ΔP, or $P_1 - P_2$), and without a difference in pressures between two points, there cannot be blood flow. The pressure difference is the energy at the beginning of the vessel, P_1, minus the energy at the end of the vessel, P_2.

Pressure energy is the driving force of the blood through the blood vessels. It is the pumping of the heart that provides the necessary **potential energy** (in the form of blood pressure) at the beginning of the system. Subsequently, this potential energy is converted into **kinetic energy** in the form of flowing blood (velocity) within the blood vessels (Table 4-1). **Hydrostatic pressure** describes the relationship between gravity, the density of the blood, and the distance between an arbitrary reference point, which is usually the heart (Table 4-2).

TABLE 4-1 Kinetic energy

Formula
Kinetic energy $= \frac{1}{2}\rho v^2$
Kinetic energy is equal to one half of the product of the density (ρ) and the velocity (v) of the blood squared.

TABLE 4-2 Hydrostatic pressure

Formula
$P = \rho g h$
Hydrostatic pressure (P) is equal to the product of the height (h) of the column of blood, the density (ρ) of the blood, and gravity (g).

> **SOUND OFF**
> In a normal blood vessel, there must be the same total energy at the end of a vessel as there is at the beginning. Though the type of energy may vary, the total (net) energy in a system never changes.

As blood flows through a vessel, it loses energy in different forms. **Viscous energy** (aka viscosity) is a form of energy loss. Viscous energy is produced when kinetic energy is converted to heat as a result of **friction**. Blood also undergoes inertial losses, which occur when blood vessels divide, forcing the blood flow to change the direction. **Inertia**, which is resistance to acceleration, is described by Newton's first law that states that an object at rest stays at rest and an object in motion stays in motion, unless acted upon by an outside force. As the ventricles contract and relax, there is a changing pressure wave in the arteries, and inertia is resistance to that change (Table 4-3).

TABLE 4-3 Energy terms related to hemodynamics and their description

Terms	Description
Potential energy	In the cardiovascular system, the potential energy is created by contraction of the heart. Also referred to as pressure energy and is equivalent to blood pressure.
Kinetic energy	Energy created by flowing blood. The potential energy is converted to kinetic energy minus the energy lost because of friction. This is equivalent to velocity.
Hydrostatic pressure	Energy that is created because of gravity. In the cardiovascular system, it is the weight of a column of blood. The heaviest pressure is at the bottom of the column because it must support the weight of blood superior to it.
Viscous energy	Energy lost as a result of friction, which occurs when structures rub against each other, and heat is created.
Inertial losses	Energy lost because of acceleration in a pulsatile system.

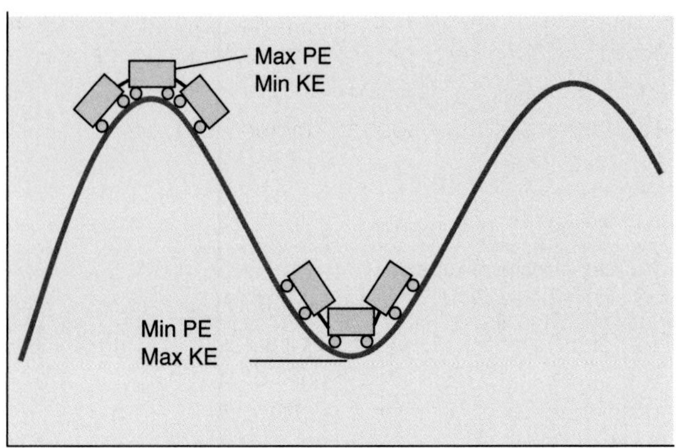

Figure 4-1 Conservation of energy. With a roller coaster, the potential and kinetic energy are transformed from one form to the other with no loss of energy. Potential energy is maximum when the roller coaster is farthest from the ground, at the same time the kinetic energy is at its minimum. As the roller coaster descends the track, it gains speed, increasing its kinetic energy, whereas it is losing potential energy as it moves closer to the ground.

It is important to note that the total energy in a system never changes (the **law of conservation of energy**). That is to say, there must be the same total energy at the end of a vessel as there is at the beginning. However, the types of energy may be different between the two points. The potential energy in a vascular system is in the form of blood pressure, from the left ventricle of the heart. The potential energy is converted into kinetic energy in the form of blood flow, the velocity of the blood. As blood flows, energy losses occur in the form of friction, causing heat to be produced. The kinetic energy plus the heat energy is equal to the potential energy that was initially found at the beginning of the system (Figure 4-1).

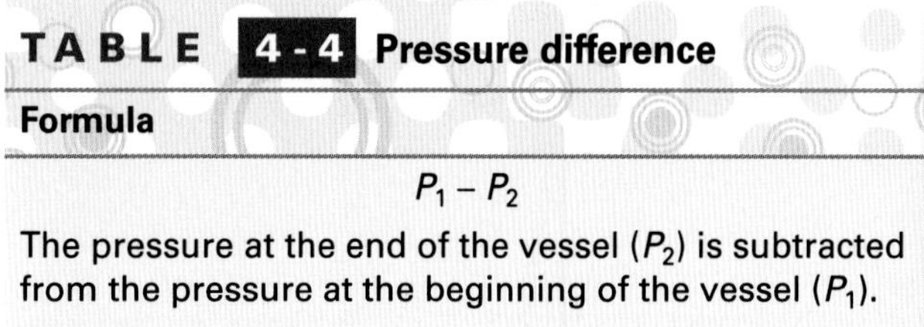

TABLE 4-4 Pressure difference

Formula
$P_1 - P_2$
The pressure at the end of the vessel (P_2) is subtracted from the pressure at the beginning of the vessel (P_1).

Pressure Difference

Flow (Q) is the volume of blood moving through a vessel per unit time. In order for there to be flow, there must be a higher pressure at one end of a blood vessel and a lower pressure at the other end. This variance in pressure is referred to as a **pressure difference** (ΔP, or $P_1 - P_2$) (Table 4-4). The amount of flow in a blood vessel is directly proportional to the pressure difference. Therefore, the bigger the difference in pressures, the more flow that occurs (Figure 4-2).

SOUND OFF
In order for there to be flow, there must be a higher pressure at one end of a blood vessel and a lower pressure at the other end. This variance in pressure is referred to as the pressure difference.

The systemic circulation begins with the left ventricle of the heart to the aorta and from the aorta to the arteries of the body. The arteries become arterioles, the vessels responsible for **vasoconstriction** and

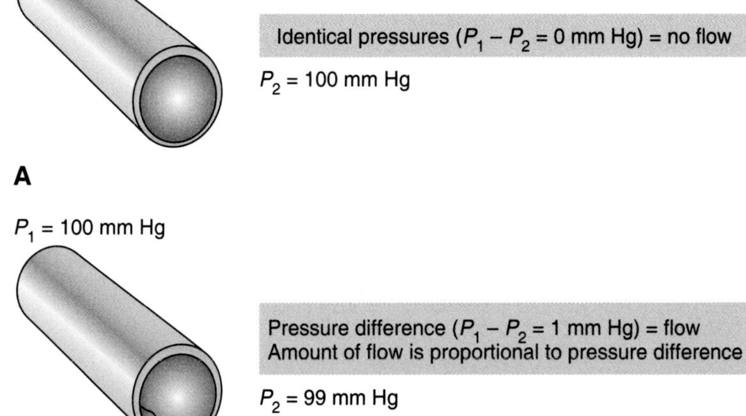

Figure 4-2 Pressure difference. In image **(A)** the pressure is the same at the beginning of the vessel (P_1 = 100 mm Hg) and at the end (P_2 = 100 mm Hg). Therefore, there is no pressure difference and therefore no flow. Image **(B)** depicts a pressure difference in which there is higher pressure at the beginning (P_1 = 100 mm Hg) than at the end of the vessel (P_2 = 99 mm Hg). Therefore, there is flow within the vessel.

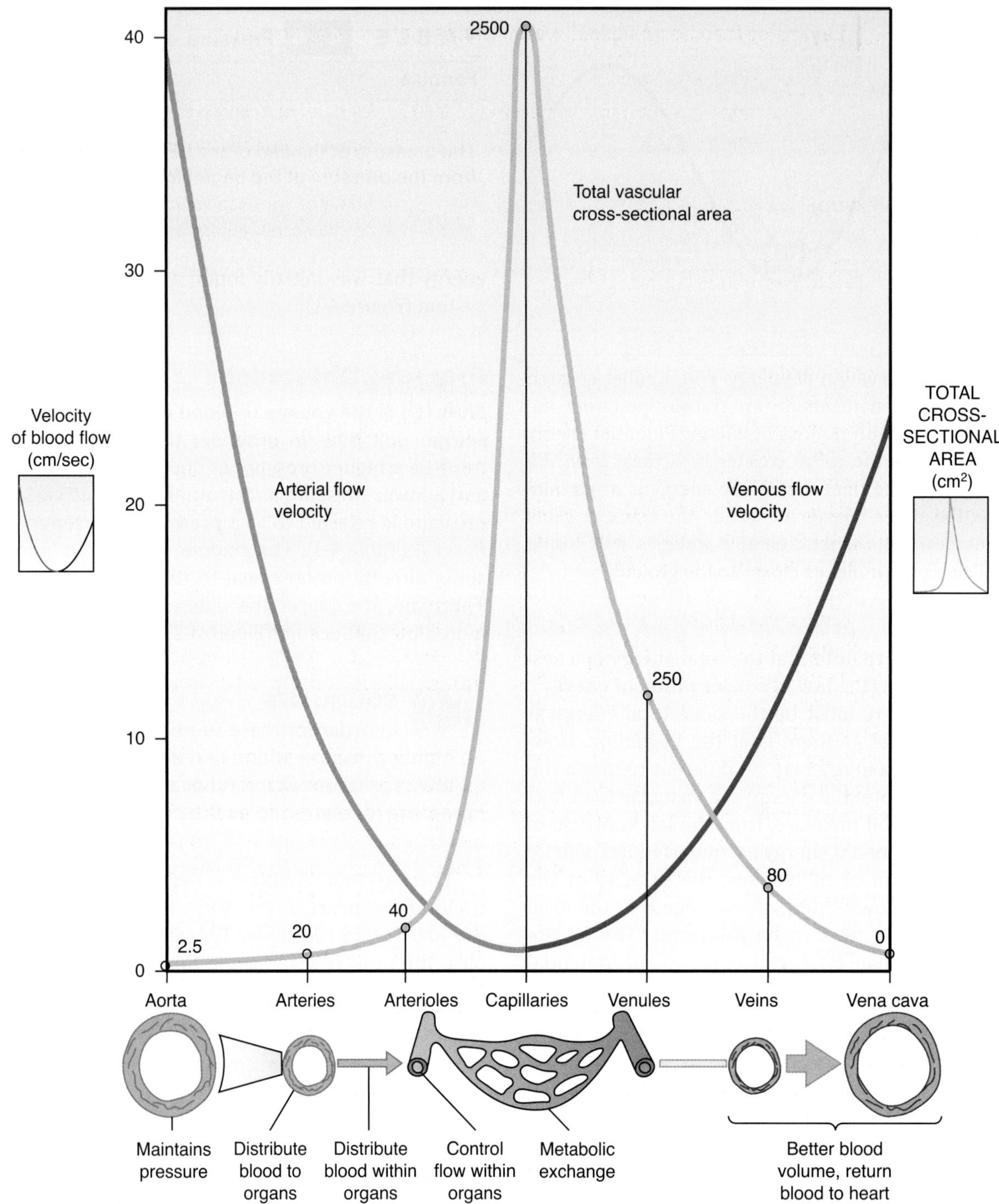

Figure 4-3 Relationship between area and velocity throughout the blood vessels of the body.

vasodilatation in the body. The arterioles lead to the vast network of tiny capillaries, where nutrient and waste exchange occur. From the capillaries, the blood flows into the larger venules and then into the even larger veins (Figure 4-3). The venous part of the systemic circulation is known for its **capacitance**, as approximately two-thirds of the blood is stored in the veins. The veins drain into the inferior vena cava or superior vena cava, both of which empty into the right atrium.

Blood Vessels and Blood Flow

Structure of Blood Vessels

SOUND OFF
It is the tunica media that differs dramatically between veins and arteries. The tunica media is typically much thicker in arteries.

TABLE 4-5 Layers of the blood vessel walls, their location, and structure

Layer	Location	Structure
Tunica intima	Inner layer (closest to passing blood)	Made of endothelium
Tunica media	Middle layer	Made of smooth muscle and elastic tissue. Thinner in veins, thicker in arteries.
Tunica adventitia (externa)	Outermost layer	Made of connective tissue and has its own blood supply via the vasa vasorum

Blood vessels are made up of muscle that enables them to expand or contract as needed. The walls of the arteries and veins are similar in that they consist of the same layers. Both arteries and veins have a **tunica intima**, **tunica media**, and **tunica adventitia** (Table 4-5). The inner layer of the vessel, a layer of endothelial cells closest to the flowing blood, is the tunica intima. The outer layer is referred to as the tunica adventitia or externa. This layer requires its own blood supply to function properly. The **vasa vasorum**, a small network of blood vessels, accomplishes this task. Between the intima and adventitia is the middle muscular layer, the tunica media. It is this layer of muscle and elastic tissue that differs dramatically between veins and arteries. As blood travels through the cardiovascular system, the arteries and veins experience differences in pressure. Arteries are unique in that they experience a pressure wave as blood is pumped from the heart. One can feel this pressure wave as a "pulse" within the arteries as the heart beats. It is because of this pressure that arteries typically have a much thicker tunica media compared with that of veins (Figure 4-4).

Types of Blood Flow

Three types of flow are found in blood vessels: **plug flow**, **laminar flow**, and **turbulent (or chaotic) flow**. Plug flow can be found in large blood vessels such as the ascending aorta and at the entrance of vessels such as the common carotid artery (CCA) (Figure 4-5). The velocity profile of plug flow is blunt as a result of the flow traveling at mostly the same velocity. With plug flow, the blood cells undergo minimal frictional losses at the vessel wall. Plug flow occurs as a result of the acceleration that occurs after **systole**. However, as the blood cells travel down the length of the vessels, friction causes the red blood cells closest to the vessel walls to decrease in velocity, whereas the fastest velocity is found at the center of the vessel. This velocity profile resembles more of a parabola or is said to have a parabolic shape (Figure 4-6). Although it is often said that *parabola* describes the shape of the flow profile, the definition for *parabolic flow* is a flow profile whose average velocity is 50% of the velocity at the center of the vessel.

SOUND OFF
Each successive layer extending from the boundary layer inward travels faster than the layer before it, with the fastest flow in the center of the vessel.

SOUND OFF
Turbulent flow does not always indicate the presence of disease. A Reynolds number greater than 2000 is considered to represent turbulence.

Laminar flow, in which the red blood cells travel in parallel, nonmixing layers, is the most common type of flow found in arteries. Laminar flow assumes that all red blood cells are parallel to the blood vessel walls. The red blood cells that are immediately adjacent to the intima of the vessel are stationary or near-stationary. This region is called the **boundary layer**. Each successive layer extending from the boundary layer inward travels faster than the layer external to it, with the fastest flow at the center of the vessel (Figure 4-7). A subcategory of laminar flow is disturbed flow. Disturbed flow is when the red blood cells are moving downstream, like laminar flow, but they are no longer parallel to the blood vessel wall because of a flow divider (a bifurcation), an obstruction (like plaque), etc. Figure 4-8 asks you to imagine traveling in a canoe down a docile river. Your canoe is parallel to the riverbanks, and you stay at the center of the river where the flow is fastest. This is representative of laminar flow. Disturbed flow is more like if there were a boulder on the side of the riverbank, you would steer the canoe around the obstruction. You are still moving downstream—it is not like you turned the canoe around and went upstream—but you are no longer parallel to the riverbank.

Turbulent, or chaotic, flow results when the red blood cells tumble in all different directions, resulting in a wide range of velocities (Figure 4-9). Going back to the canoe example, now you have turned the canoe upstream and sideways, and you started doing barrel

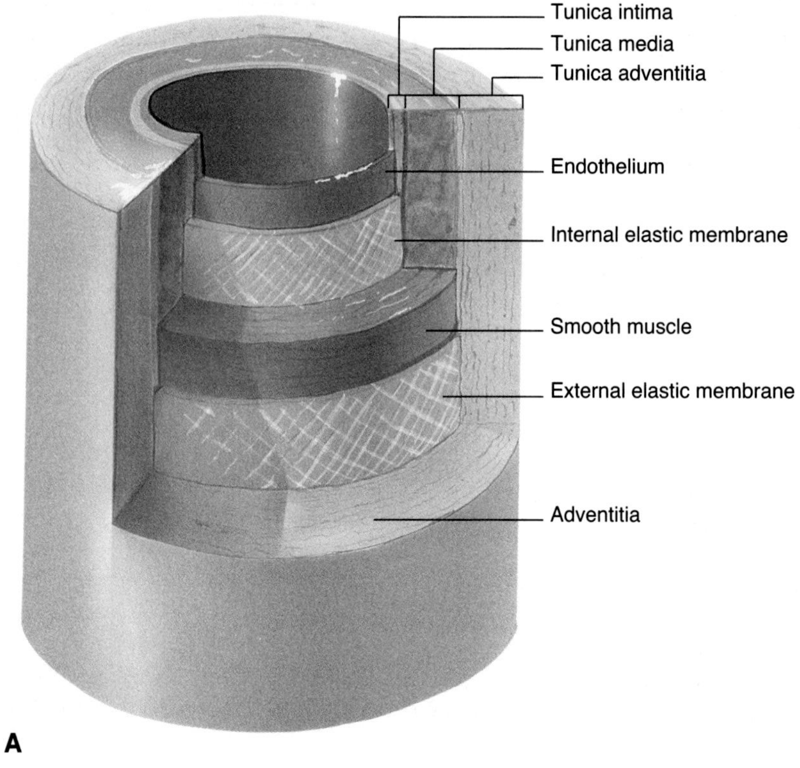

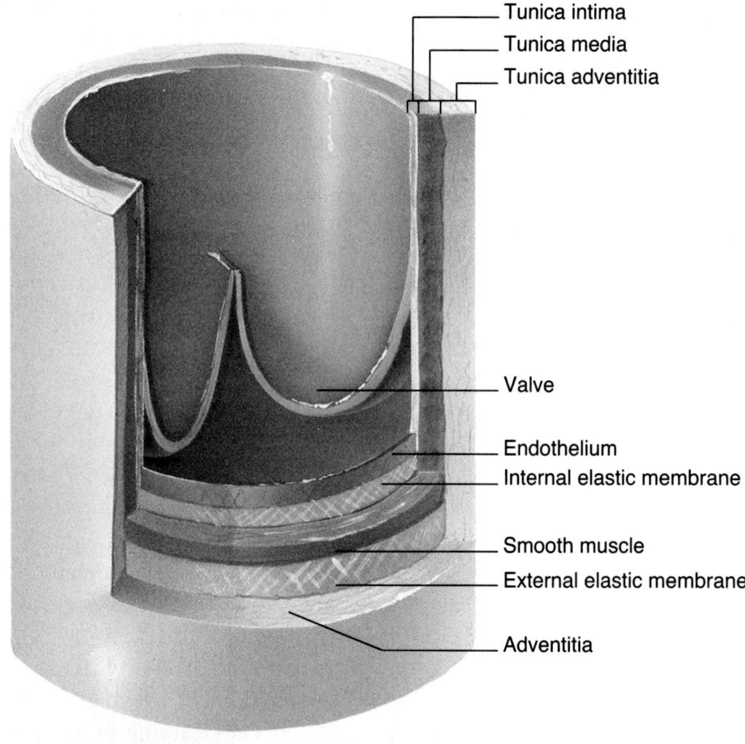

Figure 4-4 Blood vessel anatomy. Note the difference in the thickness of the tunica media between an artery **(A)** and a vein **(B)**. (Asset provided by Anatomical Chart Co.)

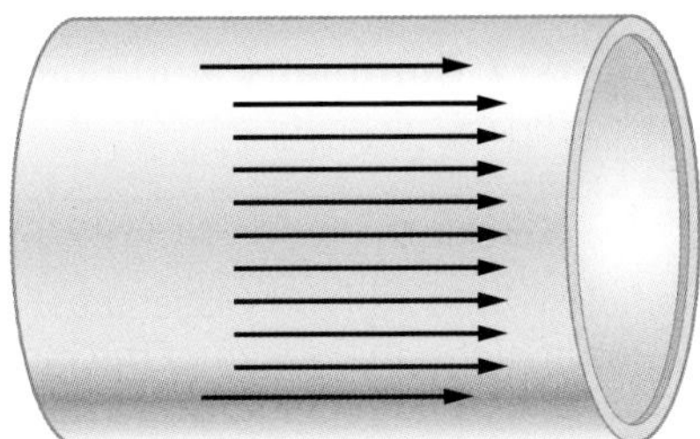

Figure 4-5 Plug flow. Plug flow is represented by blood that is mostly flowing at the same velocity (*arrows*). Plug flow occurs in large vessels and at the entrance of vessels.

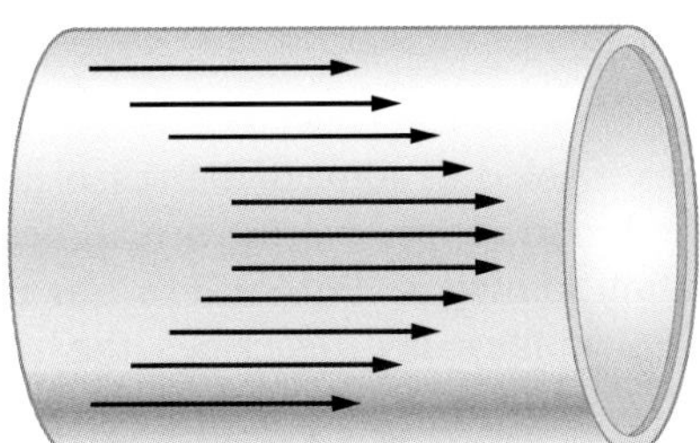

Figure 4-6 Laminar flow. Laminar flow is represented by blood that travels in nonmixing layers of different velocities, with the fastest flow in the center and the slowest flow near the vessel walls (*arrows*).

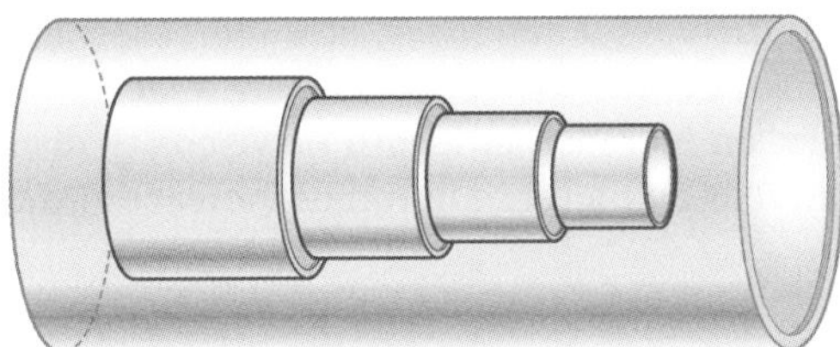

Figure 4-7 Layers in laminar flow. The layers of laminar flow are nonmixing concentric layers, with the fastest flow in the center and the slowest flow closest to the vessel walls.

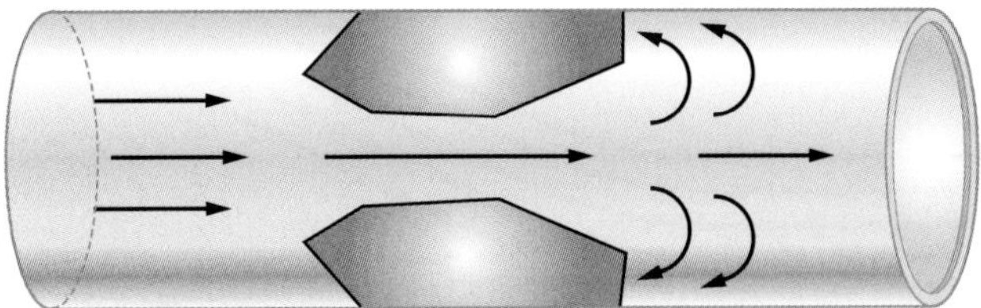

Figure 4-9 Turbulent flow and Reynolds number. Flow exiting an area of narrowing will demonstrate turbulence (*curved arrows*). Distal to the obstruction, the flow resumes its prestenotic flow pattern. Reynolds number is used to measure turbulence. Turbulence is present when Reynolds number is greater than 2000.

rolls. Although turbulent flow can indicate stenosis, turbulence alone does not always indicate the presence of disease. At some points in normal vessels, such as in the area of the carotid bulb (distal CCA), turbulence can be found (Figure 4-10). Turbulence may also occur normally from high-velocity flow and from tortuous or kinked vessels. The equation used to quantify the degree of turbulence in a blood vessel is the **Reynolds number** (Table 4-6). A Reynolds number greater than 2000 is considered to represent turbulence.

The Continuity Equation and Bernoulli's Principle

As blood flows through the body, it may encounter vessels that have a decreased area, possibly secondary to **stenosis** caused by **thrombus**. When blood flows through an area of decreased radius, the same volume of flow must travel through that area. The **continuity equation** describes the relationship between the vessel area, the velocity of blood, and the volume of blood flow. The volume flow within a blood vessel must be the same at all points along the length of the blood vessel (Table 4-7). Volume of blood flow (Q) is constant. Therefore, if the

A

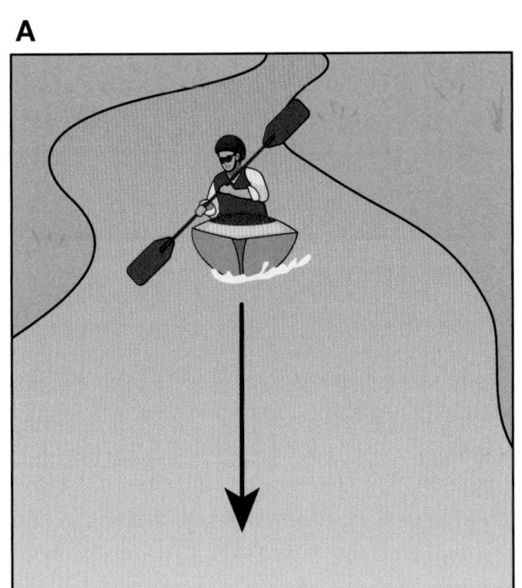

B

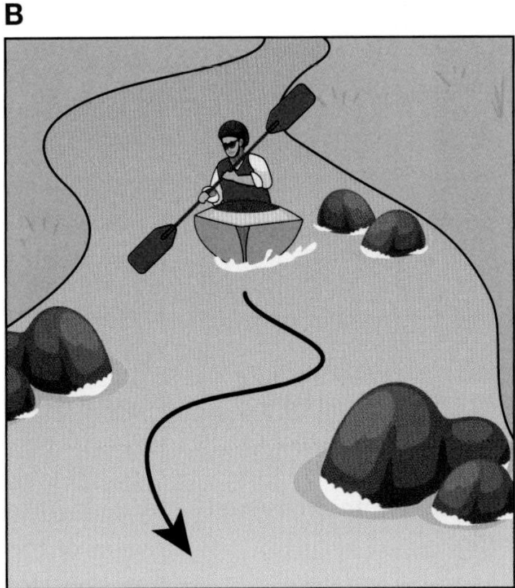

Figure 4-8 A. Laminar flow: A canoe is floating down the center of a stream. The canoe stays parallel to the shoreline. **B.** Disturbed flow: The canoe encounters a rock, causing the stream to change direction. The canoe is still floating downstream, but is no longer parallel to the shoreline. Notice the canoe is not turning backwards or turning in varying directions. That would be turbulence, or chaotic flow.

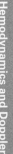

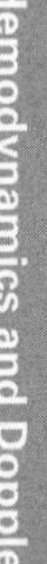

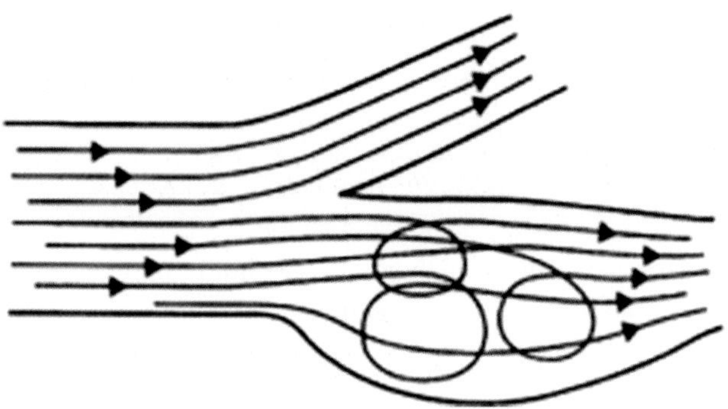

Figure 4-10 Flow stream separation. Some turbulence typically occurs at the bifurcation of blood vessels.

TABLE 4-7 Continuity equation
Formula
$Q = VA$
The volume flow within a blood vessel must be the same at any point along the length of the blood vessel. The continuity equation demonstrates the relationship between velocity (V) and area (A). Volume flow (Q) is equal to the product of velocity and area. In a nonhemodynamically significant stenosis, Q is a constant. If the area decreases, the velocity increases. Where the velocity increases, the pressure decreases.

area of the vessel decreases, as in the case of a stenosis, the velocity must increase (Figure 4-11). Putting a finger partially over the front of a garden hose demonstrates the continuity equation. The area at the outlet of the hose decreases when the finger partially covers the opening, so the velocity must increase in order to maintain the flow rate. **Bernoulli's principle** states that an increase in velocity must be accompanied by a corresponding decrease in pressure. This inverse relationship between pressure and velocity is linked to the law of conservation of energy. Subsequently, any increase in velocity is an increase in energy, and therefore the pressure must decrease to preserve the total energy (Figure 4-12). Assuming a **nonhemodynamically significant stenosis** (NHSS), once the vessel goes back to its prestenotic area, there is a decrease in velocity with a corresponding increase in pressure. Using the previous example of the water hose, although the water shooting out of the hose was at a higher velocity than it was preobstruction, at the point of the blockage, it was at a lower pressure. The simplified formula for Bernoulli's principle is provided in Table 4-8.

Poiseuille's Law

In addition to the pressure differential, there are other factors that may increase or decrease the amount of blood flowing through a blood vessel, including the length of the vessel, the radius of the vessel, and the viscosity of the blood. These factors are all tied together by an equation known as **Poiseuille's law** (Tables 4-9 and 4-10). Poiseuille's law describes the relationship between the volume of blood flow and the **resistance** to flow in a blood vessel. In its simplest form, Poiseuille's law states that flow is equal to the difference in pressure divided by the resistance to flow in the vessel (Figure 4-13). As stated by the formulas in Tables 4-9 and 4-10, if the length of the vessel or the viscosity of the blood (both of which contribute to resistance to flow) increases, there is decreased flow. Likewise, if the radius of the vessel increases, flow increases. In fact, if the radius doubles, flow increases by a factor of 16. In summary, an increase in length or viscosity decreases flow, whereas an increase in radius increases flow.

TABLE 4-6 Reynolds number
Formula
$Re = \frac{\nu^2 r \rho}{\eta}$
Reynolds number (Re) is defined as the product of the velocity of blood (ν), two times the radius (r) of the vessel, and the density (ρ) of the blood divided by the viscosity (η) of the blood. A vessel with a number over 2000 is considered to be turbulent.

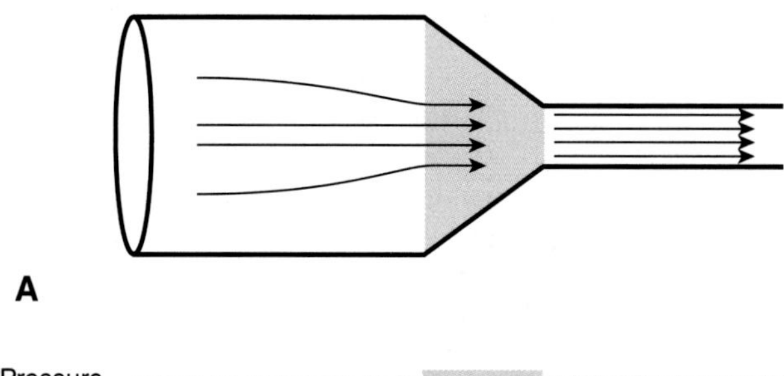

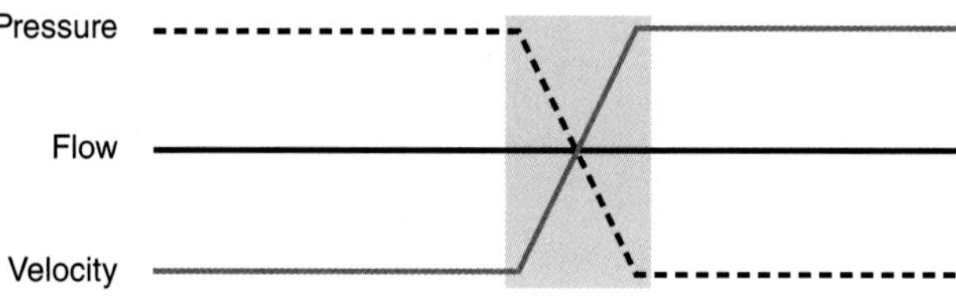

Figure 4-11 Continuity equation explains the relationship between area, pressure, and velocity. Blood flow *(arrow)* through a blood vessel **(A)**. There is an increase in velocity and a decrease in pressure as the area decreases in the region of the narrowing of the vessel **(B)**. The volume of flow does not change.

Hemodynamics and Doppler

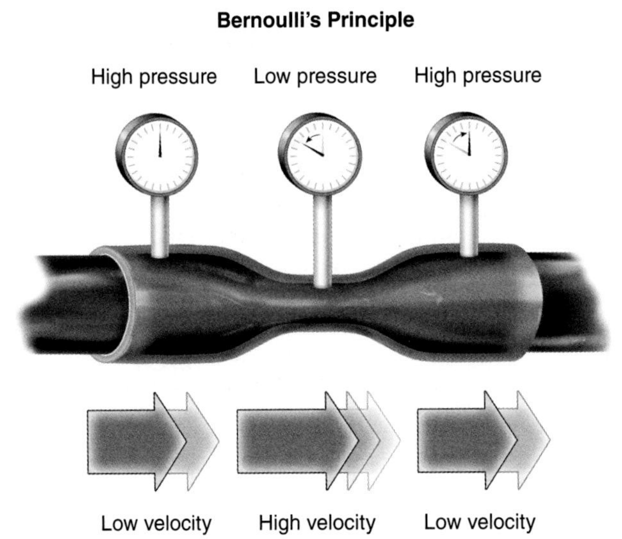

Bernoulli's Principle

High pressure Low pressure High pressure

Low velocity High velocity Low velocity

Figure 4-12 Bernoulli's principle. In the area of blood vessel that is suffering from a stenosis or decrease in area, the blood velocity increases, whereas the pressure decreases.

TABLE 4-8 Simplified Bernoulli's principle

Formula
$\Delta P = 4\nu^2$
ΔP (change in pressure) represents the pressure difference ($P_1 - P_2$) and ν is the velocity of the blood through a stenosis.

TABLE 4-9 Poiseuille's law (short form)

Formula
$Q = \frac{\Delta P}{R}$, where $R = \frac{8L\eta}{\pi r^4}$
Flow (Q) is equal to the difference in pressure (ΔP) divided by the resistance (R) to flow in the vessel. R is the resistance and L is the length of the vessel. The η in the equation represents the viscosity of the blood and r is the radius of the vessel.

TABLE 4-10 Poiseuille's law (long form)

Formula
$Q = \frac{\Delta P \pi r^4}{8L\eta}$
Combination of the two previous equations into one equation. (See Table 4-9 for explanation of abbreviations.)

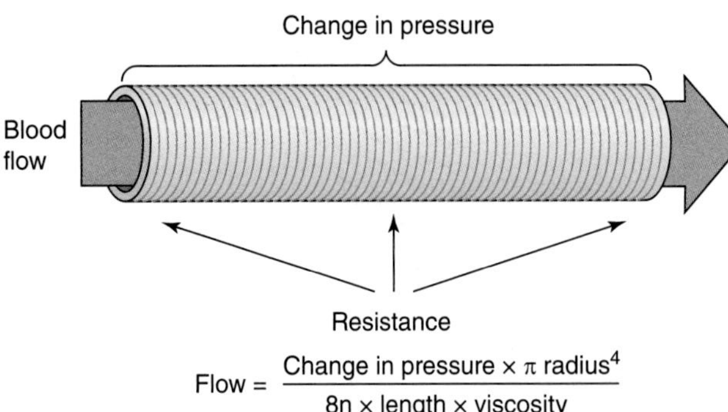

Figure 4-13 Poiseuille's law. Increasing the pressure difference between the two ends of a blood vessel increases flow. Flow diminishes as resistance increases. Resistance is directly proportional to blood viscosity and the length of the vessel and inversely proportional to the fourth power of the radius.

SOUND OFF
An increase in length or viscosity decreases flow, whereas an increase in radius increases flow.

Inertial losses occur as vessels branch and change direction. Friction, another form of resistance, is the loss of energy in the form of heat and is another impediment to flow. As the arterioles branch out into capillaries, frictional and inertial losses are responsible for the accompanying decrease in the velocity of the blood. The capillaries are tiny, typically about the width of a red blood cell. It is the small size of the capillaries that contributes to the energy loss and slow velocity of flow. However, capillaries require slow flow in order to perform their primary function, which is the exchange of nutrients and waste products.

Poiseuille's law assumes a straight (noncurved), rigid (nonelastic) pipe with a steady flow rate (nonpulsatile). Unfortunately, this does not describe the blood vessels found in the human body. Although there is no simple way to describe the cardiovascular system, Poiseuille's law demonstrates the relationships between flow and resistance. Poiseuille's law is analogous to **Ohm's law**, a principle in electronics in which flow is equal to the pressure differential divided by resistance (Table 4-11 and Figure 4-14).

SOUND OFF
A cross-sectional area loss of 60% to 75% is generally considered to be hemodynamically significant, though this percentage varies among organ systems. It is important to remember that a 75% decrease in area corresponds to a 50% decrease in diameter.

TABLE 4-11 Ohm's law

Formula
$I = \frac{V}{R}$
$Q = \frac{P}{R}$
Ohm's law is a principle in electronics (equation on the left) in which flow (*I*, or current) is equal to the pressure differential (*V*, or voltage) divided by resistance (*R*). For the vascular system (equation on the bottom), blood flow (*Q*) is equal to the pressure difference (*P*) divided by the resistance (*R*).

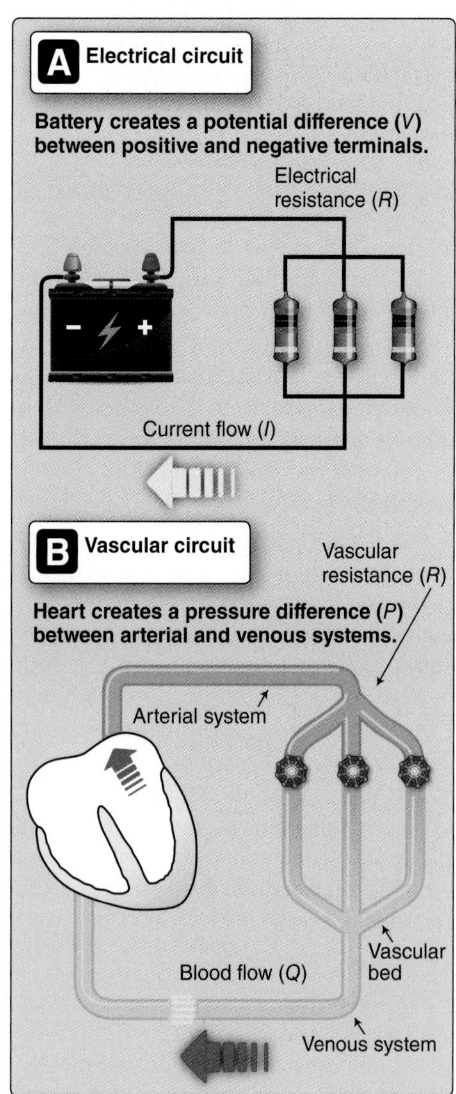

Figure 4-14 Ohm's law. Though Ohm's law is a principle of electronics, the relationship between blood flow (*Q*), pressure (*P*), and resistance (*R*) to flow can be expressed as a variation of Ohm's law.

SOUND OFF
The innervated arteriole walls can constrict or dilate in response to signals from the brain to either increase or decrease flow distally.

SOUND OFF
It is more detrimental to have more than one stenosis in a vessel than a single substantial stenosis. Thus, multiple nonhemodynamically significant stenoses can create a hemodynamically significant stenosis.

Resistance and Stenotic Flow

The theorems provided by Bernoulli and Poiseuille describe the changes in energy and blood flow that occur as blood travels. It has been previously described that flow is a constant and does not change. In other words, the heart continues to beat and pump the same volume of blood regardless of the presence of a stenosis downstream. However, there can be a stenosis so severe that it compromises flow to a certain part of the body. A **critical stenosis**, also referred to as a **hemodynamically significant stenosis**, is one in which there is decreased distal flow or pressure. A critical stenosis leads to a significant pressure difference after the stenosis (aka poststenosis). A cross-sectional area loss of 75% is generally considered to be hemodynamically significant, though this percentage may vary among vessels. It is important to remember that a 75% decrease in area corresponds to a 50% decrease in diameter. Though spectral Doppler will be discussed on page 112, Figure 4-15 demonstrates the spectral changes in the presence of a hemodynamically significant stenosis (Figure 4-15).

Blood vessels may be connected end to end (in series) or flow into multiple parallel channels (in parallel) (Figure 4-16). The **effective resistance**, the resistance of the distal bed, is the sum of the individual resistances when multiple vessels are connected in series (Table 4-12). When vessels are connected in parallel, the effective resistance is reduced, as there are more channels or paths for flow to exploit (Table 4-13 and Figure 4-17). Arterioles, because of their muscular walls, are the main contributors to the resistance in the cardiovascular system. The **innervated** arteriole walls can constrict or dilate in response to signals from the brain to either increase or decrease flow distally.

SOUND OFF
Remember that multiple vessels in parallel offer less total resistance to flow. In the body, if a major artery is blocked, it becomes the path of highest resistance; thus, the blood will choose collateral vessels because they become the path of least resistance.

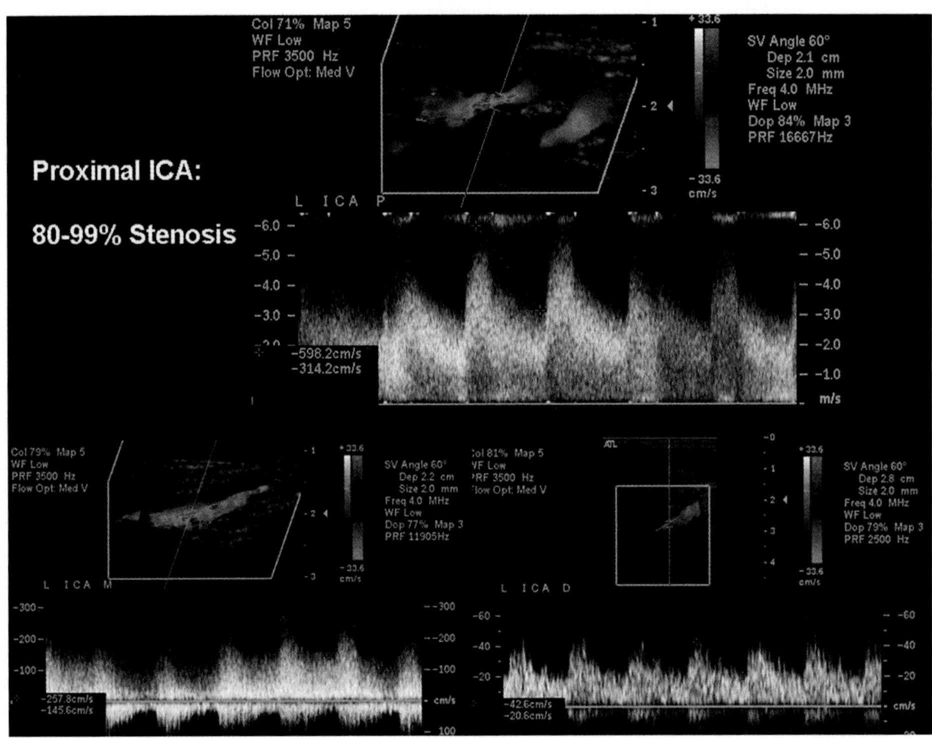

Figure 4-15 Duplex of a hemodynamically significant stenosis. A stenosis of 80% to 99% of the ICA with poststenotic turbulence.

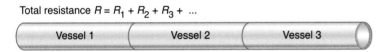

Total resistance $R = R_1 + R_2 + R_3 + \ldots$

Vessel 1 Vessel 2 Vessel 3

A

Total resistance $R = \frac{1}{R_1} + \frac{1}{R_2} + \frac{1}{R_3} + \ldots$

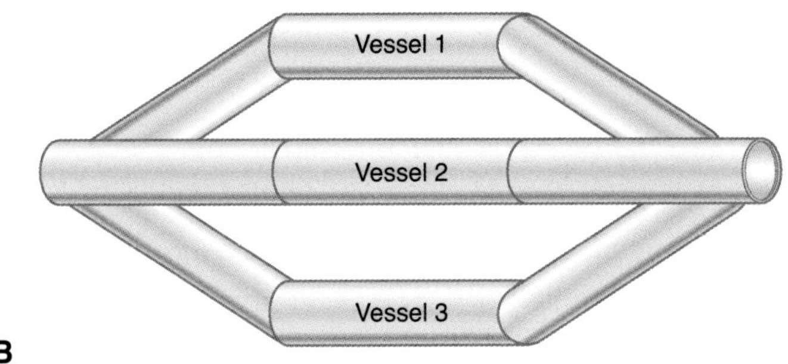

B

Figure 4-16 Vessel arrangement and effective resistance. Blood vessels may be connected end to end **(A)** or flow into multiple parallel channels **(B)**. The effective resistance, the resistance of the distal bed, is the sum of the individual resistances when multiple vessels are connected in series **(A)**. The equation that represents vessels in series is: $R = R_1 + R_2 + R_3 \uparrow$. When vessels are connected in parallel **(B)**, the effective resistance is reduced, as there are more channels or paths for the flow to go, or $R + 1/R_1 + 1/R_2 + 1/R_3 \uparrow$.

TABLE 4-12 Vessels in series

Formula
$R = R_1 + R_2 + R_3 + \uparrow$
The effective resistance (R), the resistance of the distal bed, is the sum of the individual resistances when multiple vessels are connected in series.

TABLE 4-13 Vessels in parallel

Formula
$R = 1/R_1 + 1/R_2 + 1/R_3 + \uparrow$
The effective resistance (R) is reduced, as there are more channels or paths for blood to access.

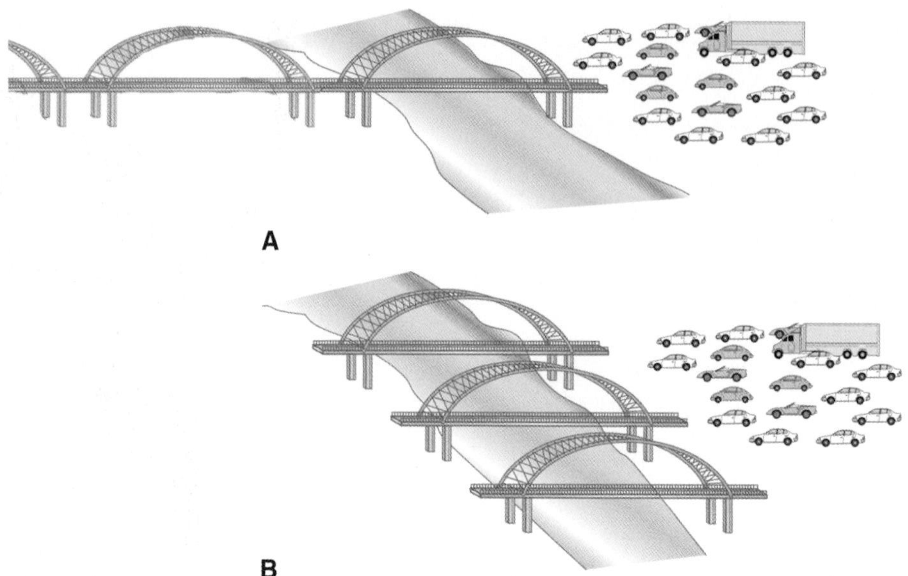

Figure 4-17 Example of effective resistance. A simple comparison for in-series and in-parallel vessels is that of trying to leave an island that has only one long bridge. When many cars are trying to leave the island at the same time on one long bridge "in series," the resistance to the flow of traffic is high **(A)**. When more bridges are opened **(B)**, the cars are able to travel out of the city quite rapidly "in-parallel," because there is little or low resistance to the flow of traffic.

At the region of an NHSS, the velocity of the blood cells must increase in order to maintain the same volume flow. The region of increased velocity is accompanied by a decrease in pressure through this region, as described by Bernoulli's principle. As the blood exits the region of narrowing and enters a suddenly expanded vessel, there is turbulence as the blood exists the stenosis. This turbulence eventually dissipates, and downstream the flow returns to its previous prestenotic state. Although there may be a small amount of energy loss in the region of turbulence, in an NHSS, there is not a significant drop in volume flow or pressure distally. Important to remember is that with a stenosis, it is more detrimental to have more than one stenosis in a vessel than a single substantial lesion. This is true because there is more energy loss with two stenoses in series. This concept relates to what happens with vessels connected in a series, in which the total resistance is the sum of the segmental resistances. Because a decrease in radius causes increased resistance to flow, there is an increase in total resistance when there is more than one stenosis in a vessel. Therefore, it is possible that multiple nonhemodynamically significant lesions will act as a critical lesion.

Blood will always follow the path of least resistance. This concept is like the mapping software on a cellphone—if a major highway is blocked because of a car accident, the mapping software will direct drivers to exit the highway before the accident and drive through side streets, eventually rejoining the highway past the accident location. In the body, if a major artery is blocked, it becomes the path of highest resistance, whereas the **collateral blood vessels** become the path of least resistance. These collaterals will dilate to allow more flow, decreasing the resistance. It was mentioned previously that multiple vessels in parallel offer less total resistance to flow. This is what happens with collaterals. The higher pressure at the level of a stenosis causes the collateral vessel to open up, and the blood follows the lower-resistance path. Distal to the stenosis, the collateral vessel eventually rejoins the main artery. In chronic disease, if the collateral network is extensive enough, the net flow distal to the stenosis may actually be normal (Figure 4-18). Collaterals are formed over time and in response to chronic change. They are typically not found in the presence of an acute obstruction.

> **SOUND OFF**
> The farther from the heart, the more weight there is to support. Therefore, in someone who is standing, the highest hydrostatic pressures are located at body parts closest to the ground, such as the feet and ankles.

Venous Hemodynamics and Hydrostatic Pressure

As blood leaves the capillaries, it enters the larger venules. The veins that are located between the capillaries and the right atrium of the heart get progressively wider, thus offering lower resistance to flow. The pressure in the venules is very low, about 15 millimeters of mercury **(mm Hg)**, but still higher than the pressure in the right atrium, which is typically 0 to 8 mm Hg. Assuming that the person is supine, this small, but still significant

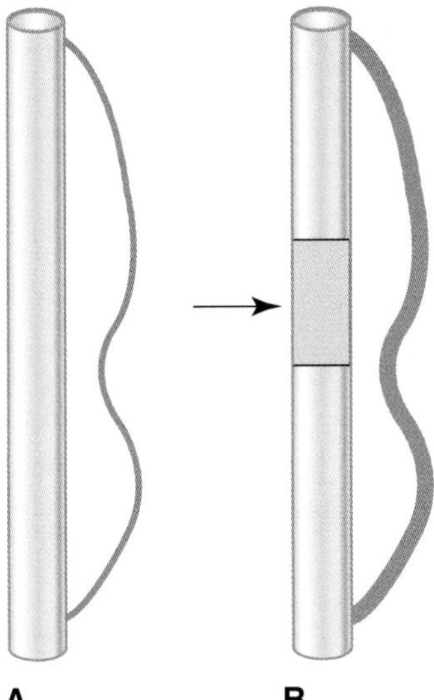

Figure 4-18 Collateral flow. **A.** In the presence of normal unobstructed flow, a collateral is a relatively high pressure vessel because of its small radius, whereas the larger vessel provides the normal low-pressure pathway. **B.** In the presence of an obstruction (*arrow*), the larger vessel becomes the high-resistance pathway. The increased pressure causes the collateral to dilate, thereby increasing its radius and decreasing its pressure. The collateral becomes the path of least resistance.

difference in pressure is a pressure difference, and, therefore, there exists forward flow (toward the heart).

When someone is in the standing position, gravity acts on the blood in the form of hydrostatic pressure. As mentioned in the "Hemodynamics" section, hydrostatic pressure is the weight of a column of fluid relative to a reference point. In humans, that reference point—the point at which the hydrostatic pressure is zero—is the heart. Below the heart, the weight of this column of blood increases with the distance from the heart (Figure 4-19). Blood in a vertical tube acts in the same way, that is, the farther from the heart, the more weight is there to support. Therefore, when erect, the highest hydrostatic pressures are located at more distal parts of the body, such as the feet and ankles. Hydrostatic pressure is the reason that venous stasis ulcers are found at the ankles and not on the thighs.

Recall that hydrostatic pressure can be calculated by using the density of the blood, gravity, and the height of the measuring point, or the distance from the heart (Table 4-2). Note in the formula that height is the only variable; the rest are constants. If the point at which you are measuring is below the heart, the hydrostatic pressure increases and will be a positive number. Conversely, if a point is measured above the heart, such as an outstretched arm over the head, the hydrostatic pressure will decrease and will be a negative number (Figure 4-20). It should be noted that the hydrostatic pressure above the arm could be said to be zero. When

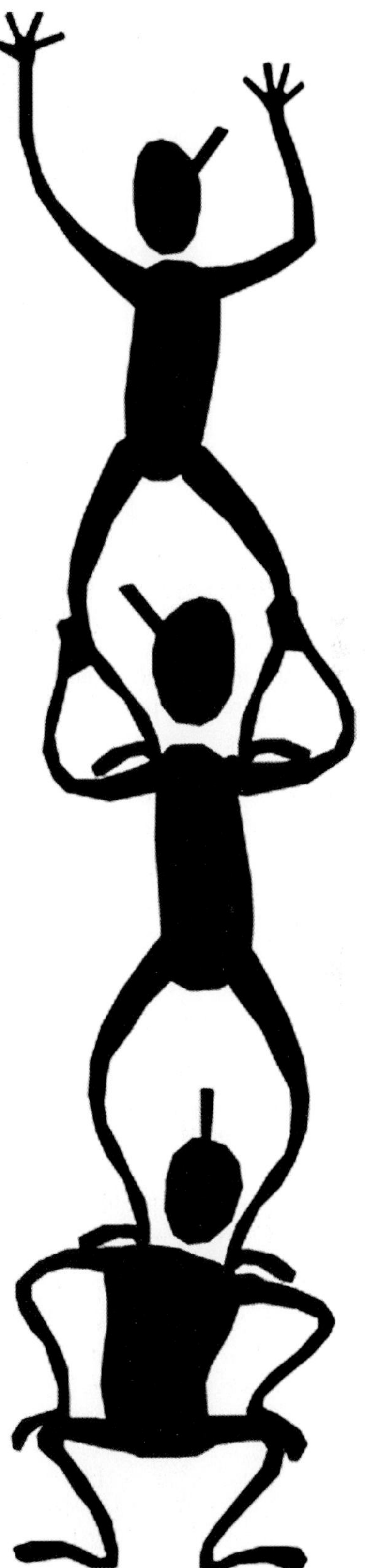

Figure 4-19 Hydrostatic pressure. This image demonstrates the effect of hydrostatic pressure. When three people are standing on each other's shoulders, the person at the bottom has to support the most weight, whereas the person at the top has it relatively easy.

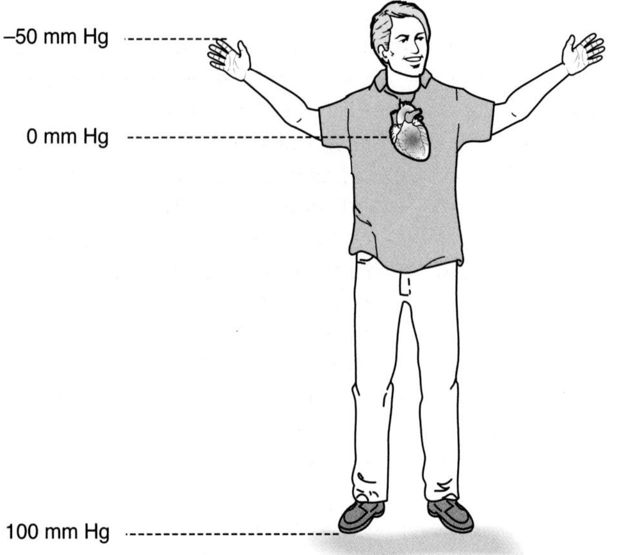

Figure 4-20 Hydrostatic pressure and the heart. If the point that you are measuring is below the heart, the hydrostatic pressure will be positive. Conversely, if a point is measured above the heart, such as an outstretched arm over the head, the hydrostatic pressure will be negative.

an arm is raised over the head, blood drains out of the veins in the arm because of gravity. The veins collapse, and the hydrostatic pressure in the veins is minimal (Figure 4-21). However, most authors state that above the heart, the hydrostatic pressure is negative.

TABLE 4-14 Mechanism of venous return to the heart

Mechanism	Explanation
Pressure difference	There is a small pressure difference between the venules and the right atrium of the heart.
Venous valves	Functional venous valves keep the blood flowing in the proper direction: toward the heart.
Calf muscle pump	Contraction of the calf muscles propels blood from the soleal veins in the calf toward the heart.
Intrathoracic pressure changes	Inspiration and expiration change the intrathoracic pressure, causing venous flow into the heart

Appropriate venous return to the heart requires several mechanisms to work properly (Table 4-14). First, as mentioned in the "Hemodynamics" section, a pressure difference exists between the venules and the right atrium. Second, there are intrathoracic pressure changes. With deep inspiration, flow ceases below the diaphragm, whereas blood above the diaphragm empties into the thorax. With exhalation, the blood flow enters the chest

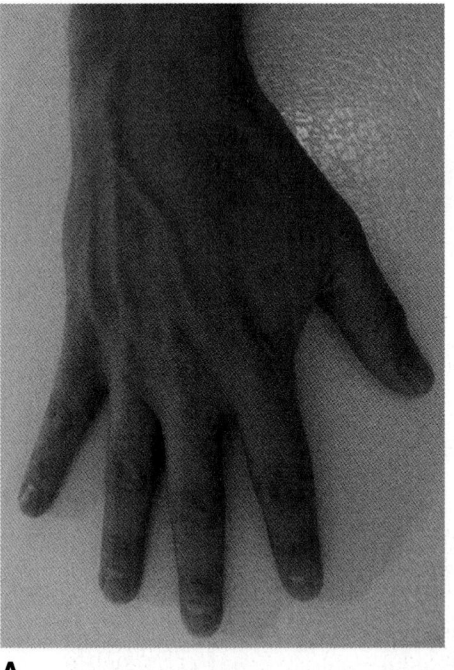

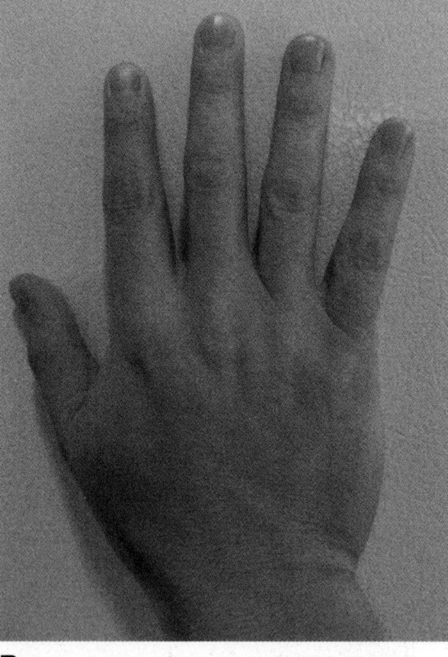

A **B**

Figure 4-21 Change in hydrostatic pressure in the extremities as a result of position. **A.** When the arm is held below the heart, hydrostatic pressure increases and veins dilate within the hand and fill with blood. **B.** When the hand is raised over the head, the hydrostatic pressure is negative and the veins collapse.

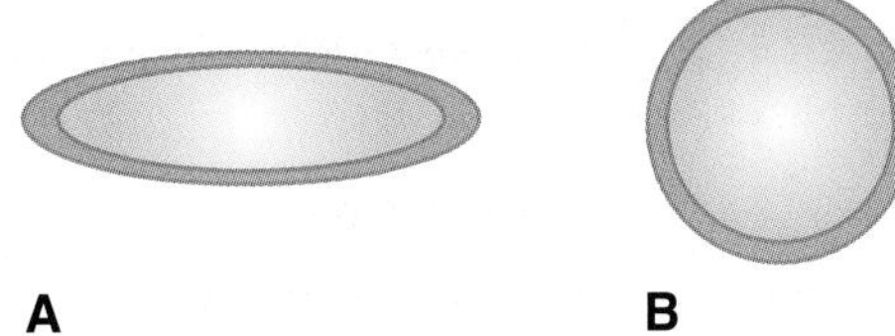

Figure 4-22 Transmural pressure. **A.** In the supine position, the vein takes on an elliptical shape owing to low transmural pressure. **B.** In the standing position, the vein takes on a circular shape owing to high transmural pressure.

from below the diaphragm. The third mechanism is the venous valves, which are folds of endothelial tissue inside of the veins. These valves provide a method to ensure forward flow by only permitting the flow of blood in one direction—to the heart. The **calf muscle pump** provides the final mechanism. The soleal veins inside the calf muscle store venous blood. When the calf muscles are used, blood is forced into the veins.

There is pressure not only inside the veins, but outside the veins as well in the form of **extrinsic pressure. Transmural pressure** is the difference between the pressure inside the vein (intravascular pressure) and the surrounding tissue (extrinsic pressure). With low transmural pressure, which may occur when a patient is lying supine, the force outside the vein exceeds the pressure inside the vein, and the vein collapses and has an elliptical shape. When the patient stands and the hydrostatic pressure increases, the transmural pressure increases and the vein assumes a circular shape (Figure 4-22).

Flow in the veins should not be pulsatile, except for the systemic veins in close proximity to the heart. Instead, veins should be **respirophasic** or show variations that relate to respiration. **Pulsatility** in the peripheral veins may indicate disease affecting the right side of the patient's heart, and thus should be documented. Lack of respiratory **phasicity**, referred to as continuous flow, may be an indicator of intrinsic thrombus or extrinsic compression between the vessel being sampled and the heart (Figure 4-23).

Pulsatility and Phasicity

Unlike veins, arteries should be pulsatile in nature, with a distinct **systole** and **diastole** that correspond to both the flow from the heart and to the distal vascular bed. Flow was formerly described by the shape of its waveform on spectral Doppler as triphasic, biphasic, or monophasic. A consensus article by Kim et al. (2020) published recommended terminology for arterial and venous flow to have a uniform guideline regarding waveform definitions. In that guideline, triphasic and biphasic are replaced by multiphasic because of the inconsistencies in defining triphasic versus biphasic flow (Figure 4-24). Although this is a generalization, and more detail is outside the scope of this book, flow that is multiphasic tends to a high-resistance bed, with typically little diastolic flow evident and possibly some flow reversal in diastole. Examples of multiphasic flow would be seen in blood vessels that supply the face or resting legs. Monophasic flow usually provides blood to a low-resistance bed. A low-resistance bed is a bed that demands constant flow in all phases of the cardiac cycle. Examples of a normally low-resistance bed are the internal carotid artery (ICA) that feeds the brain and the renal artery that supplies oxygenated blood to the kidney (Figure 4-25).

> **SOUND OFF**
> The shape of the waveform may be an indicator of disease that is more distal or more proximal to the sampling point.

> **SOUND OFF**
> Arterial phasicity is always about the resistance in the distal bed. It is important to know what the normal arterial phasicity is for the vessel being sampled.

The shape of the waveform may be an indicator of disease that is more distal or more proximal to the

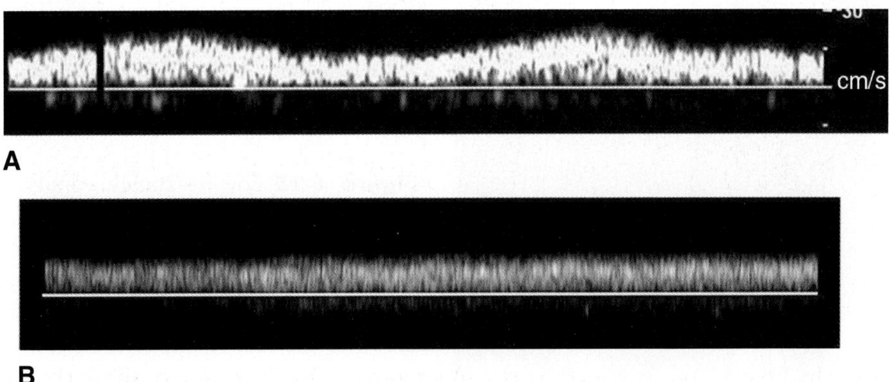

Figure 4-23 Phasicity of the peripheral venous form. **A.** Phasic flow indicates respiratory variability. **B.** Continuous flow implies intrinsic or extrinsic obstruction between the sampled vessel and the heart.

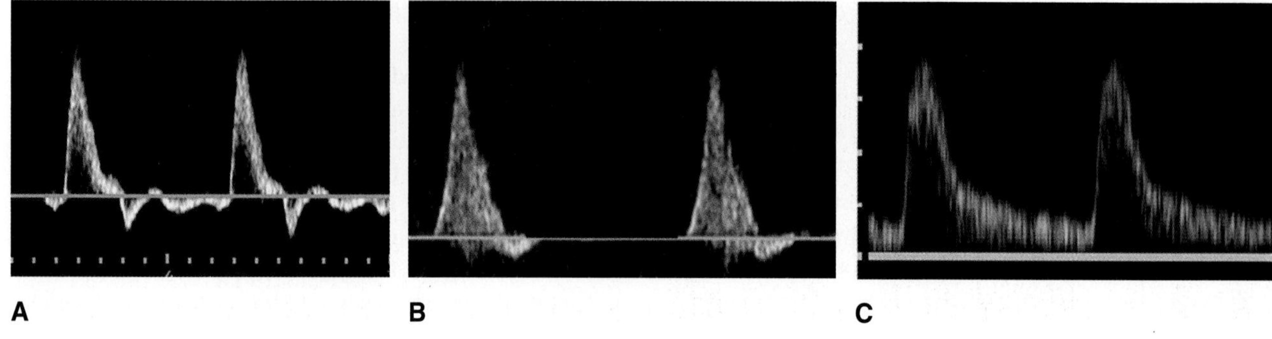

Figure 4-24 Types of arterial flow. **A.** and **B.** Multiphasic flow. **C.** Monophasic flow.

sampling point. In the presence of a stenosis, the distal arterioles will dilate, thereby allowing more oxygenated blood to get to the periphery. The increase in the diameter of the vessels is accompanied by a pressure drop. For example, the lower extremity arteries at rest are normally high-resistance vessels. However, if there is a superficial femoral artery (SFA) obstruction, there will be the dilatation of the distal arterioles, with a corresponding change to monophasic flow in the spectral waveform of the SFA.

Arterial phasicity is always about the resistance in the distal bed. For example, in the resting patient, monophasic flow is always abnormal in the lower extremities. If monophasic flow is seen in the lower extremity arteries of the resting patient, it indicates persistent dilatation downstream, which is an abnormal condition. Conversely, blood vessels that normally have low-resistance waveforms, such as the ICA, should never exhibit a high-resistance pattern. If high-resistance flow is noted in the ICA, it would be an ominous sign indicating a distal high-pressure state, as seen with distal occlusion or near occlusion, cerebral edema, or brain death.

An additional noteworthy waveform shape that can be indicative of pathology is referred to as **tardus parvus** (literally interpreted as "slow small"), which is seen in the presence of a proximal obstruction (Figure 4-26). Tardus parvus, also called **dampened** waveforms, are identified by a delay in the upstroke of the systolic component of the waveform (time to peak). Most arteries have flow that initially accelerates rapidly, causing a sharp systolic upstroke. An increased acceleration time, represented by a prolonged systolic upstroke, is a sign that there is an obstruction and that obstruction is located more proximal to the point of sampling. It is important to remember that a proximal obstruction causes distal arteriolar dilatation; therefore, tardus parvus waveforms are monophasic in nature. Tardus parvus waveforms always indicate that there is an obstruction proximal to the point of sampling.

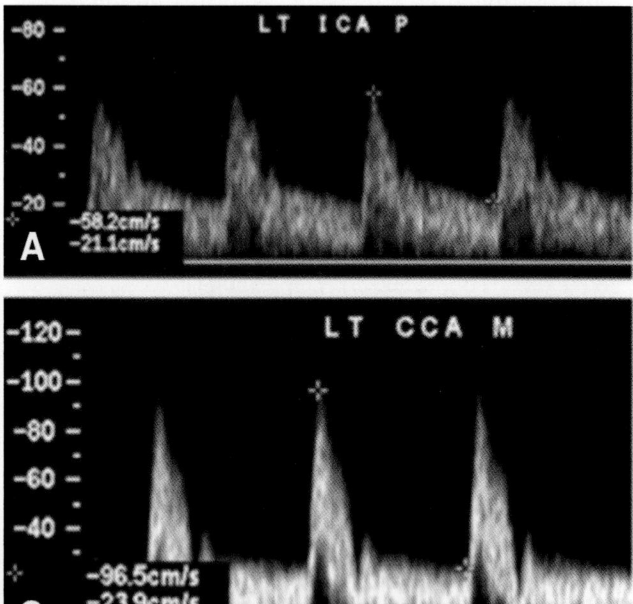

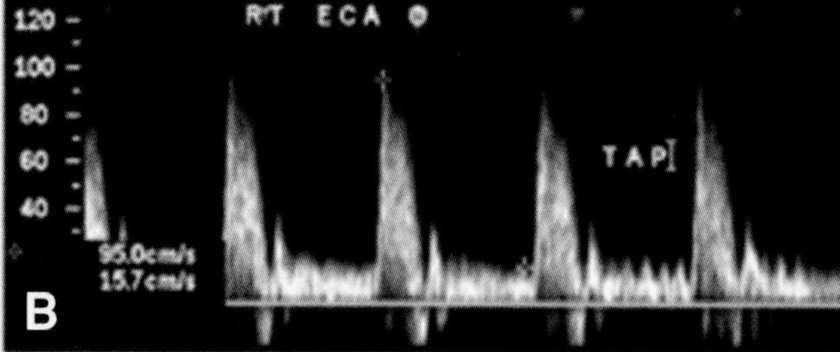

Figure 4-25 Low-resistance versus high-resistance patterns. **A.** The ICA, which supplies blood to the brain, demonstrates a low-resistance, monophasic blood flow pattern, with continuous flow throughout the cardiac cycle. The external carotid artery (ECA), which supplies blood to the face, demonstrates a high-resistance, multiphasic blood flow pattern **(B)**. The CCA is also considered low-resistance but has a waveform that is a combination of the two vessels it feeds, the ECA and ICA **(C)**.

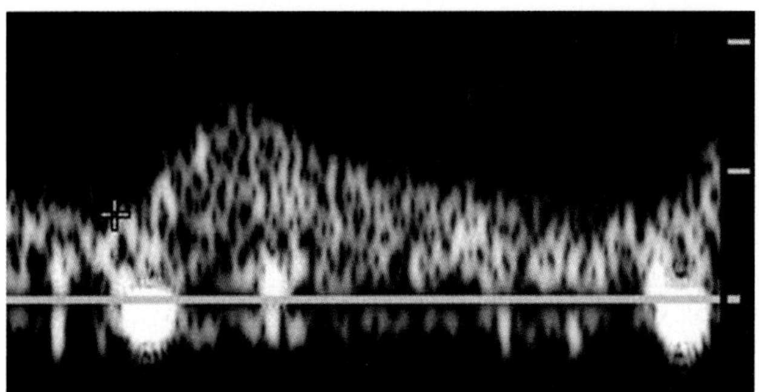

Figure 4-26 Tardus parvus waveform. This image of a tardus parvus (dampened) waveform demonstrates a prolonged systolic upstroke (increased acceleration time).

SOUND OFF
An increased acceleration time, represented by a prolonged systolic upstroke, is a sign that there is an obstruction and that obstruction is located more proximal to the point of sampling.

SOUND OFF
Exercise causes arteriolar dilatation, which results in larger diameter blood vessels, and therefore a lower-resistance distal bed with a corresponding increase in blood flow.

Effects of Exercise on Flow

In the resting patient, the peripheral lower extremity arteries are of normally high resistance owing to distal arteriolar constriction. With exercise, there is an increased demand for oxygen by the muscles. This increase in demand causes arteriolar dilatation, which results in larger diameter blood vessels and therefore a lower resistance distal bed with a corresponding increase in blood flow. In the normal patient, there is little pressure change in the distal lower extremities as a result of this arteriolar dilatation. The patient with arterial obstructive disease may have normal resting pressures, but the increased demand for oxygen that occurs with exercise may be more than the blood vessels are able to supply, causing a pressure drop distally.

SOUND OFF
When a reflector is moving toward the transducer, the reflected frequency will be higher than the transmitted frequency. Likewise, when a reflector is moving away from the transducer, the reflected frequency will be lower than the transmitted frequency.

DOPPLER PRINCIPLES

The Doppler Effect

The effect of differing frequencies with motion was first identified by Christian Doppler and is thus called the **Doppler effect**. When sound impinges on a stationary reflector, the reflected frequency is identical to the transmitted, or incident, frequency. However, when a reflector is moving toward the transducer, the reflected frequency will be higher than the transmitted frequency. Likewise, when a reflector is moving away from the transducer, the reflected frequency will be lower than the transmitted frequency (Figure 4-27). The difference between the transmitted and reflected frequencies is called the **frequency shift** or Doppler shift. A positive frequency shift occurs when a reflector is moving in a direction toward the transducer. A negative frequency shift occurs when a reflector is moving in a direction that is away from the transducer. The frequency shift can be calculated by utilizing the **Doppler equation** (Table 4-15 and Figure 4-28).

SOUND OFF
If the frequency shift is a positive number, then there is a positive shift and flow is moving toward the transducer. Likewise, if the frequency shift is a negative number, then there is a negative shift and flow is moving away from the transducer.

When the transmitted frequency is subtracted from the reflected frequency, the result is a number that is approximately 1/1000th of the operating frequency. The

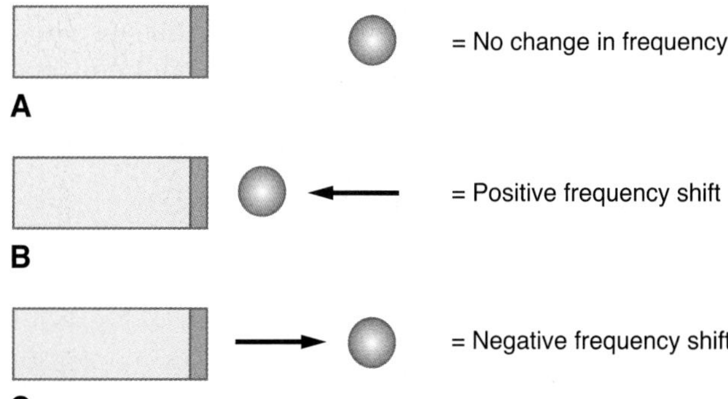

Figure 4-27 Frequency shifts and moving reflector. **A.** With a stationary reflector, the reflected frequency is equal to the incident frequency, resulting in no change in frequency. **B.** With a reflector moving toward the source, the reflected frequency is greater than the incident frequency, resulting in a positive frequency shift. **C.** With a reflector moving away from the source, the reflected frequency is less than the incident frequency, resulting in a negative frequency shift.

TABLE 4-15 The Doppler equation

Formula
$$F_D = \frac{2f\nu \cos\theta}{c}$$ In the formula, the frequency shift (F_D) is measured in Hertz by the ultrasound machine. The frequency shift is the difference between the incident frequency and the reflected frequency. The product of the operating frequency (f) of the transducer multiplied by 2, the velocity (ν) of the blood, and the cosine ($\cos\theta$) of the Doppler angle is divided by the propagation speed (c) of sound through soft tissue.

resultant value is in the audible range of sound, meaning that all that is needed to hear the frequency shift is a set of speakers or headphones. If the resultant value is a positive number, then there is a positive shift and flow is moving toward the transducer. Likewise, if the resultant value is a negative number, then there is a negative shift and flow is moving away from the transducer (Figure 4-29).

Although the frequency shift is measured by the machine, it is the velocity of the blood that is of interest to the imager and not the frequency shift itself. The ultrasound system measures the frequency shift but calculates the velocity (Table 4-16).

Doppler works because the incident sound reflects off the red blood cells in the blood. Red blood cells are small, normally about 7.0 μm. Because of their size, they are **Rayleigh scatterers**. Rayleigh scatterers are very small compared with the incident wavelength. As frequency increases, the intensity of the scatter increases proportionally to the fourth power of the frequency; therefore, a small increase in frequency results in a dramatic increase in scatter (Figure 4-30). Higher frequency transducers may provide stronger Doppler signals, but at the expense of the attenuation. Therefore, the higher the frequency, the more scatter there is, and therefore, the more attenuation. Remember that scatter is a form of attenuation. Therefore, if the energy is scattered, it is not transmitted deeper into the tissue. There is always a trade-off between improved resolution and penetration.

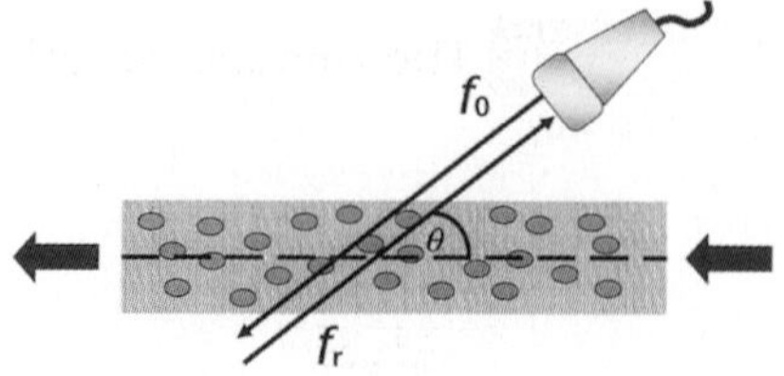

Figure 4-28 Doppler shift diagram. Calculation of the Doppler shift requires knowledge of the transmitted frequency (f_0), the reflected frequency (f_r), the angle of incidence (θ), and the speed of sound. See texts for details.

SOUND OFF
Although higher frequency transducers offer stronger Doppler signals, the higher the frequency, the more scatter there is, and therefore, more attenuation.

SOUND OFF
As the Doppler angle increases, the cosine of the angle decreases.

In the Doppler equation, it is not the Doppler angle that is utilized in the equation but it is rather the cosine of the angle (Table 4-17). As the Doppler angle increases, the cosine of the angle decreases, that is, the Doppler angle and the frequency shift are inversely proportional. The Doppler angle must be known in order to more accurately calculate the velocities, although in echocardiography a 0° angle is always assumed. Table 4-17 reveals that the cosine of 0 is 1. If "1" is plugged into the

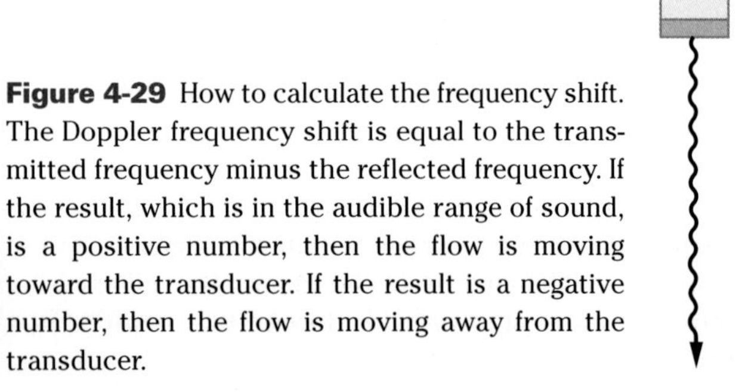

Figure 4-29 How to calculate the frequency shift. The Doppler frequency shift is equal to the transmitted frequency minus the reflected frequency. If the result, which is in the audible range of sound, is a positive number, then the flow is moving toward the transducer. If the result is a negative number, then the flow is moving away from the transducer.

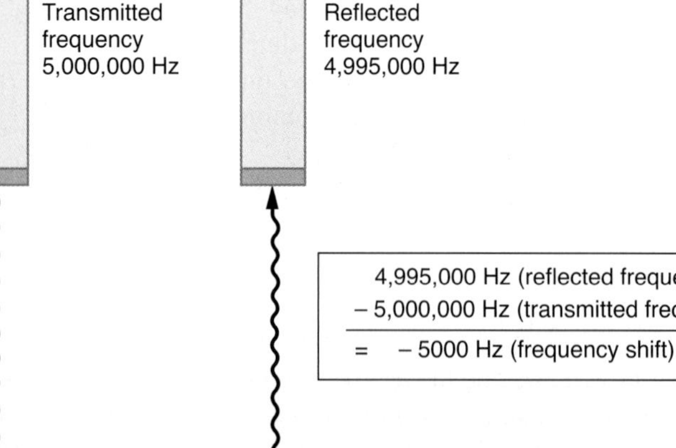

TABLE 4-16 The Doppler equation solving for velocity

Formula
$$\nu = \frac{cF_D}{2f\cos\theta}$$ Velocity (ν) is equal to the product of the propagation speed of sound through soft tissue (c) and the frequency shift (F_D), divided by the product of the operating frequency (f) multiplied by 2 and the cosine ($\cos\theta$) of the Doppler angle.

TABLE 4-17 Cosines of the angles

Angle(°)	Cosine of the Angle
0	1.0
30	0.87
45	0.71
60	0.50
90	0.00

Doppler equation, the equation would not change at all. Therefore, the most accurate frequency shift (and therefore the most accurate velocity) will come from a 0° angle. Because of the inverse relationship between the Doppler angle and the cosine of the angle, as the angle increases, the frequency shift decreases. Therefore, the highest frequency shift comes from a 0° angle. No frequency shift is obtained at a 90° angle; at an angle of 90°, the cosine of 90 is 0 and therefore the frequency shift is 0.

Some Doppler devices are **nondirectional**, or unable to distinguish between positive or negative frequency shifts. In order to determine the direction of flow, Doppler devices use **phase quadrature** to determine whether there is a positive shift flow toward the transducer or a negative shift flow away from the transducer. Phase quadrature permits **bidirectional Doppler** that is able to display positive versus negative shifts. There are two ways of obtaining a Doppler signal: **continuous-wave Doppler** and **pulsed-wave Doppler**.

SOUND OFF
CW devices do not pause to listen to the return echo, nor do they calculate how long it takes for the echo to return. Therefore, CW devices have no range resolution nor the ability to determine how far away the reflectors are from the transducer.

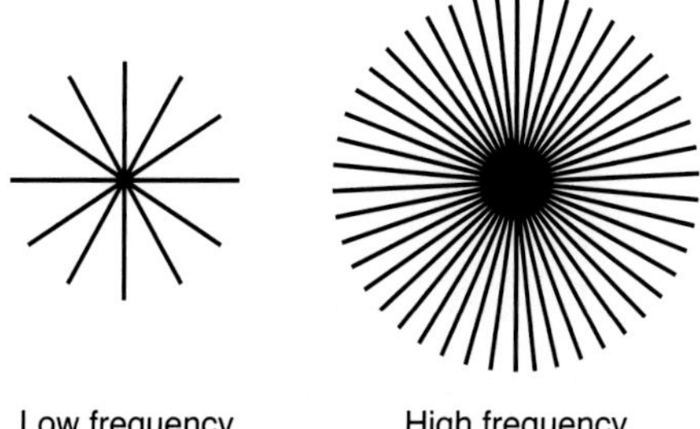

Figure 4-30 Scatter. The higher the frequency, the more scatter there is. Scatter, a form of attenuation, keeps the beam from penetrating. The more energy that is scattered, the less there is to penetrate deeper in the body.

Continuous-Wave Doppler

A continuous-wave (CW) Doppler device consists of two elements: One element is used by the system to constantly transmit sound, and the other is used to constantly receive sound. CW devices are constructed this way because the piezoelectric elements used by the system to create ultrasound cannot send and receive at the same time. CW devices do not pause to listen to the return echo, nor do they calculate how long it takes for the echo to return. Therefore, CW devices have no **range resolution** or the ability to determine how far away the reflectors are from the transducer (Figure 4-31). It is for this reason that CW transducers themselves do not provide a 2D image, only a spectral Doppler waveform (see the section "Analyzing the Spectral Waveform").

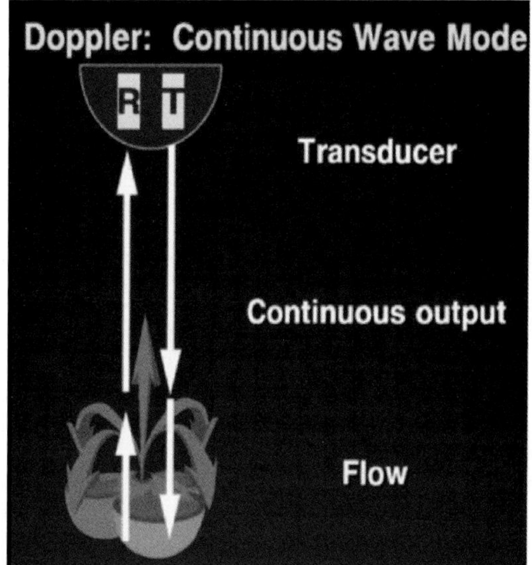

Figure 4-31 Continuous-wave Doppler. Continuous-wave Doppler uses one element to receive (*R*) and one to transmit (*T*). By continuously transmitting and receiving Doppler-shifted echoes, it is possible to quantify velocities of any magnitude, although it lacks the capability of determining the range information and therefore specific depth of that velocity.

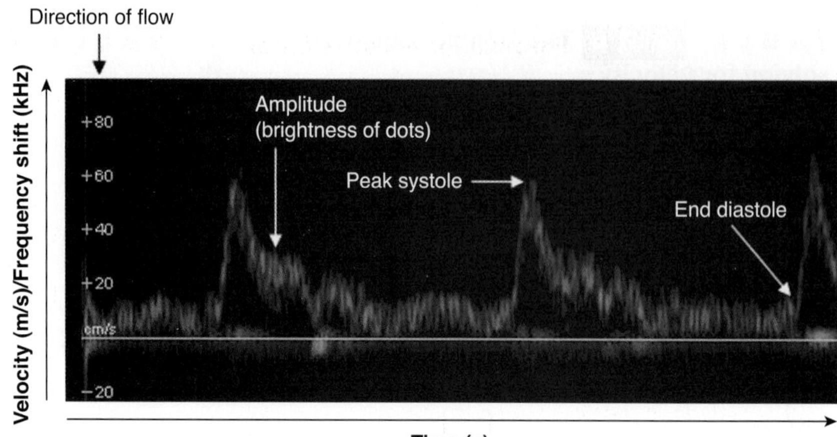

Figure 4-32 Spectral waveform. The spectral display provides the following information: time, velocity, frequency shift, flow direction, and amplitude.

The **sample volume**, which is the region that is being measured using Doppler, is very large with CW. Any blood vessel that lies within the sample volume will be measured and displayed in the signal. With CW, the operator is not able to select a specific vessel. This dilemma can present problems when there are several vessels within the sample volume.

The CW transducer is driven by an **oscillator** that provides a continuous voltage to the transmitting element. With CW transducers, the oscillating voltage is equal to the operating frequency. If the oscillator vibrates at 3,000,000 times per second, the CW transducer operates at 3 MHz. The signal processor in the machine compares the transmitted and received frequencies, and their difference is sent to a loudspeaker and/or spectrum analyzer. It is also important to remember that there is no damping with a CW transducer; if the sound is being transmitted continuously, damping is not needed. The continuously transmitting CW device has a 100% transmit time. Therefore, the duty factor of a CW device is 100% or 1.

> **SOUND OFF**
> With CW, the device has a 100% transmit time, which means that the duty factor is 100% or 1.

> **SOUND OFF**
> FFT is a technique used by the ultrasound machine to interpret the complex mix of frequency shifts in the spectral Doppler signal and thus offers the ability to measure velocities.

Analyzing the Spectral Waveform

The signal that is received by the transducer is a complex mix of frequency shifts and time. The signal undergoes processing before it is displayed to improve the analysis of Doppler information. Spectral analysis dismantles the complex signal and breaks it down by frequency. The resultant waveform is a visual, quantifiable representation of what is happening in the blood vessel at a given point in time. The mathematical technique used to break down the signal and produce a spectral waveform is called **fast Fourier transform** (FFT). Accurate velocity measurements are needed to be able to quantify the level of disease and perform other assessments, and it is FFT that accomplishes this task. The spectral display provides the following information: time, velocity, frequency shift, flow direction, and amplitude (Figure 4-32).

Time is displayed on the spectral display along the horizontal or *x*-axis. Tick marks represent seconds, so it is possible to calculate events as they occur over a specific period of time. The number of seconds displayed at one time can be adjusted by changing the **sweep speed** of the Doppler instrument (Figure 4-33).

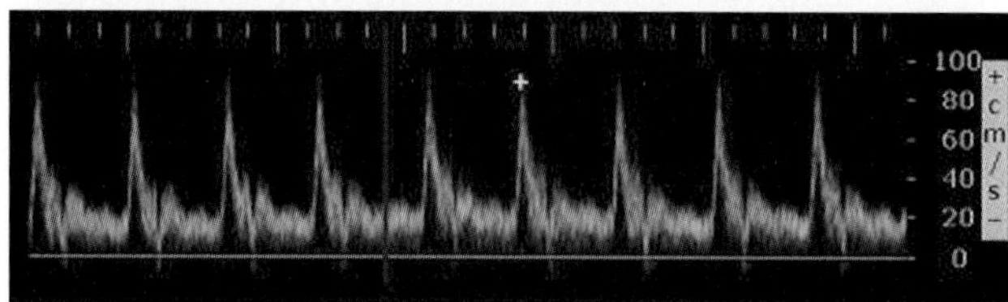

A

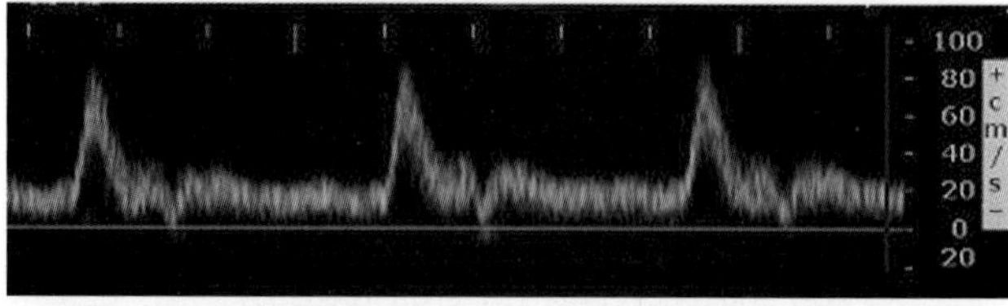

B

Figure 4-33 Changing the sweep speed. The sweep speed can be changed to display more **(A)** or fewer **(B)** waveforms on the screen at one time.

TABLE 4-18 Formula for resistive index

Formula
$$RI = \frac{A - B}{A}$$ In this formula of the resistive index (RI), peak systolic velocity (*A*) is subtracted from the end diastolic velocity (*B*) and then divided by the peak systolic velocity.

TABLE 4-19 Formula for pulsatility index

Formula
$$PI = \frac{A - B}{\text{mean}}$$ In this formula of the pulsatility index (PI), peak systolic velocity (*A*) is subtracted from the end diastolic velocity (*B*) and then divided by the *mean* or average of the velocities between peak systole and end diastole.

SOUND OFF
Time is displayed on the spectral display along the horizontal or *x*-axis, whereas velocities are presented on the vertical or *y*-axis.

As stated in the "Doppler Effect" section, it is the frequency shift that is measured by the machine; however, it is the velocity information that is of the greatest interest. Therefore, today's spectral displays commonly display only velocity information. Velocities are presented on the vertical or *y*-axis. On some machines, it may also be possible to display frequency shift information, but to reduce interoperator variability, angle-corrected velocities are commonly used (except in echocardiography and transcranial Doppler, which typically do not use angle correction).

Measurement of the flow velocity generally enables the sonographer to measure peak systolic and end diastolic measurements that are, in turn, used to quantify the degree of disease within vessels. In addition to the peak systolic and end diastolic velocities, the mean velocity is used for some applications. The mean velocity is derived by tracing the spectral waveform from the end-diastole of one heartbeat to the end-diastole of the next heartbeat. Examples of measurements that are obtained on a spectral waveform include the **resistive index** (RI) and the **pulsatility index** (PI). The RI is used to quantitate the resistiveness of the distal vascular bed (Table 4-18 and Figure 4-34). An example of the use of RI is the analysis of the liver and kidneys in cases of transplant. The PI is used to determine how pulsatile a vessel is over time (Table 4-19 and Figure 4-35). The PI is often used in obstetrics for the evaluation of the fetal brain and the umbilical cord. Both of these measurements estimate the relative difference between systole and diastole.

SOUND OFF
When using autotrace to obtain the spectral waveform measurements (Figure 4-36), always double check the tracing. Autotrace may provide an inaccurate result if the patient has an irregular heartbeat, if the gain is too low or too high, if the wall filter is set incorrectly, etc. Most manufacturers let the operator adjust the parameters as to how the autotrace is obtained (one heartbeat, average of multiple heartbeats, etc).

Figure 4-34 Resistive index. This image demonstrates the measurement obtained for the resistive index.

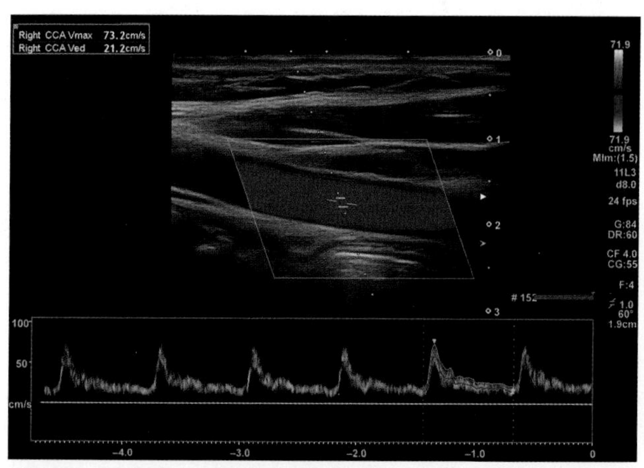

Figure 4-35 Pulsatility index. This image demonstrates the measurement obtained for the pulsatility index.

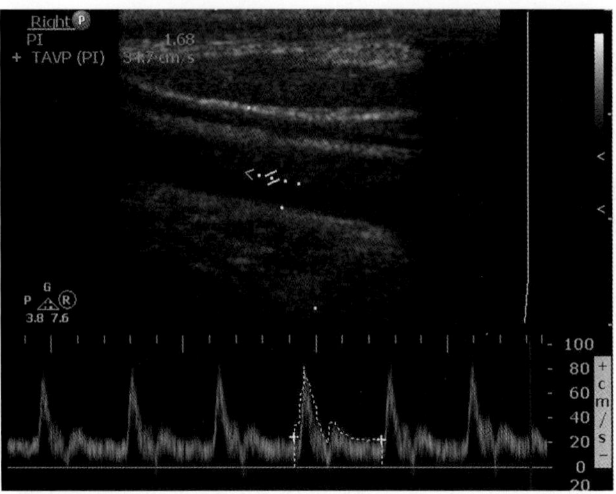

Figure 4-36 Autotrace. Ultrasound machines have automated waveform tracing that automatically calculates PSV, EDV, RI, PI, S/D ratio, and other measurements as required. Automation can be a time saver but allows for inaccuracies if the operator is not trained to know when the autotrace performed incorrectly, as might occur in different situations (irregular heartbeat, wall filter set incorrectly, etc).

The flow direction is displayed on the spectral display as flow being above or below the baseline. Note that the newer term for the "baseline" is the *zero-flow baseline*, although it may not yet be in widespread use. Flow on the one side of the zero-flow baseline is a "positive shift," and flow on the other side represents a "negative shift." The flow can be inverted for convention so that flow always appears above the zero-flow baseline, even when it represents a negative shift. The spectral display also allows for the display of the pathologic reversal of flow. An example of the pathological reversal of flow occurs in the ICAs when cerebral edema is present or in the fetal umbilical artery when there is severe placental insufficiency.

When trying to determine whether the flow is "toward" or "away" from the transducer, the practitioner must search for the minus (negative) symbol that precedes the velocity on the spectral velocity scale. Some machines display the word *inverted* instead of a minus symbol to denote that the display has been inverted (Figure 4-37).

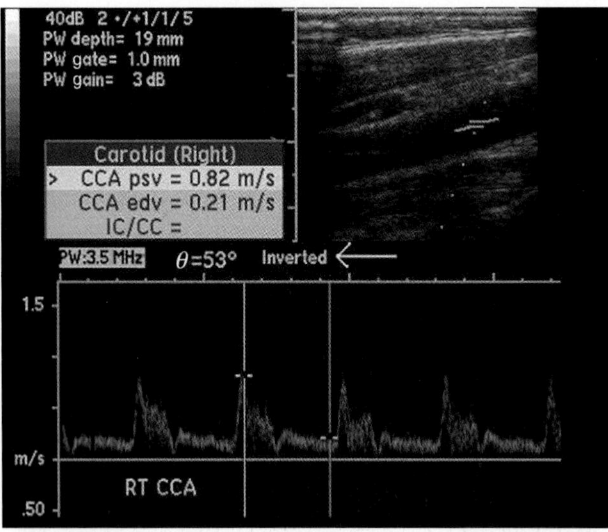

A

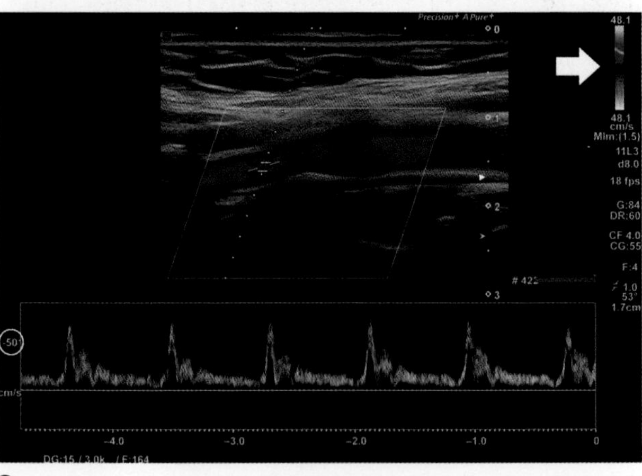

C

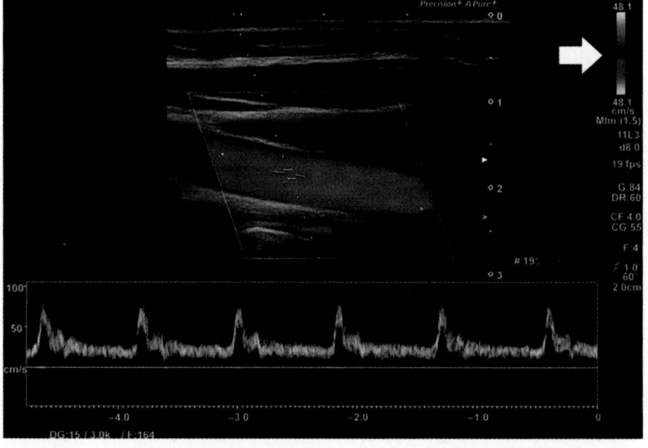

B

Figure 4-37 Demonstration of a negative frequency shift. **A.** Some manufacturers signify negative frequency shifts by displaying the word *inverted* (*thin arrow*) above the spectral waveform. **B.** This image shows blood flow with a positive Doppler shift. The color scale is that of the blue-away, red-toward (BART) scale. Notice the color gate is steered to the right, the vessel is red (flow is toward the probe), and the spectral Doppler indicates a positive Doppler shift. **C.** To image further in this blood vessel, the color gate is now steered left. Notice the color scale has inverted, with a red-away, blue toward (RABT) scale (*thick arrow*). There is an option on most ultrasound machines to automatically invert the color scale when the steering on the spectral Doppler flips, as occurred between images **(B)** and **(C)**. On the spectral Doppler, the manufacturer signifies a negative frequency shift by placing a minus sign in front of the number (*yellow circle*). Blood flow is still going toward the left side of the screen (in this case, the patient's head), but the direction of flow (toward the probe or away from the probe) changes as the steer changes from right to left.

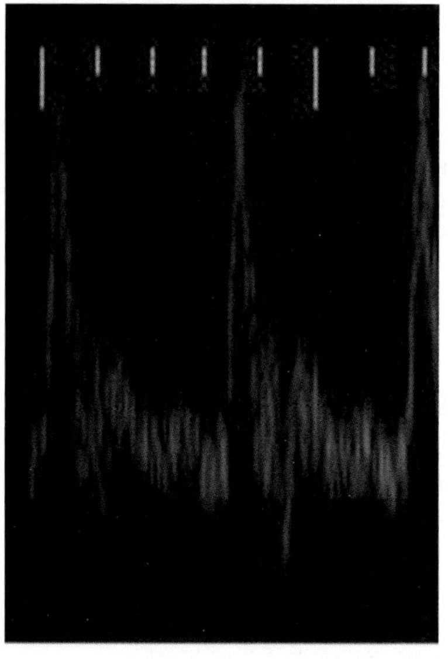

A

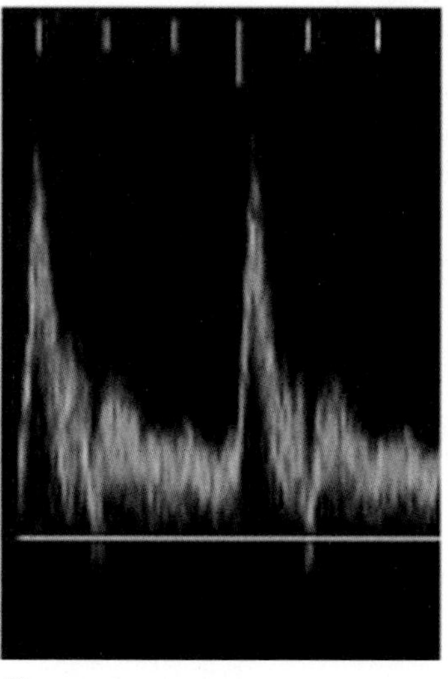

B

Figure 4-38 Amplitude of the Doppler signal. **A.** The less bright the envelope of the spectral waveform, the fewer the red blood cells that make up the image. **B.** The brighter the envelope, the more red blood cells that make up the signal. The brightness of the spectral waveform can also be changed by adjusting the spectral gain.

If velocity is on the *y*-axis and time is on the *x*-axis, the amplitude of the signal is represented by the brightness of the dots in the spectral envelope or the ***z*-axis**. The brighter the dots of the spectral waveform, the more red blood cells that make up the signal (Figure 4-38).

SOUND OFF

In a normal vessel, a small sample volume is typically used in order to sample only the highest velocities in the center of the vessel.

The envelope of the spectral waveform represents how many red blood cells are traveling at that velocity at a specific period of time (Figure 4-39). The wider the range of velocities in a sample at a given point of time, the thicker the envelope. In a normal vessel, a small sample volume is typically used in order to sample only the highest velocities in the center of the vessel. A large sample volume that encompasses both the fast central flow and all the progressively decreasing velocities toward the edges will represent many different velocities (Figure 4-40). The area under the envelope is called the **spectral window**. A flow sample in which the red blood cells are traveling at almost identical speeds, as in the case of laminar flow with a small sample volume, will demonstrate a thin envelope. Conversely, analyzing one instance of time in turbulent flow or the use of a large sample volume will demonstrate a wide range of velocities. These scenarios therefore demonstrates a filling-in of the spectral envelope. This is termed **spectral broadening**. As mentioned in the "Types of Blood Flow" section, turbulence is not always pathologic. Turbulence is normal and expected in some instances, such as in the area of the carotid bulb. However, if turbulence is seen where laminar flow is expected, further investigation is warranted. The spectral window disappears in the presence of spectral broadening. CW flow uses a large sample volume and samples many vessels (at a variety of velocities) at the same time. Therefore, CW waveforms will typically demonstrate spectral broadening (Figure 4-41).

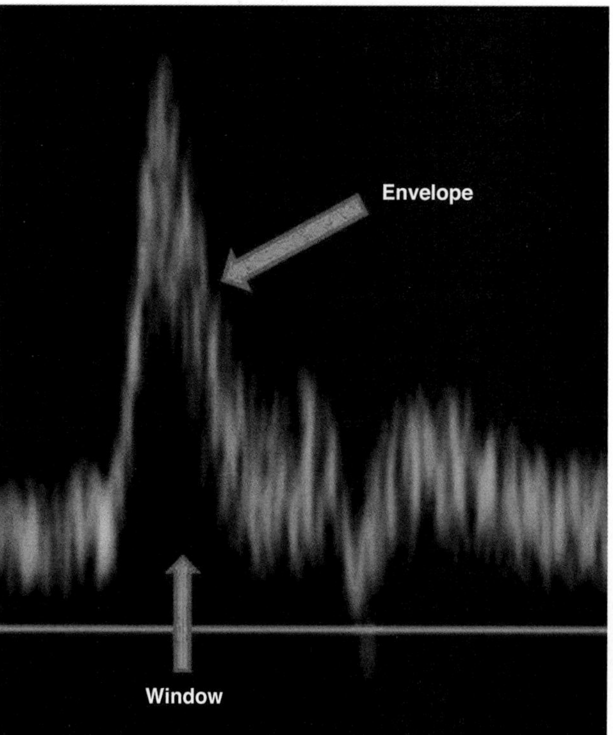

Figure 4-39 The envelope and window of the spectral display. The envelope (*envelope*) of the waveform represents how many red blood cells are traveling at that velocity at a specific period of time. The spectral window (*window*) is the area under the envelope.

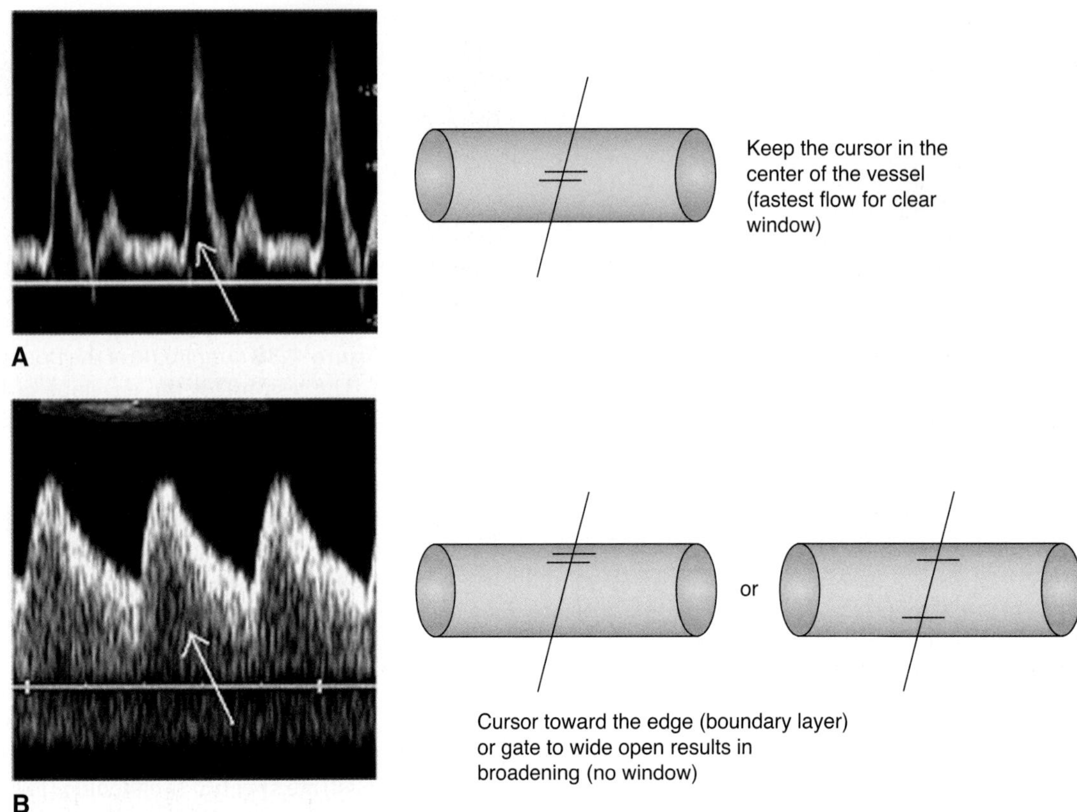

Figure 4-40 Sample volume size and appearance of the spectral waveform. **A.** A small sample volume placed in the center of a vessel where flow is the fastest will result in a clear window (*arrow*). **B.** A large sample or one taken near a vessel wall will demonstrate spectral broadening of the window (*arrow*).

Pulsed-Wave Doppler

Pulsed-wave (PW) Doppler functions much like PW grayscale imaging in that it transmits pulses of sound and waits for the sound to return in order to determine the depth of the returning echoes (Figure 4-42).

Unlike CW, PW Doppler allows the operator to select the depth at which the Doppler measurements will be taken. The operator places a **range gate** over the vessel to be sampled, and the area within that "gate"—the sample volume—is where the PW Doppler signal is

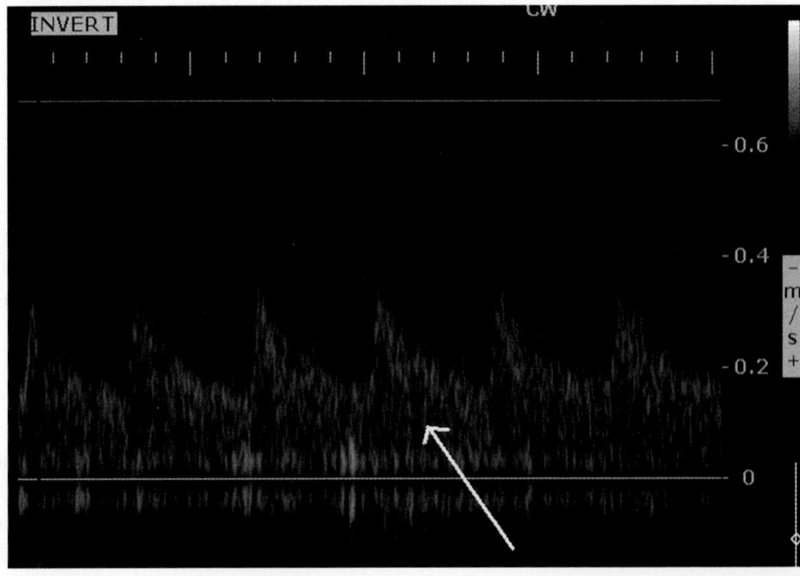

Figure 4-41 Spectral broadening with CW Doppler. Note the filling in of the spectral window (*arrow*).

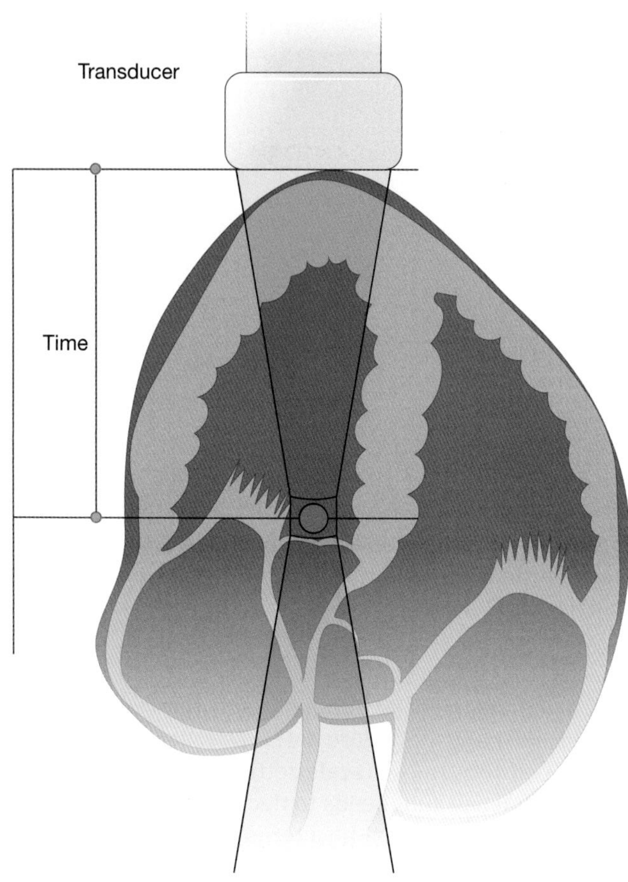

Figure 4-42 Pulsed-wave Doppler. Pulsed wave, also referred to as PW Doppler, much like pulsed-wave grayscale imaging, transmits pulses of sound and waits for the sound to return in order to determine the depth of the returning echoes. By transmitting a brief pulse of ultrasound and listening to returning echoes from a specific depth, it is possible to measure velocities, though at the cost of not being able to quantify very high velocities.

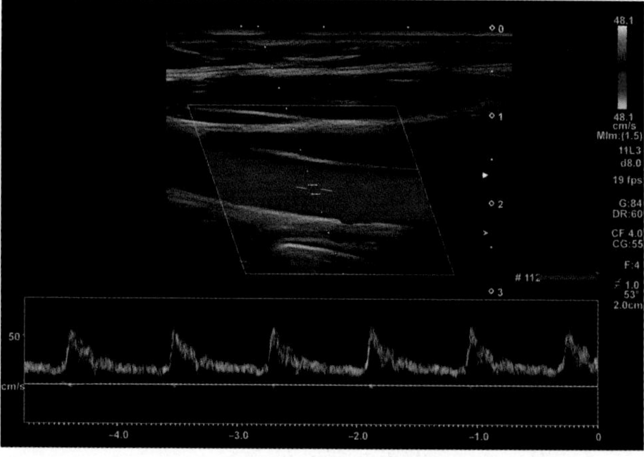

A

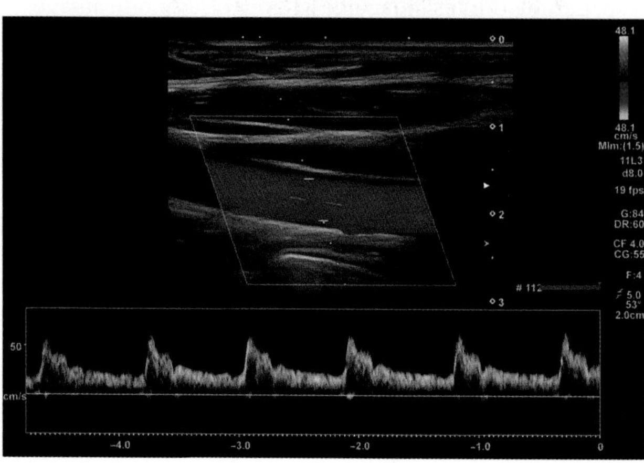

B

Figure 4-43 Controlling the size of the sample volume. **A.** A small pulsed-wave sample volume placed in the center of the vessel. Notice the spectral waveform has a thin envelope and no spectral broadening. **B.** The sample volume can also be larger if needed, especially important if searching for flow in an abnormal or difficult-to-scan blood vessel. The spectral waveform will have a thicker envelope with spectral broadening.

obtained. The operator can select the size of the sample volume by adjusting a gate control on the machine, which permits many different size sample volumes (Figure 4-43). Grayscale imaging devices typically use 2 to 3 cycles per pulse to produce a B-mode image. PW Doppler devices typically transmit anywhere from 5 to 30 cycles per pulse. This higher pulse length provides a more accurate sampling of the blood.

SOUND OFF

PW Doppler devices typically transmit anywhere from 5 to 30 cycles per pulse.

PW Doppler also utilizes **angle correction**. Angle correction is used with PW Doppler in order to more accurately calculate velocities from frequency shifts. When performing Doppler studies, it is rare that the beam is parallel to the flowing blood (ie, 0° angle of flow). Therefore, angle-correction is used to inform the machine what the flow angle is, so that velocities can be accurately calculated. Angle-correction is further discussed in this chapter (see the section "Review of Doppler Controls").

PW Doppler devices also permit **duplex** imaging in which the B-mode image is on the display at the same time as the Doppler signal (Figure 4-44). Duplex imaging allows for the real-time adjustment of the Doppler cursor while observing the grayscale image. With duplex imaging, the Doppler and 2D information must be obtained separately. The acquisition of the grayscale information alternates with obtaining the Doppler information, which is called time-sharing. This switching back and forth occurs quickly but does affect the frame

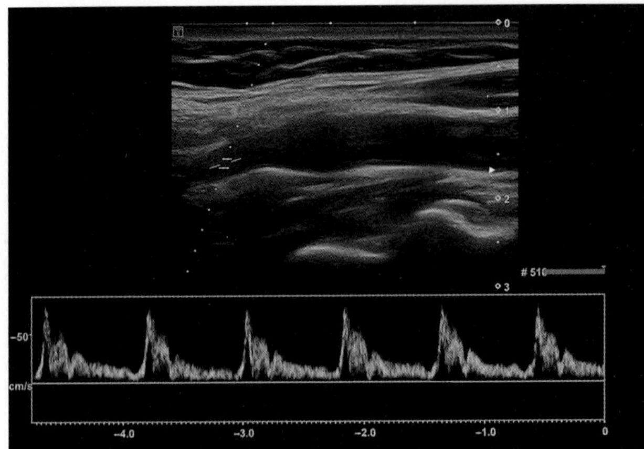

Figure 4-44 Duplex Doppler. Pulsed-wave Doppler devices also permit duplex imaging, where the B-mode image is on the display at the same time as the Doppler signal. The B-mode (also called grayscale or 2D) image can be frozen or live at the time the spectral waveform is obtained.

rate in a negative way, because it decreases the temporal resolution. **Triplex** imaging is combined grayscale, spectral, and color Doppler information on the screen (Figure 4-45).

SOUND OFF

With duplex imaging, the grayscale (B-mode) image is on the display at the same time as the Doppler signal. Triplex imaging is combined grayscale, spectral, and color Doppler.

PW Doppler has a major limitation called **aliasing**. Aliasing is a wraparound of the Doppler signal, in which the positive shifts are displayed as negative shifts (Figure 4-46). The highest frequency shift that can be measured is equal to one-half of the **pulse repetition frequency** (PRF) that is known as the **Nyquist limit**. PRF is the number of pulses per second. For example, if the PRF is 2500 Hz, a frequency shift greater than 1250 Hz will alias. Aliasing occurs because the Doppler signal must be measured at such a rapid rate. If the PRF is too low, as in the case of a deep blood vessel, the blood

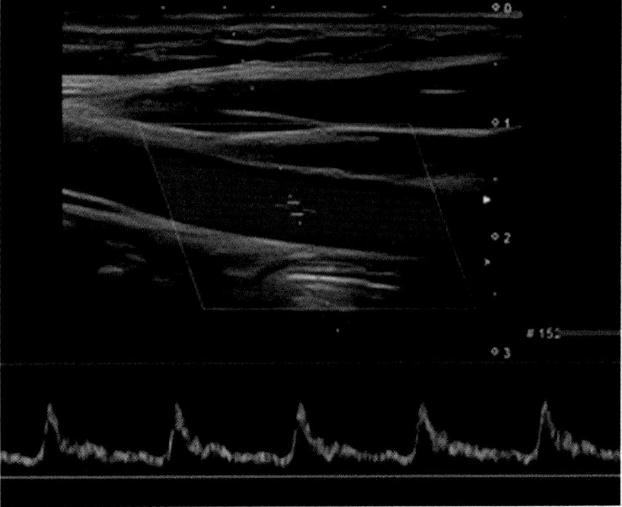

Figure 4-45 Triplex image. This triplex image demonstrates ovarian blood flow with color Doppler, pulsed-wave Doppler, and B-mode.

cannot be sampled fast enough, and the signal is displayed erroneously (Figure 4-47). In order to eliminate aliasing, either the PRF (**scale** setting) needs to increase or the frequency shift needs to decrease. Table 4-20 lists the parameters that can be altered to assist in eliminating aliasing, and Table 4-21 has some sample problems related to aliasing.

SOUND OFF

The highest frequency shift that can be measured is equal to one-half of the PRF, which is known as the Nyquist limit. Aliasing occurs because the Doppler signal must be measured at such a rapid rate.

SOUND OFF

PW Doppler has a minimum of one crystal in the transducer, and CW Doppler has a minimum of two crystals in the transducer.

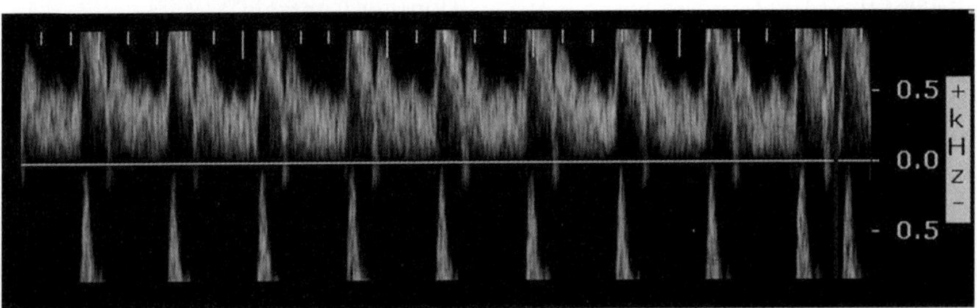

Figure 4-46 Aliasing of the spectral signal. Pulsed-wave Doppler has a major limitation: aliasing. Aliasing is a wraparound of the Doppler signal, where the positive shifts are displayed as negative shifts.

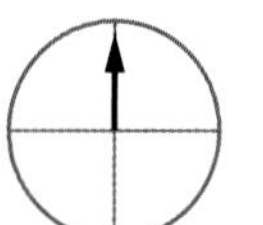
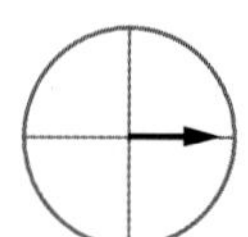
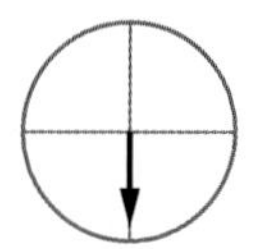
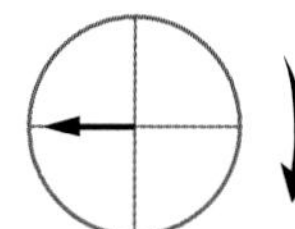

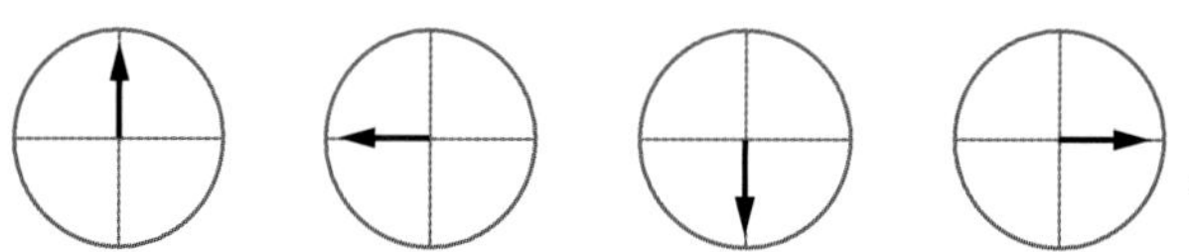

Figure 4-47 Explanation of aliasing. **A.** When the second hand is observed at 15-second intervals, it appears that the hand is moving in a clockwise direction. **B.** However, when the second hand is observed at 45-second intervals, it appears that the clock is running backwards. This apparent reversal, or aliasing, is caused by too infrequent sampling (every 45 instead of every 15).

In summary, there are certain advantages and disadvantages to both PW and CW Doppler (Table 4-22). The chief advantage of PW Doppler over CW Doppler is the ability to select a specific depth to sample by utilizing the range gate, thereby offering the user the ability to sample a specific vessel at a specific point. Another advantage of PW Doppler over CW Doppler is the ability to angle-correct in order to more accurately calculate the velocity of the blood. Though CW Doppler needs two crystals to simultaneously send and receive, the simplest PW Doppler device needs only one crystal to perform this task. However, it must wait for the prior pulse to return before sending the next pulse.

TABLE 4-20 Tools to eliminate aliasing

- Increase the PRF (scale) setting
- Decrease the sample depth
- Decrease the frequency
- Increase the Doppler angle
- Use continuous-wave transducer

TABLE 4-21 Examples of questions relating to aliasing

Question	Explanation
At what frequency shift would aliasing occur if the PRF is 6 kHz?	Aliasing occurs when the frequency shift exceeds the Nyquist limit, which is one-half of the PRF. If the PRF is 6 kHz, divide that by two to get a Nyquist Limit of 3 kHz, or 3000 Hz. In this example, a frequency shift exceeding 3 kHz would cause aliasing
You are scanning a blood vessel using PW Doppler and there is a velocity high enough to cause aliasing. You tried lowering the baseline and increasing the scale, to no avail. What other option(s) are available?	Try lowering the operating frequency and increasing the Doppler angle. If that does not resolve the aliasing, CW Doppler is the only option remaining.
At what frequency shift does CW Doppler demonstrate aliasing?	There is no aliasing with CW Doppler

TABLE 4-22 Advantages and disadvantages of continuous-wave Doppler and pulsed-wave Doppler

Instrument	Advantage	Disadvantage
Continuous-wave Doppler	• There is no aliasing • Able to measure very high velocities	• Operator cannot select vessel to sample • The signal may have come from any vessel inside the large sample volume • Must assume 0° angle
Pulsed-wave Doppler	• Depth of sample volume is operator selectable • User is able to select a specific vessel and sample volume size • Allows for angle-correction to more accurately measure velocities	• Limited by aliasing • Limited depth and velocity range

Review of Doppler Controls

Numerous controls are used to manipulate the spectral waveform to aid in diagnosis and interpretation. The range gate, already mentioned in previous sections, is on the cursor used in PW Doppler and placed in the vessel where sampling is desired. The size of the sample volume, the area within the range gate, may be controlled by increasing or decreasing the size of the gate. With CW Doppler, the sampling depth cannot be selected. However, there is a user-controllable cursor that is placed over the area to be sampled. The sample volume, which is not user controllable with CW Doppler, is larger than PW Doppler and may encompass several blood vessels.

Angle-correction is used with PW Doppler to more accurately calculate the velocities from the frequency shifts. The cosine (θ) portion of the Doppler equation is for the angle-correction component (Table 4-15), in which "θ" is the angle between the Doppler beam and flow. If performing Doppler on a vessel that lies at a 0° angle to the beam, then no angle-correction is needed. The 0° angle also provides the most accurate velocity measurements. However, in most clinical practices angles between 30° and 60° are often used. The higher the Doppler angle, the greater the degree of potential error in the measurement. Angles greater than 60° exhibit an unacceptably high rate of velocity measurement error, and therefore should be avoided. When using a linear transducer, the Doppler cursor can be steered to center, left or right. Some machines enable the operator to specify the angle of the steer (eg, 15° vs. 20°). The advantage of steering is that it permits the operator to keep the angle-correction at or below 60° by changing the steer angle. In transducers where the steer angle itself cannot be adjusted, the operator may have to "heel" or "toe" the transducer to properly angle-correct. The operator must always try to avoid a 90° angle to flow when sampling a vessel (Figure 4-48). Table 4-23 provides some vital Doppler rules to remember.

SOUND OFF
The deeper the blood vessel, the lower the PRF, and subsequently the higher the risk of aliasing.

The scale, or Doppler PRF setting on the machine, represents the sampling rate of the Doppler. The sampling rate must be fast enough in order to accurately plot the frequency shifts, or aliasing will occur. The Doppler PRF (scale) is determined by the sample volume depth. The deeper the blood vessel, the lower the PRF, and subsequently the higher the risk of aliasing. Likewise, when sampling vessels with high frequency shifts (which are directly related to the velocities), the PRF needs to be increased to keep sampling at an adequate rate. If the frequency shift is greater than one half of the PRF (the Nyquist limit), then aliasing will occur. When sampling vessels with slow or hard-to-find flow, the PRF needs to be decreased in order to make the waveform bigger on the screen. A small waveform relative to the spectral display window is poor technique and does not allow for accurate measurements when needed. Typically, the spectral waveform should occupy two thirds of the spectral display window (Figure 4-49).

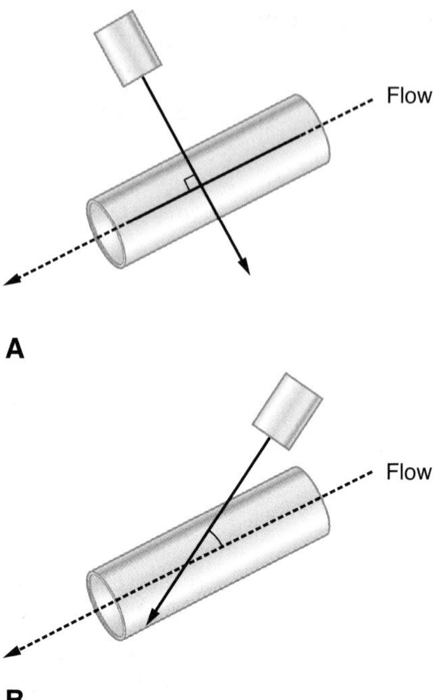

Figure 4-48 Proper steering of the Doppler gate. **A.** Notice that steering 90° to flow produces an "X," as in "incorrect." **B.** The correct angle should be equal to or preferably less than 60°.

Occasionally, when a vessel with a high velocity or a deep vessel needs to be imaged, the PRF cannot sample at a sufficient rate. Some ultrasound systems solve this dilemma with the use of a high PRF (HPRF) setting, which allows the machine to ignore the **depth ambiguity** problem. When the machine goes into HPRF mode, multiple range gates appear on the screen, signifying that the machine is not sure where the pulse is coming from, and could have originated from anywhere along the Doppler cursor (Figure 4-50).

TABLE 4-23 Doppler rules

Rules of Doppler—Know These!
• 0° is the most accurate angle—the degree of error increases as the angle increases • Never use an angle greater than 60° • At 90° the Doppler shift is at its lowest • At 0° the Doppler shift is at its highest

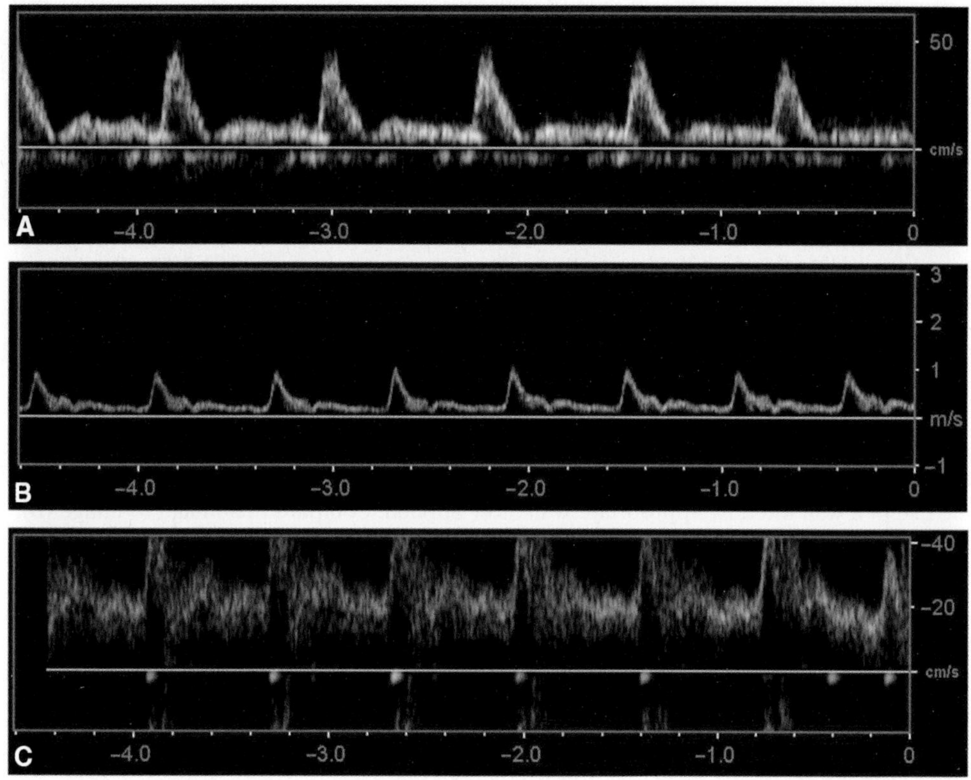

Figure 4-49 Adjusting the pulse repetition frequency (PRF). **A.** Scale or PRF set so that the waveform takes up approximately two-thirds of spectral window. **B.** Scale or PRF too high, and thus the waveform is too small. **C.** Scale or PRF too low, causing aliasing.

SOUND OFF
When using the wall filter, care must be taken to not eliminate useful diastolic information from the spectral display.

The **wall filter** is a Doppler control used to eliminate the low-frequency signals caused by wall or heart valve motion. Movement of the heart muscle or vessel walls causes a low-frequency, high-amplitude signal that appears on the spectral display as low-level acoustic **noise**, or **clutter**. Noise takes away from the image and does not contribute useful information and is therefore filtered out with the wall filter. Other names for the wall filter are high-pass and wall-thump filter. In general sonography and vascular imaging, wall motion is not a common concern, so the wall filter is kept low. In cardiac imaging, a high wall filter is

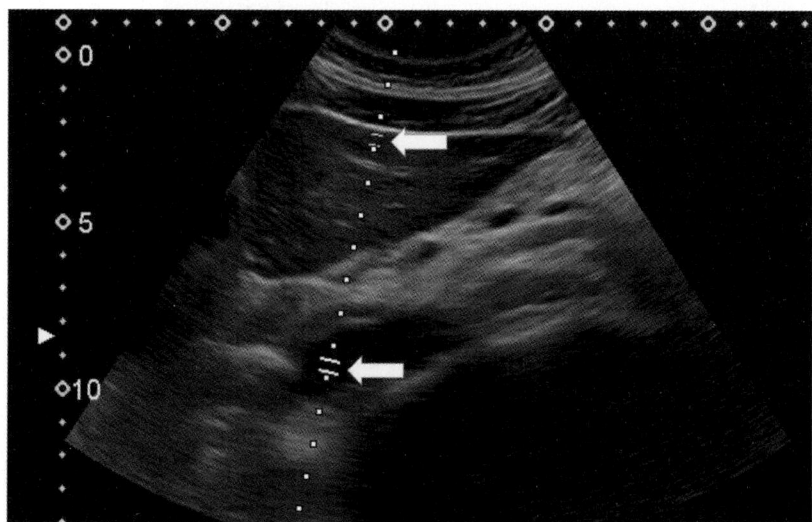

Figure 4-50 High-pulse repetition frequency (HPRF) setting. HPRF occurs when the scale is set so high that depth ambiguity occurs. Extra "fake" gates (*arrows*) are placed along the spectral cursor to signify the lack of depth information.

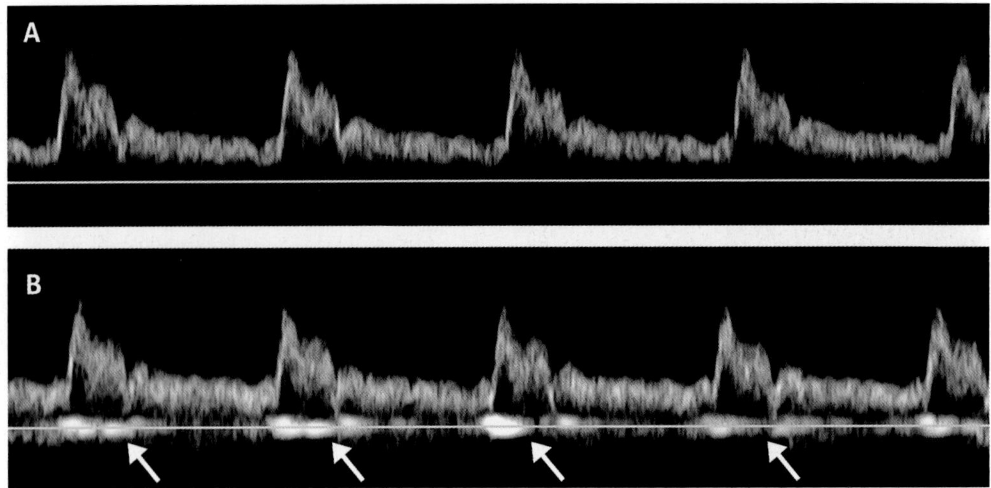

Figure 4-51 The use of a wall filter. **A.** Appropriate wall filter applied. Compare this image to image **(B)**. **B.** The hyperechoic noise along the zero-flow baseline is called **clutter** (*arrows*). Clutter should be removed with a wall filter (high-pass) setting that does not eliminate important diastolic information.

used to counteract the low-frequency, high-amplitude signal coming from the movement of the heart muscle and valves. Caution should be used when applying the wall filter so that useful diastolic information is not inadvertently removed from the spectral display (Figure 4-51).

Just as the PRF of the Doppler is separate from the PRF of the B-mode image, the gain of the spectral display can be set independent of the B-mode gain. The brightness of the envelope of the spectral display corresponds to the amplitude of the Doppler shift. If the spectral signal is weak, the gain can be increased to improve visualization of the signal. If the spectral gain is too high, it may cause over-measurement of the spectral waveform, so it is imperative that the gain be set to an appropriate level. Spectral gain that is too high will also cause spectral broadening, and the window underneath the envelope will be lost (Figure 4-52).

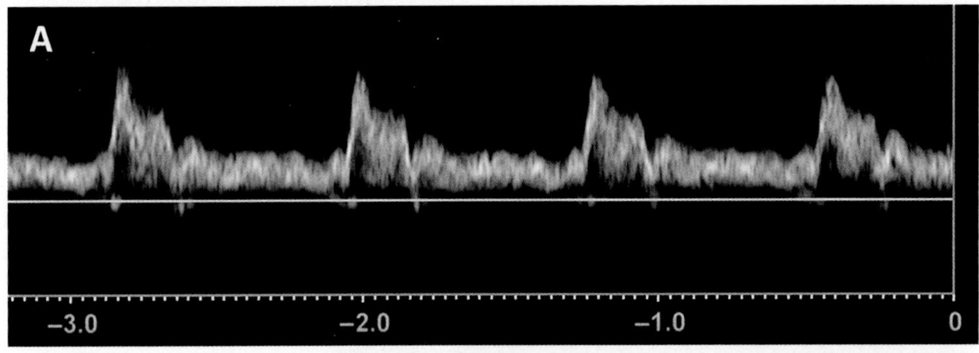

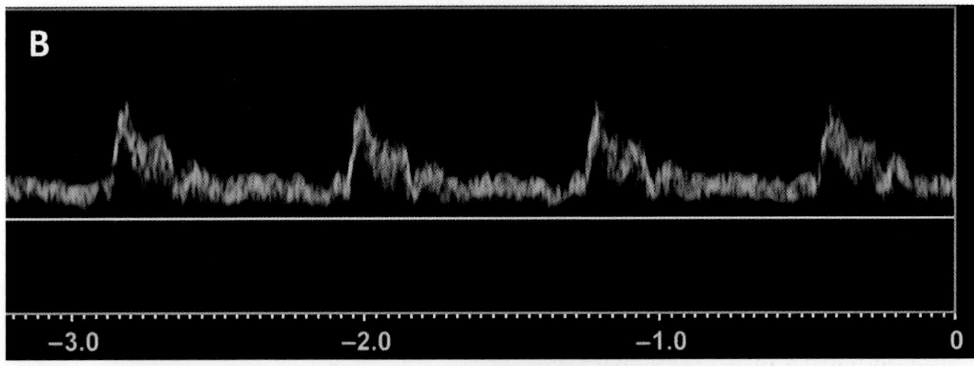

Figure 4-52 Spectral gain. **A.** Overgaining the spectral display will result in overmeasurement of the velocities and spectral broadening. **B.** Decreasing the spectral gain eliminates the spectral broadening.

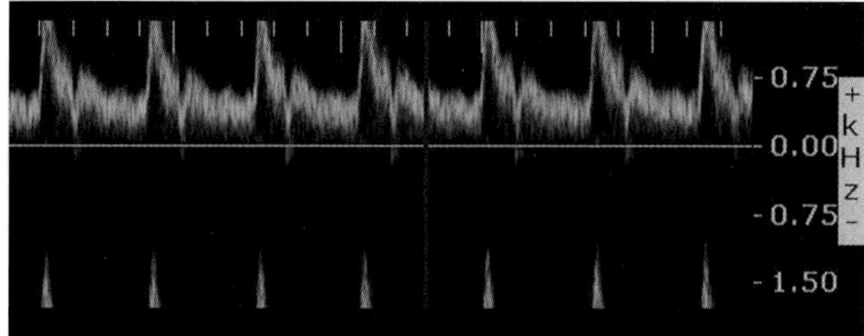

A

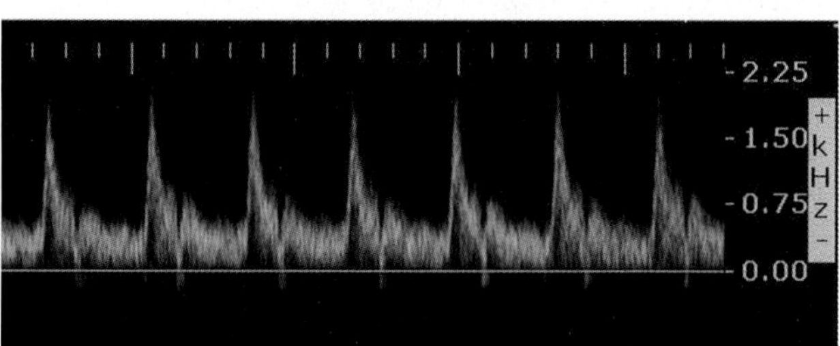

B

Figure 4-53 Adjusting the zero-flow baseline. If the zero-flow baseline is too high **(A),** there appears to be aliasing. Lowering the zero-flow baseline will eliminate the appearance of aliasing. With the zero-flow baseline lowered, the aliasing disappears **(B)**. Keep in mind that if the frequency shift, 2000 Hz in this case **(B)**, is greater than one half the pulse repetition frequency, then there is still aliasing, even if you appear to eliminate it by lowering the zero-flow baseline.

The **zero-flow baseline**, (or **baseline)**, is the movable dividing line that separates positive from negative Doppler shifts. Its location is determined by the operator based on the study being performed, although if the zero-flow baseline is too high, aliasing may be seen. Lowering the zero-flow baseline will resolve this problem, although if the Doppler shift is greater than the Nyquist limit, aliasing will still be present even if lowering the zero-flow baseline appears to eliminate the problem (Figure 4-53).

Color Doppler Imaging

Color Doppler imaging (CDI), which is a PW technique, is the color representation of the Doppler shift information superimposed on the grayscale image. CDI provides information pertaining to both the direction and mean velocity of the flow. **Autocorrelation** is the processing technique used to obtain the color flow information, but it does not have the accuracy of FFT. Therefore, CDI only provides mean velocity information, and not maximum/minimum velocities.

SOUND OFF
Autocorrelation is the processing technique used to obtain color flow information.

CDI also uses a larger gate than spectral Doppler, a gate that is made up of many scan lines proportional to the width of the gate. Color information is obtained at many points along each scan line and each pulse packet is checked for movement by searching for frequency shifts. Moving reflectors are specified as a color and nonmoving reflectors are specified as a shade of gray.

The **ensemble length**, also known as the **packet size**, is the number of pulses per scan line within the color gate. The higher the ensemble length, the more sampling points along each scan line, and therefore, the higher the sensitivity of the color signal. High ensemble lengths increase the ability to detect slow flow and offer a more accurate mean velocity. Unfortunately, this is at the expense of the frame rate that is decreased with high ensemble lengths. The ensemble length can be as low as 3 pulses per scan line but is typically around 10 to 20 pulses per scan line. Another disadvantage of high ensemble lengths is the machine's inability to detect rapidly changing hemodynamic events secondary to the longer acquisition time. CDI is inherently slow, and large gates and/or high ensemble lengths slow it down even further. For the best frame rate, the smallest color gate should always be employed (Table 4-24).

SOUND OFF
The ensemble length can be as low as 3 pulses per scan line but is typically around 10 to 20 pulses per scan line.

SOUND OFF
In cardiac imaging, the color scale is thought of as *BART*: *b*lue *a*way, *r*ed *t*oward. However, for other studies, the color scale can be inverted so that blue is toward and red is away.

The color Doppler scale shows direction of flow as a color or range of colors on each side of a black baseline. Black within a color display means that either there was no Doppler shift present in that location (as a result of either a 90° angle to flow or no flow), or the shift was so low that it was eliminated by wall filters. In general

TABLE 4-24 Ensemble length and color Doppler

Results of Higher Ensemble Lengths
• More pulses per scan line • More sensitive to slow flow • More accurate mean velocity • Slower frame rate (temporal resolution)

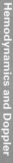

and vascular imaging, the color scale is often set by convention, so that red represents arteries and blue represents veins. In cardiac imaging, the color scale can be remembered by using the acronym **BART**: *b*lue *a*way, *r*ed *t*oward. However, the color scale can be inverted, so that blue is toward and red is away (**RABT**). The preferred color scale setting may vary from lab to lab.

> **SOUND OFF**
> There are three main components of color imaging: hue, saturation, and brightness (or luminance).

The color scale is most commonly presented in **velocity mode**, where the colors are vertically oriented for positive/negative shifts. An older cardiac imaging mode, no longer widely used, is **variance mode** (Figure 4-54), where colors are represented vertically and shades of green are oriented horizontally to denote the presence of turbulence.

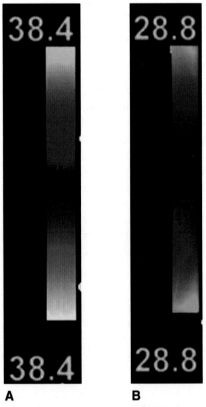

Figure 4-54 The color Doppler scale. **A.** In a blue-away, red-toward (BART) velocity scale, flow toward the transducer is displayed in red, above the baseline (*the black line separating the colors*), whereas flow away from the transducer is displayed in blue, below the baseline. If the scale is inverted, the colors will be red-away, blue-toward (RABT). The scale shown is a RABT color scale. **B.** This image is the variance color scale. Although no longer commonly used, the green in the scale signifies turbulence.

There are three main components of the color imaging: **hue**, **saturation**, and **brightness** (or **luminance**). The hue of a color is the color itself as determined by its wavelength. A color can be made to appear lighter by adding white to it. Saturation is how much white is added compared to the original color. The less white in the color, the more saturated it is. Pink, for example, is less saturated than red. The brightness of the color is how intense the color is and related to the amplitude of the signal. One of the more challenging aspects of CDI is identifying direction of color flow just by looking at the image and the color scale. Figure 4-55 shows a novel way of determining direction of flow.

> **SOUND OFF**
> Increasing the persistence setting reduces the effect of noise and makes it easier to follow small vessels. The drawback of high persistence is a decrease in the frame rate.

Color Aliasing

As a PW technique, CDI is bound by the same limitation as PW spectral Doppler. Therefore, aliasing can occur. Aliasing on CDI is represented by a wraparound of the color scale (Figure 4-56). As with spectral Doppler, aliasing can be eliminated by increasing the PRF, or scale. Appropriate setting of the color PRF allows for setting the proper sensitivity to flow. Low PRF color settings are used for slow or difficult-to-demonstrate flow, and high PRF settings are used for fast flow and also to eliminate aliasing. In addition to PRF, color Doppler also has a gain setting, and it is imperative that the gain is set properly. If the color gain is set too high, the result is color noise throughout the color gate, and color "bleeding" or "blossoming" outside of the vessel (Figure 4-57). If the color gain is set too low, the vessel will not be adequately filled with color.

In the presence of very slow flow, or if small vessels are being analyzed, it may be helpful to average multiple frames instead of displaying only one frame of color information at a time. Increasing the **color persistence** setting reduces the effect of noise and makes it easier to follow small vessels. The drawback of high persistence is a decrease in the frame rate.

When both grayscale and color information are present within the same pixel, **color priority** is a setting on the machine that allows the operator to set a threshold for displaying color pixels instead of grayscale pixels. A pixel—the smallest component of a sonographic image—can be either a color or shade of gray, not both at the same time. Priority sets the threshold that the amplitude (ie, brightness of the shade of gray) will have to exceed in order for grayscale pixels to be displayed rather than color pixels. Below that threshold, color pixels will be

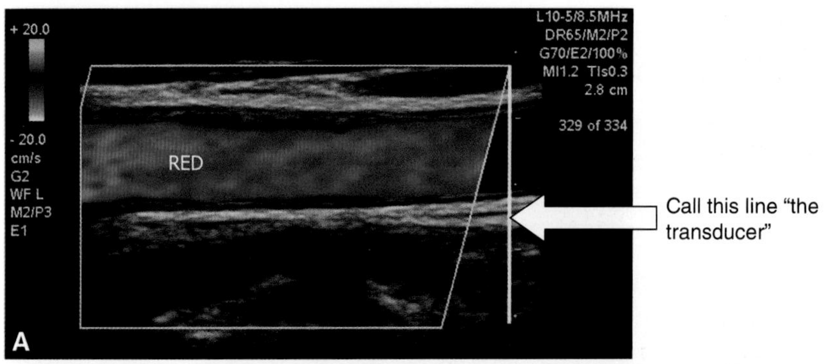

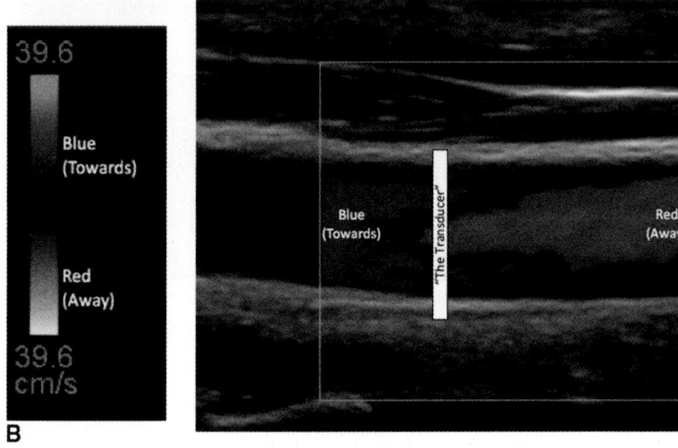

Figure 4-55 How to determine the direction of flow. **A.** With a steered gate, draw a line from the overhanging corner of the Doppler gate. Call this "the transducer" for the sake of this demonstration. Notice how the blood flow in this vessel is red. Look at the color scale: red is "away from the transducer." Therefore, flow is moving in a direction away from the line that represents the transducer, or toward the left of the screen. **B.** When there is a non-steered-gate, first look at the color scale. In this case, red is "away" and blue is "toward." Now imagine a line in the center of the vessel, where blue changes to red. Call this line "the transducer." Look at the blue and move your finger on the image toward the "transducer." Move your finger on the red part of the image away from the "transducer." See the direction of flow? In this example it is left to right on the image. Blue is toward the imaginary "transducer" and red is away.

placed. If the priority is set too low, then image noise or artifacts within the vessel will be displayed instead of color pixels. A higher priority setting is useful in filling a vessel with color when there is a low signal-to-noise ratio.

Tissue Doppler Imaging

Specifically used for cardiac imaging, **tissue Doppler imaging** (TDI) is another CDI technique. Flowing blood typically produces a low-amplitude, high-velocity signal. However, myocardial wall motion produces a high-amplitude, low-velocity signal. Instead of using a high-pass filter to filter out the signal from the wall motion, TDI uses a low-pass filter to eliminate the signal from the blood and only show color information representing the wall motion. TDI is still limited by frequency shifts at 90° angles; but because the myocardial walls are oriented 0° to the beam in some views, this is not a limitation. TDI can be performed with color Doppler and spectral Doppler display modes (Figure 4-58).

Figure 4-56 Color Doppler aliasing. Aliasing on color Doppler imaging is represented by a wraparound of the color scale. The arrow is pointing to the aliasing appearing within the blood vessel.

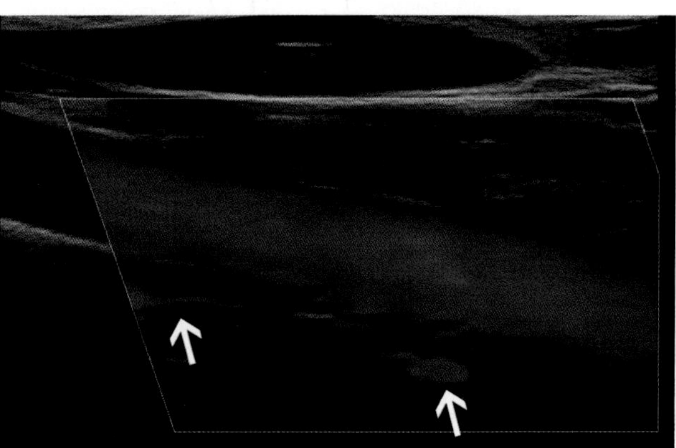

Figure 4-57 The color "bleeding" or "blossoming" artifact (*arrows*) occurs when the color gain is set too high. Decreasing the color gain reduces the artifact.

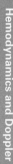

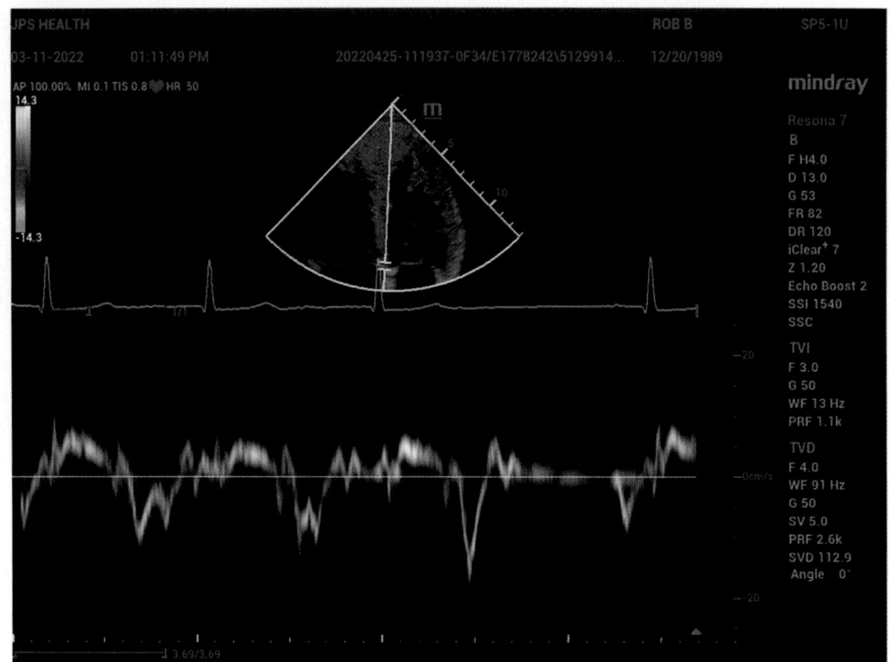

Figure 4-58 Tissue Doppler imaging of the heart from a normal subject (Image courtesy of Mindray North America).

> **SOUND OFF**
> Both an advantage and a disadvantage of power Doppler is its sensitivity. Because power Doppler is very sensitive, it is ideal for slow, small vessels, but it also makes it more susceptible to patient or organ motion.

Power Doppler

PW spectral and color Doppler are limited by flow at 90° angles, because the frequency shift on which the flow information is based is equal to 0 at that critical angle. **Power Doppler**, also termed *color Doppler energy, amplitude Doppler,* or *color power angio*, ignores the frequency shift information and focuses only on the amplitude, or strength, of the shift. Power Doppler is only able to display amplitude information and does not provide information on velocity or direction of flow (Figure 4-59). Power Doppler is almost completely independent of angle, which makes it useful for evaluating slow flowing and/or tortuous vessels. Both an advantage and a disadvantage of power Doppler is its sensitivity. Because power Doppler is very sensitive, it is ideal for

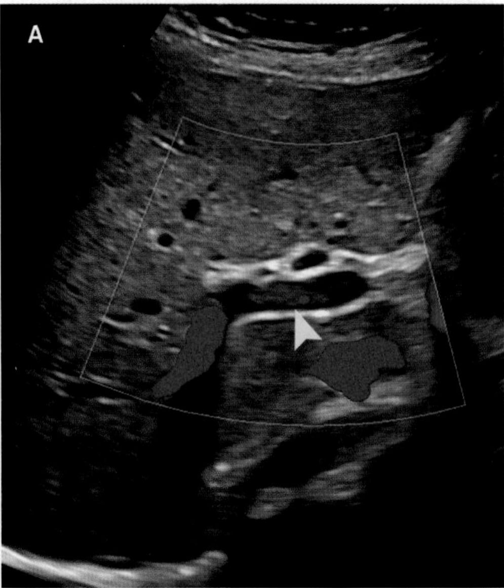

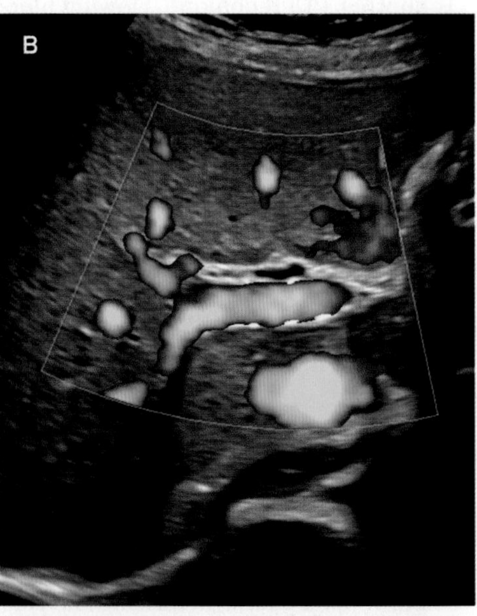

Figure 4-59 Comparison of color flow and power Doppler. **A.** Transverse image of the porta hepatis (liver). There is no Doppler shift at a 90° angle, so no flow appears in the portal veins (*yellow arrowhead*). **B.** Power Doppler is almost completely independent of angle, so in this image the portal veins are visualized well.

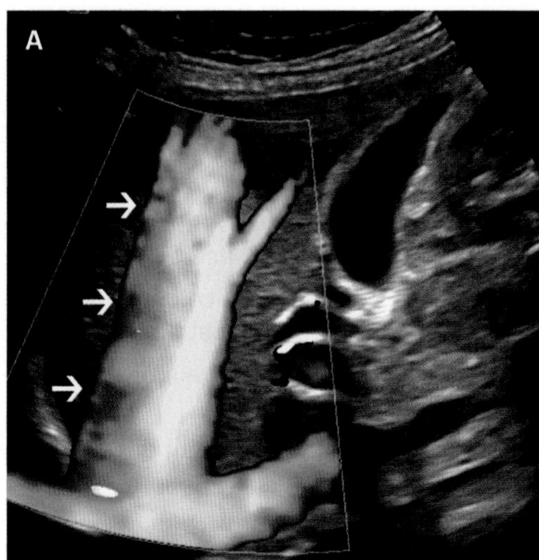

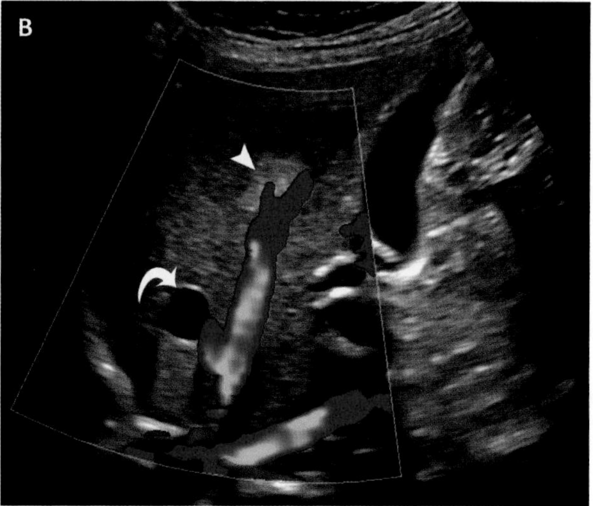

Figure 4-60 **A.** Power Doppler image of the liver in long-axis. Flash artifact (*arrows*) is obscuring pathology, seen on color Doppler imaging. **B.** Color Doppler image of the liver demonstrating a liver neoplasm (*arrowhead*) and a cyst (*curved arrow*) that were missed owing to the flash artifact.

slow, small vessels, but it also makes it more susceptible to patient or organ motion. **Flash artifact** occurs when power Doppler is being used and the signal created by nearby motion obscures part of the image (Figure 4-60).

Cardiac Strain and Strain Rate

Cardiac strain and strain rate are used for measuring myocardial function. **Strain** is the changing of the shape of the muscle as it lengthens and contracts. Strain and strain-rate analysis permit evaluation of the deformation of the cardiac wall to evaluate for ventricular function. **Speckle tracking** is the method used to obtain the strain information. By observing the "dots" that represent the myocardial tissue, the machine can measure the movement of the tissue in the longitudinal, radial, and circumferential axes (Figure 4-61).

Doppler Artifacts

Table 4-25 provides a summary of several common Doppler artifacts and how to correct them.

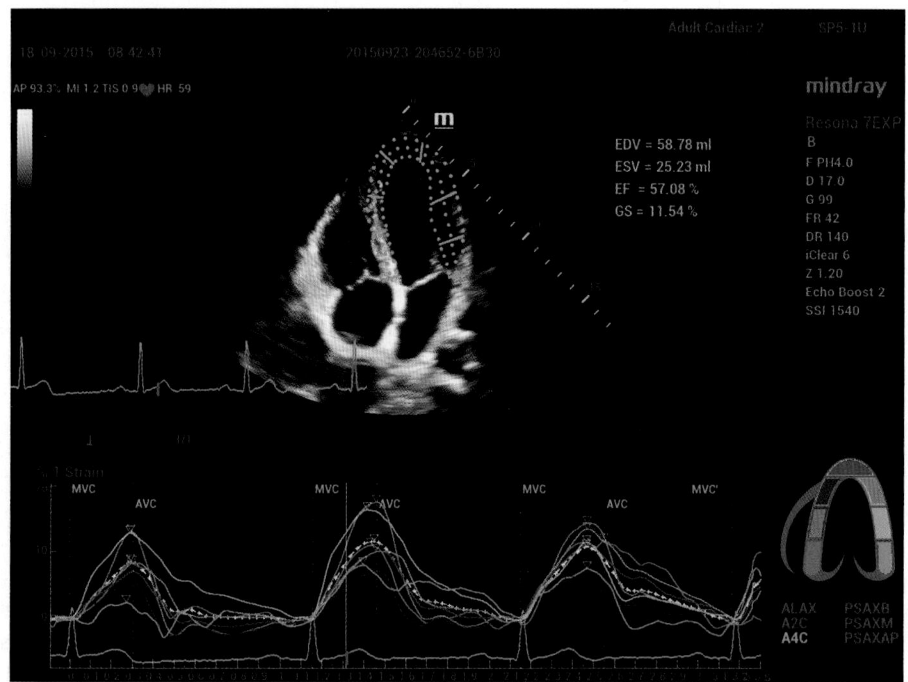

Figure 4-61 Left ventricular strain derived from a three-dimensional data set (Image courtesy of Mindray North America).

Hemodynamics and Doppler

TABLE 4-25 Doppler artifacts, their definitions, and means to fix the image

Artifact	Definition	Quick Fix
Clutter (Figure 4-51)	Acoustic noise along the zero-flow baseline that is eliminated with high-pass wall filters	Increase wall filter
Aliasing (Figure 4-56)	Pulsed-wave artifact caused by insufficient sampling of flow	Increase PRF, decrease frequency shift, or use CW
Mirror image (Figure 4-62)	Reproduction of spectral or color information opposite a strong reflector	Decrease color/spectral gain or angle (must be <90°)
Color bleeding (Figure 4-57)	Overgained color or spectral waveform causing signal to be larger than it should be	Decrease gain or transmit power
High PRF (depth/range ambiguity, Figure 4-50)	HPRF setting in PW Doppler means the PW is emulating a CW probe and is unsure of where echoes came from	Change depth or Doppler angle
Flash artifact (Figure 4-60)	Excessive color signal in surrounding tissue caused by movement during power Doppler	If possible, eliminate source of motion (eg, with a breath hold)

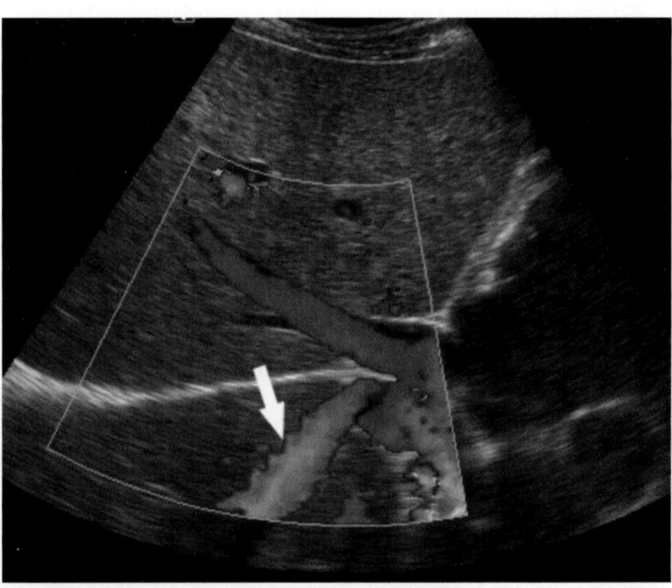

Figure 4-62 Color Doppler mirror image. The arrow is indicating a mirror image of the hepatic vein.

REVIEW QUESTIONS

1. What provides the potential energy in the cardiovascular system?
   a. Distal arterioles
   b. Blood flowing through the vessels
   c. Beating heart
   d. Venous system

2. A "color" (red, blue, green) is called a __________.
   a. saturation
   b. hue
   c. dialect
   d. luminance

3. What is the name of the blunted flow profile that is seen at the entrance of large vessels?
   a. Plug flow
   b. Laminar flow
   c. Turbulent flow
   d. Chaotic flow

4. What does increasing the PRF/scale setting on a spectral Doppler do?
   a. Increases the potential of aliasing
   b. Decreases the potential of aliasing
   c. Makes the spectral waveform appear larger
   d. Optimizes the system to detect slow flow

5. Which of the following is seen with CW instrumentation?
   a. Transducer frequency matches that of the oscillator
   b. Sample depth can be determined by a range gate
   c. Very short pulses are used
   d. Aliasing limits velocity measurements

6. When is the Doppler shift highest?
   a. When the beam is at a 45° angle to flow
   b. When the beam is perpendicular to the direction of flow
   c. When the beam is parallel to the direction of flow
   d. Doppler shift is unrelated to the beam angle

7. Which of the following will eliminate aliasing?
   a. Decreasing the PRF
   b. Increasing the Nyquist limit above the frequency shift
   c. Increasing the sample depth
   d. Increasing the frequency shift above the Nyquist limit

8. When a reflector moves toward the transducer, what will happen to the reflected frequency?
   a. Increase
   b. Decrease
   c. Stay the same
   d. It is not possible to predict

9. From a hemodynamics standpoint, which of the following has to be increased in order to see an increase in flow volume?
   a. Pressure difference
   b. Resistance
   c. Vessel length
   d. Viscosity

10. Adjusting which of the following will have no effect on the measured frequency shift?
   a. Flow velocity
   b. Operating frequency
   c. Amplitude
   d. Propagation speed

11. Which of the following is representative of Ohm's law?
   a. $V = IR$
   b. $I = R/V$
   c. $R = I/V$
   d. $R = VI$

12. What is the point at which Reynolds number predicts turbulence?
   a. 500
   b. 1200
   c. 2000
   d. 4000

13. In order to maintain volume flow as a constant, if the area of a vessel increases what must happen to the velocity?
   a. It increases
   b. It decreases
   c. It does not change with changes in area
   d. Not enough information

14. Venous blood returns to the heart from the lower extremities through all of the following EXCEPT:
   a. Calf muscle pump
   b. Inspiration
   c. Expiration
   d. Venous valves

15. In a standing patient, where is the hydrostatic pressure the highest?
   a. In the feet
   b. In the arms
   c. In the abdomen
   d. Near the heart

16. A stenosis of 75% in area is equal to what percent of stenosis in diameter?
   a. 25%
   b. 50%
   c. 75%
   d. 100%

17. An arterial waveform that has flow above and below the zero-flow baseline is properly referred to as
   a. Monophasic
   b. Tardus parvus
   c. Low-resistance
   d. Multiphasic

18. Which of the following will be seen with a stationary reflector?
   a. There is a higher reflected frequency compared with the incident frequency
   b. There is a lower reflected frequency compared with the incident frequency
   c. The incident frequency is equal to the reflected frequency
   d. The reflected intensity is higher than the incident intensity

19. What happens as the frequency of the transducer increases?
    a. Penetration ability is increased
    b. The amount of scatter is increased
    c. The frequency shift is decreased
    d. The amount of attenuation is decreased

20. What occurs as the Doppler angle is increased?
    a. It decreases the frequency shift
    b. It increases the frequency shift
    c. It increases the risk for aliasing
    d. It improves the accuracy of the velocity calculation

21. What component of the ultrasound machine is used to detect positive versus negative frequency shifts?
    a. Analog Doppler
    b. Oscillator
    c. Fourier transformer
    d. Phase quadrature

22. Which of the following is true for CW Doppler devices?
    a. It only needs to have one piezoelectric element
    b. It must have at least two piezoelectric elements
    c. It must have three piezoelectric elements
    d. No piezoelectric elements are needed for CW Doppler

23. Which of the following will result in aliasing?
    a. Too low an operating frequency
    b. Increased sampling of the blood flow
    c. Undersampling of the blood flow
    d. Too high a Doppler angle

24. Which mathematical processing technique is used to analyze the data and produce a spectral waveform?
    a. Amplitude shifting
    b. Autocorrelation
    c. Amplitude sampling
    d. Fast Fourier transform

25. Which of the following represents the resistive index?
    a. Peak systolic velocity minus the end diastolic velocity divided by the mean velocity
    b. End diastolic velocity minus the peak systolic velocity divided by the peak systolic velocity
    c. Peak systolic velocity minus the end diastolic velocity divided by the peak systolic velocity
    d. Peak systolic velocity minus the end diastolic velocity divided by the end diastolic velocity

26. What does the brightness of the dots that make up the spectral display represent?
    a. The number of red blood cells present
    b. The velocity of the signal
    c. The frequency shift
    d. The amount of turbulence present

27. Which of the following describes the principle that an object at rest will stay at rest unless acted on by an outside force?
    a. Laminar flow
    b. Inertia
    c. Friction
    d. Bernoulli

28. In order to add more spectral Doppler waveforms to the display, what setting on the machine should be adjusted?
    a. PRF
    b. Sweep speed
    c. Heart rate
    d. Gain

29. Which of the following may result if the spectral Doppler gain is too high?
    a. Too much output power sent into the patient
    b. Undermeasurement of the velocities
    c. Overmeasurement of the velocities
    d. An image that is too dark

30. The Doppler shift is lowest at what angle to flow?
    a. 0°
    b. 45°
    c. 60°
    d. 90°

31. Which signal processing technique used for color Doppler is not as accurate as, but is faster than the technique used for spectral Doppler?
    a. Zero crossing
    b. Phase quadrature
    c. Autocorrelation
    d. Fast Fourier transform

32. A low-pass filter is used for what Doppler imaging technology?
    a. CW Doppler
    b. Power Doppler
    c. Color Doppler
    d. Tissue Doppler imaging

33. Which type of Doppler does not rely on the frequency shift but instead relies on the amplitude (strength) of the shift?
    a. Spectral Doppler
    b. Power Doppler
    c. Color Doppler imaging
    d. CW Doppler

34. What is it called when the 2D image, color Doppler image, and spectral Doppler are displayed simultaneously?
   a. Duplex mode
   b. Triplex mode
   c. Phase quadrature mode
   d. Multiplex mode

35. What is the duty factor of CW Doppler?
   a. 100%
   b. 100
   c. 0.01
   d. 1%

36. Which of the following is true about CW Doppler?
   a. The measured frequency shifts come from a user-selected depth
   b. A range gate is placed in the vessel to be sampled
   c. There is a large sample volume that obtains signals from all vessels within
   d. Pulses of sound are sent into the tissue to measure the frequency shifts

37. When compared to 2D (grayscale) imaging, which of the following color Doppler statements is true?
   a. There is improved frame rate
   b. There is worse temporal resolution
   c. There are fewer pulses per scan line
   d. There is a higher frame rate

38. Which of the following statements is true?
   a. Aliasing occurs with color Doppler
   b. CW Doppler is unable to measure very high frequency shifts
   c. PW Doppler has no range resolution
   d. Power Doppler cannot be obtained at a 90° angle

39. Which of the following frequency shifts would exhibit aliasing if the PRF is 5000 Hz?
   a. 1.0 kHz
   b. 2.5 kHz
   c. 3.0 kHz
   d. 2.7 Hz

40. Which of the following is true about the frequency shift?
   a. It increases with an increase in Doppler angle
   b. It is typically greater than 20,000 Hz
   c. It is inversely related to operating frequency
   d. It is in the audible range of sound

41. What can be said about the ensemble length of color Doppler?
   a. It is less than 3 pulses per scan line
   b. It is more than 100 pulses per scan line
   c. It is about 10 to 20 pulses per scan line
   d. It is typically 0

42. What happens if blood flow is sampled in the center of laminar flow?
   a. There will be a higher velocity than if sampled toward the edges
   b. There will be a slower velocity than if sampled toward the edges
   c. It will be made up of many different velocities
   d. It will be turbulent

43. Which of the following is **false** about color Doppler imaging?
   a. It is prone to aliasing
   b. It obtains mean velocity information
   c. It uses autocorrelation as its signal processing technique
   d. It allows for measurement of peak systolic and end diastolic velocities

44. Which of the following is a property of power Doppler?
   a. Able to obtain velocity information and direction of flow
   b. Signal is obtained by detecting amplitude of shift
   c. It is prone to aliasing
   d. Limited by perpendicular angle of incidence

45. Assuming flow is constant, what happens in a region of blood vessel narrowing?
   a. There is a significant pressure increase
   b. There is an increase in the velocity along with a corresponding increase in pressure
   c. There is an increase in the velocity along with a corresponding decrease in pressure
   d. Velocity and pressure are unchanged

46. Which of the following is true about the spectral Doppler envelope?
   a. It is thin when there are many different velocities
   b. It is thin with CW Doppler
   c. It is thickened in the center of a laminar flow vessel
   d. It is thickened in the presence of turbulence

47. What is the term for the pressure difference between the inside of a vein and the tissue outside?
   a. Hydrostatic pressure
   b. Autocorrelation
   c. Transmural pressure
   d. Kinetic energy

48. What will a proximal stenosis look like on the spectral waveform?
   a. Reversal of flow in diastole
   b. Delay in the systolic upstroke
   c. Triphasic waveform
   d. Aliasing

49. The low velocity component is missing on a spectral waveform. Which of the following should be adjusted to fix this?
   a. Gain
   b. Scale
   c. High-pass filter
   d. Frequency

50. In the exercising patient, the distal arterioles are dilated. What type of flow pattern would most likely be demonstrated on spectral Doppler within the proximal vessels?
   a. Monophasic flow
   b. Multiphasic flow
   c. Reversal of flow
   d. Respiratory phasicity

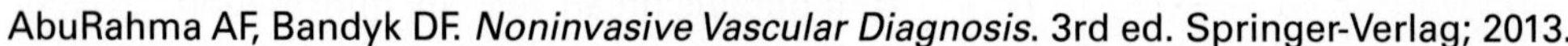

SUGGESTED READINGS

AbuRahma AF, Bandyk DF. *Noninvasive Vascular Diagnosis*. 3rd ed. Springer-Verlag; 2013.

Belloni FL. Teaching the principles of hemodynamics. *Adv Physiol Educ*. 1999;22(1):S187–S202.

Bushberg JT, Seibert JA, Leidholdt Jr. EM, Boone JM. *The Essential Physics of Medical Imaging*. 4th ed. Wolters Kluwer; 2021.

Daigle RJ. *Techniques in Non-Invasive Vascular Diagnosis*. 5th ed. Summer Publishing; 2023.

Edelman SK. *Understanding Ultrasound Physics*. 4th ed. ESP Inc.; 2012.

Fox TF. Arterial hemodynamics for the vascular sonographer. *Vasc Ultrasound Today*. 2008;8(13):159–176.

Gaiser R, Fox TB. *Vascular Technology Examination PREP*. 2nd ed. McGraw Hill; 2021.

Hedrick WR. *Technology for Diagnostic Sonography*. Mosby; 2013.

Kim Esther SH, Sharma AM, Scissons R, et al. Interpretation of peripheral arterial and venous Doppler waveforms: A consensus statement from the Society for Vascular Medicine and Society for Vascular Ultrasound. *Vasc Med*. 2020;25(5):484–506.

Kremkau FW. *Diagnostic Ultrasound: Principles and Instruments*. 10th ed. Saunders; 2020.

Kupinski A. *The Vascular System* (Diagnostic Medical Sonography Series). 3rd ed. Wolters Kluwer; 2022.

Miele F. *Ultrasound Physics and Instrumentation*. 6th ed. Miele Enterprises; 2022.

Milnor WR. *Hemodynamics*. 2nd ed. Williams & Wilkins; 1989.

Oh JK, Seward TB, Tajik AJ. *The Echo Manual*. Wolters Kluwer; 2007.

Pellerito J, Polak JF. *Introduction to Vascular Ultrasonography*. 7th ed. Elsevier; 2020.

Rumwell C, McPharlin M. *Vascular Technology: An Illustrated Review*. 5th ed. Davies; 2014.

Taylor KJ, Burns PN, Wells NT. *Clinical Applications of Doppler Ultrasound*. Raven Press; 1988.

Thrush A, Hartshorne T. *Vascular Ultrasound: How, Why, and When*. 3rd ed. Elsevier; 2009.

Zierler RE, Dawson D. *Duplex Scanning in Vascular Disorders*. 5th ed. Wolters Kluwer; 2015.

5

Quality Assurance and Lab Accreditation

Outline

Introduction

A quality assurance program in the sonography department is critical to system accuracy and patient care. It must be completed on a routine schedule. Preventative maintenance may be performed semiannually or annually. Several testing phantoms exist to ensure correct equipment operation. The primary objective for completing quality assurance is the confirmation that image quality is optimal and that subtle changes in function are detected.

Key Terms

axial resolution—the ability to accurately identify reflectors that are arranged parallel to the ultrasound beam

contrast resolution—the ability to differentiate tissues with similar shades of gray

Doppler phantom—the test object used to evaluate the flow direction, the depth capability or penetration of the Doppler beam, and the accuracy of the sample volume location and measured velocity

dropout—defect in image that appears as a shadow emanating from the very top of the image

elevational plane—the resolution in the "third dimension" of the beam or the slice-thickness plane

gold standard—the test that all other tests are compared to for statistical analysis. Considered to be the "best test" for that type of exam

horizontal calibration—the ability to place echoes in the proper location horizontally and perpendicular to the sound beam

lab accreditation—a voluntary process that acknowledges an organization's competency and credibility according to standards and essentials set forth by a reliable source

lateral resolution—the ability to accurately identify reflectors that are arranged perpendicular to the ultrasound beam

preventative maintenance—a methodical way of evaluating equipment's performance on a routine basis to ensure proper and accurate equipment function

quality assurance program—a planned program consisting of scheduled equipment-testing activities that confirm the correct performance of equipment

quality improvement—a continuous process of evaluation, feedback, and skills development that occurs in the ultrasound lab

registration—the ability to place echoes in the correct location

sample volume—the area within the range gate where Doppler signals are obtained

sensitivity—the ability of a system to display low-level or weak echoes

slice-thickness phantom—the test object that evaluates the elevational resolution, or the thickness portion, of the sound beam perpendicular to the imaging plane

tissue-equivalent phantom—the test object that mimics the acoustic properties of human tissue and is used to ensure proper equipment performance

vertical depth calibration—the distance from the transducer

QUALITY ASSURANCE

The practice of modern medicine is supposed to be evidence based, meaning based on research backed by scientific proof. A sonography lab is only as accurate as the equipment within that lab and the people performing and interpreting the studies produced. For that reason, a **quality assurance (QA) program** is essential for ensuring that a lab is producing quality work and ensuring high-quality accuracy and patient care. An ultrasound lab QA program should include the development of an accredited lab, which includes equipment testing performed by biomedical engineers, maintenance and documentation of appropriate sonographer credentials, and evaluation of statistical data related to lab performance. A quality improvement (QI) program should also be part of an ultrasound lab. A QI program is essential to ensure that sonographers perform to a set standard and that their work is evaluated routinely by the interpreting physician or other designee. Lab accreditation organizations recommend a QA program to maintain the standard for lab quality set by the guidelines of that accreditation body.

> **SOUND OFF**
> A QA program is essential for ensuring that a lab is producing quality work and discovering deficiencies in equipment. QI is related to the quality of the scans produced and ensures continuous feedback and training.

QA programs in ultrasound labs include annual testing performed by a biomedical engineer or similarly trained service person (see the Performance Testing section). In addition, there are everyday duties that the sonographers should be performing, such as inspecting the machines and transducers for physical damage. This includes the probe housing, cable connector, face of the transducer, and the power cord of the machine. Any problems with the probe, image, or machine should be reported and the equipment should be taken out of service. Table 5-1 lists the items that should be checked along with the frequency of inspection. Documentation of any testing or repairs that are performed should be kept by the lab supervisor.

TABLE 5-1 Quality assurance of equipment

QA Parameter	Frequency
Transducers: damaged, absent or separated strain reliever; missing insulation from cord; damaged/cracked housing; damaged face of the transducer; dropout or other problem with the image	Check equipment before every patient and report and image anomalies seen during scanning
Ultrasound machine: damaged display (color, brightness, etc); broken/locked brakes; damaged power cord; dust or grime (caked gel, blood, etc); buttons not working as expected; trackball problem	The machine should constantly be kept clean and free of dust; report any equipment malfunctions immediately
Machine: if user-accessible, filters should be vacuumed routinely	Monthly
Entire system: performance testing by a biomedical engineer or similarly trained service person	Annually

SOUND OFF
The American College of Radiology (ACR) describes the quality control (QC) tests that must be performed annually as well as peer-review requirements on their website at https://accreditationsupport.acr.org/support/home

STATISTICAL ANALYSIS

Labs that track performance should measure the statistics related to the quality of the lab. Table 5-2 is a list of metrics that a lab might use, including sensitivity, specificity, accuracy, etc. The data that determine these metrics are typically derived by comparing the ultrasound examination with a "gold standard." The gold standard for the purposes of medical imaging is that test by which all other tests are compared. For example, venous ultrasound is the gold standard for deep venous thrombosis (DVT) of the lower extremities, but first it had to prove it was at least as good as venography, but less invasive and without ionizing radiation. When there is a test that needs to be compared, a set number of studies are performed with both tests. The results are compared for **true positive** (both tests agree that the result is positive), **true negative** (both tests agree that the result is negative), **false positive** (the ultrasound thinks that the test is positive, but the gold standard reports it as negative), and **false negative** (the ultrasound thinks that the test is negative, but the gold standard reports it as positive). These results can be summed up in one table, called a **chi square** (Figure 5-1).

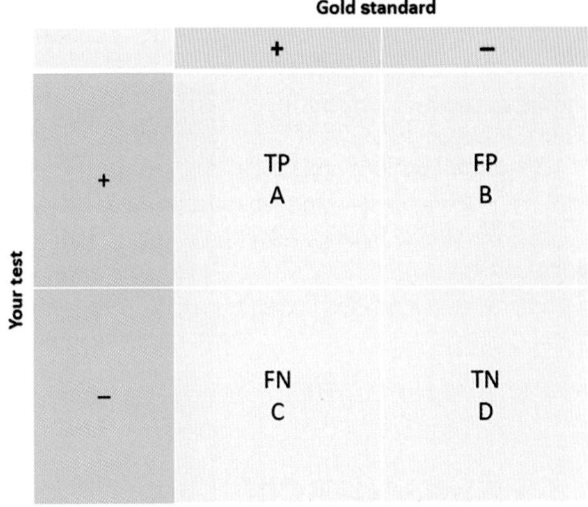

Figure 5-1 Chi square used in statistical analysis.

To calculate metrics using the chi square, first evaluate the results and compare them with the gold standard. Once the data are known, plug the results into the chi square and then do the math in Table 5-2. Figures 5-2 and 5-6 present a memory tip used by several authors in which the numerator in the equation is highlighted in some

TABLE 5-2 Statistical definitions

Term	Description
Gold standard	The imaging test that is considered the most accurate test for that particular study (eg, sonography is considered the gold standard to rule out deep venous thrombosis)
Sensitivity	How good is the test at finding positive exams? Aka the true positive rate. $$\text{PPV} = \frac{A}{A + C}$$
Specificity	How good is the test at deciding if an exam is normal? Aka the true negative rate. $$\text{PPV} = \frac{D}{D + B}$$
Positive predictive value (PPV)	How many abnormal (positive) exams your imaging test correctly identifies as positive? $$\text{PPV} = \frac{A}{A + B}$$
Negative predictive value (NPV)	How many normal (negative) exams your imaging test correctly identifies as normal? $$\text{PPV} = \frac{D}{D + C}$$
Accuracy	How good is a test overall? In other words, is the test good at finding positive and negative results? $$\text{Accuracy} = \frac{A + D}{A + B + C + D}$$
Reliability	Is the test consistent? Does it consistently provide accurate results?

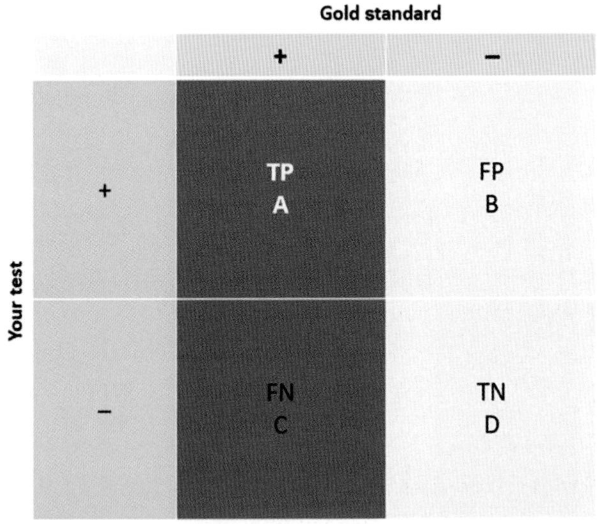

Figure 5-2 Chi-square equation for sensitivity.

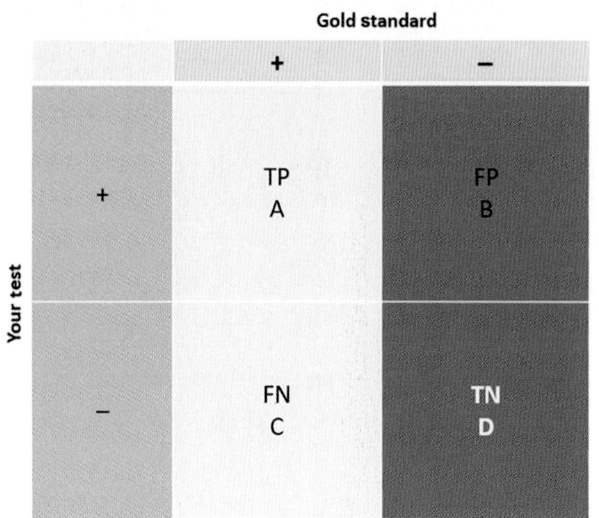

Figure 5-3 Chi-square equation for specificity.

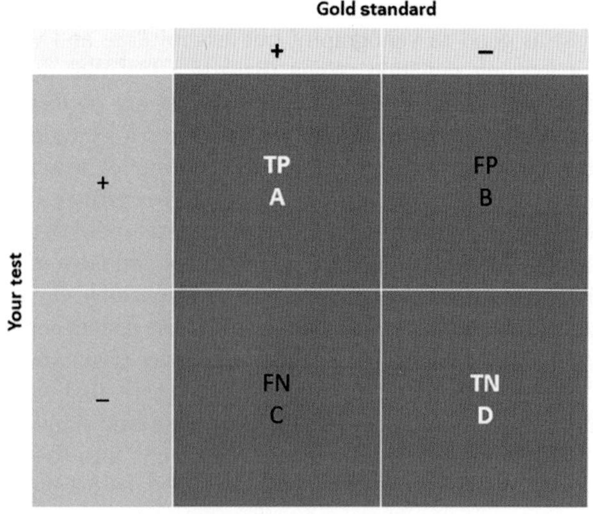

Figure 5-4 Chi-square equation for accuracy.

Figure 5-5 Chi-square equation for positive predictive value.

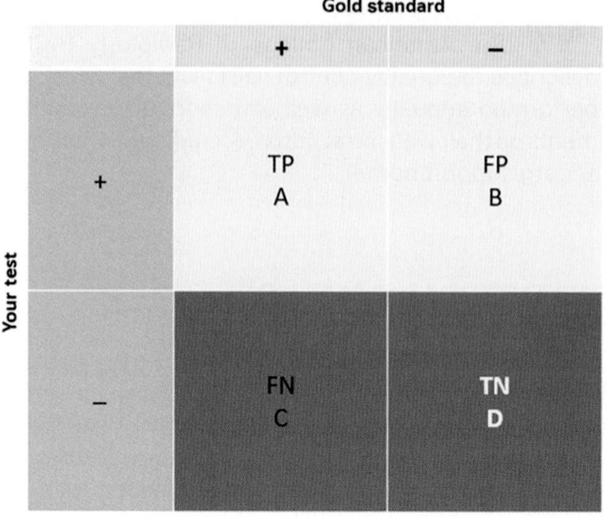

Figure 5-6 Chi-square equation for negative predictive value.

fashion (in this book, a bold, white font) and the denominators to be summed are highlighted (in this book, by an orange color). For example, sensitivity (Figure 5-2) shows the true positive (A) box in a bold, white font, and the true positive (A) and false negative (C) boxes are orange. Therefore, the equation is A/(A + C).

Example 1: Calculate the positive predictive value (PPV) if the number of true positives is 100 and the number of false positives is 80. Using the equation for PPV, the result is 100/180 = 0.56 (56%).

Example 2: Calculate the sensitivity of a test if the number of true positives is 100 and the number of false negatives is 20. Using the equation for sensitivity, the result is 100/120 = 0.83 (83%).

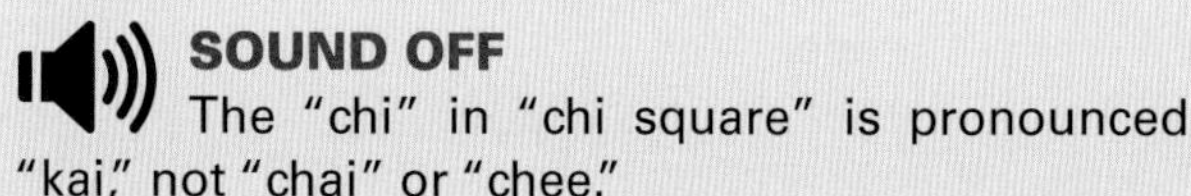

SOUND OFF

The "chi" in "chi square" is pronounced "kai," not "chai" or "chee."

PREVENTATIVE MAINTENANCE

Each sonography department should have a well-planned and formatted **preventative maintenance** program for every piece of imaging equipment in the lab. Every transducer and machine must be evaluated routinely. The AIUM suggests that all ultrasound equipment be kept in good working order and be evaluated and calibrated annually. Routine electrical evaluations should be conducted by sonographers to ensure that electrical cords are intact and do not present an electrical hazard to the sonographer or the patient. Routine cleaning of the machine's vents and outer surfaces should be performed to assure that the equipment is in an optimal working condition. Each machine should also be cleaned with an approved

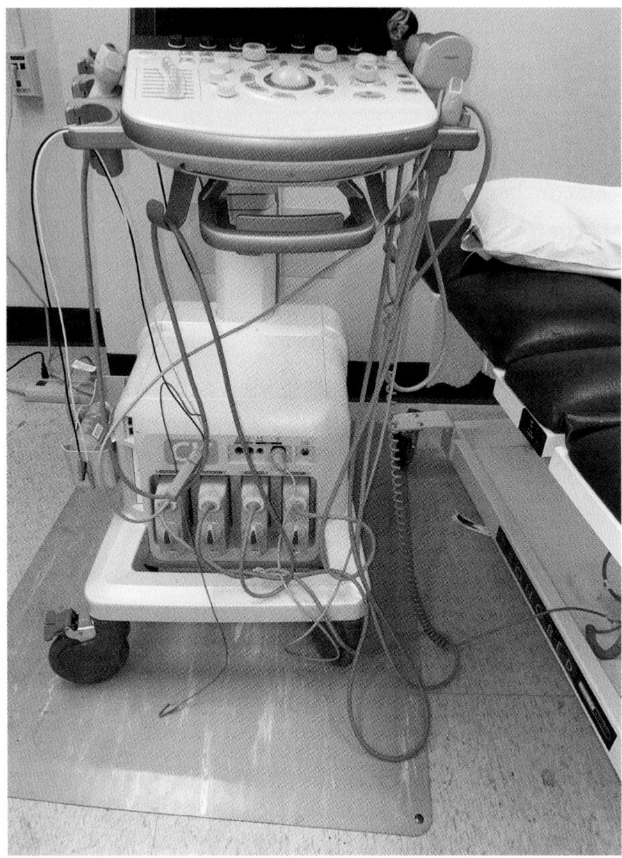

Figure 5-7 Tangled and dangling probe cords, sometimes called "cord spaghetti."

disinfectant before and after completing portable sonographic examinations. The prevention of the spread of infection is further discussed in Chapter 6. Dropping a transducer is potentially damaging, but caution should be given to avoidance of running over the cable. A heavy ultrasound machine running over the thin wires in the cable could be very detrimental to the probe and therefore the image, and unfortunately, it happens all too often. Hang cables properly (ie, not on the floor and no "cord spaghetti," Figure 5-7) and watch for the transducer and power cords when moving the equipment. If a transducer cable is on the wrong side of the wheel when you go to move a machine, get down and feed the probe around the wheel; don't run over it again to free it.

As mentioned in the Quality Assurance section, a record of each inspection, evaluation, and calibration must be maintained in the sonography department. When a sonographer notices that a transducer or equipment is out of calibration or produces nondiagnostic images, the service engineer must be contacted to evaluate the equipment. The equipment should not be used until the service engineer has corrected the problem. The sonographer is also responsible for maintaining a comprehensive QA program for the department. Accrediting agencies publish specific guidelines identifying standards for QA in an ultrasound lab.

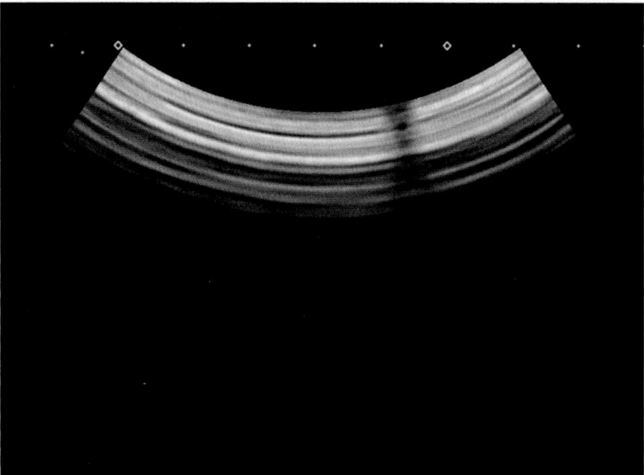

Figure 5-8 Dropout in an ultrasound image.

EQUIPMENT MALFUNCTION AND TROUBLESHOOTING

All equipment malfunctions should be reported immediately. If an issue is identified that may be a potential hazard for the sonographer or the patient, the machine should be removed from operation and stored away from the patient care area until an engineer can assess the status of the equipment. For example, frayed cords or cracked transducer housing could be a potential electrical hazard for both the sonographer and the patient, and thus should be immediately removed from the patient care setting. Transducers with dropout (Figure 5-8) should be serviced or replaced as the shadow caused by the bad element or damaged wire is detrimental to image quality. The AIUM recommends that transducers be serviced by qualified service providers and that the manufacturers provide guidance on proper operation, and how to identify when there is a defect with the transducer that could adversely affect the image or safe operation.

SOUND OFF

If an issue is identified that may be a potential hazard for the sonographer or the patient, the machine should be removed from operation and stored away from the patient care area immediately.

Most manufacturers have established technical support that can troubleshoot the problem via telephone. The user's manual for the machine may also be helpful in troubleshooting minor problems or assisting in the correct operation of an equipment feature. More complicated malfunctions require the on-site evaluation of the equipment by a service engineer.

PERFORMANCE TESTING

The daily operation of sonography equipment should be observed by the sonographer and errors or concerns

TABLE 5-3 Imaging properties

Imaging Property	Description	Interpretation
Axial resolution	The ability to accurately identify reflectors that are arranged parallel to the ultrasound beam	Correct placement and measurement of the reflectors indicate that the spatial pulse length is consistent with the manufacturer's requirements.
Lateral resolution	The ability to accurately identify reflectors that are arranged perpendicular to the ultrasound beam	Correct placement and measurement of the reflectors indicate that the beamformer and transducer's elements are working correctly.
Dead zone	Tests the ability of reflectors to be accurately imaged within the first centimeter or so of the sound beam as it leaves the transducer's face	When the dead zone area shifts deeper, the pulsing of the system or a transducer element may be compromised. Use of a standoff pad removes superficial structures from the dead zone.
Registration	The ability to accurately identify a pin with accuracy in size and location (vertical distance and horizontal distance) Note: Range accuracy is also called vertical depth calibration	Accuracy of measurement is vital to the successful diagnostic capabilities of an imaging system. Each vertical and horizontal pin must be accurately represented in size and location.
Sensitivity and uniformity	The ability of the system to detect echoes (including weak echoes) and display them uniformly with the same brightness on the monitor	Transducer failure or output variations can cause the loss of echo sensitivity and image uniformity. With the correct time-gain compensation, similar reflectors should appear the same on the monitor, regardless of their depth.

reported immediately. Daily operational tasks may include evaluating the electrical cords and transducer cords for fraying or tears in the wire casing; the face of the transducer for cracks or chips; nonfunctioning or sticking keys on the keyboard; for a nonmobile trackball; and obvious caliper malfunctions, or erroneous measurements.

Detailed and specific performance testing should be completed on a routinely scheduled basis, because the gradual degradation of the sonographic image may be difficult to detect. Performance testing includes scheduled activities that evaluate the accuracy of the system's imaging capabilities (Table 5-3). Imaging capabilities include **axial resolution** and **lateral resolution**, **vertical depth** and **horizontal calibration**, and overall **registration** of data. If the image appears to be adding or deleting echoes to the image or the transducer appears to have a bad element or functions erratically, then service should be scheduled immediately and the machine or transducer taken out of service.

SOUND OFF
Tissue-mimicking aka tissue-equivalent, or grayscale phantoms are used to evaluate a machine's grayscale sensitivity and contrast resolution at varying frequencies and depths.

Tissue-mimicking phantoms, also called tissue-equivalent or grayscale phantoms, are used to calibrate ultrasound imaging equipment. Phantoms are used by biomedical engineers as part of a lab's QA program. Phantoms include calibration and slice-thickness test objects, tissue-mimicking phantoms, and **Doppler phantoms** or test objects. Each test object or phantom has a specific purpose and may have one or more imaging parameters that it can evaluate. Calibration test objects evaluate the measurement accuracy of the machine. Tissue-mimicking or grayscale phantoms are used to evaluate a machine's grayscale **sensitivity** and **contrast resolution** at varying frequencies and depths. Sensitivity is the machine's ability to detect weak echoes. Contrast resolution is the ability to differentiate tissues with similar shades of gray. Tissue-mimicking phantoms are often combined with calibration test objects to create a general-purpose phantom. Slice-thickness test objects show the thickness of the elevational plane. Anthropomorphic phantoms, which look like the body part they are trying to represent, also provide a way to image structures in non living tissue but are more related to learner training rather than equipment testing.

SOUND OFF
Doppler phantoms are used to evaluate the flow direction, the depth capability or penetration of the Doppler beam, and the accuracy of sample volume location and measured velocity.

Doppler phantoms are used to evaluate the flow direction, the depth capability or penetration of the Doppler beam, and the accuracy of **sample volume** location and measured velocity. Each phantom is supplied with testing directions and interpretation results. Detailed records should be kept in a log with each transducer and imaging system. Any variances over the recommended allowance must be reported and investigated by a service engineer. A detailed log of every service call or malfunction should be maintained for each imaging system. The next section describes the different phantoms that may be used to test and calibrate the ultrasound machine.

Tissue-Equivalent Phantom

The **tissue-equivalent phantom**, also referred to as a tissue-mimicking or grayscale phantom, is used to test the accuracy and grayscale imaging of ultrasound imaging systems (Figure 5-9). The phantom, which is made up of an aqueous gel and graphite particles, transmits sound at 1540 m/s and thus attenuates at a rate similar to that of soft tissue. Stainless steel pins are strategically located throughout the phantom so that accurate identification and location can be recorded. Structures mimicking cysts and solid masses may also be positioned in the phantom, depending on the manufacturer and the purpose of the phantom (Figures 5-10 and 5-11).

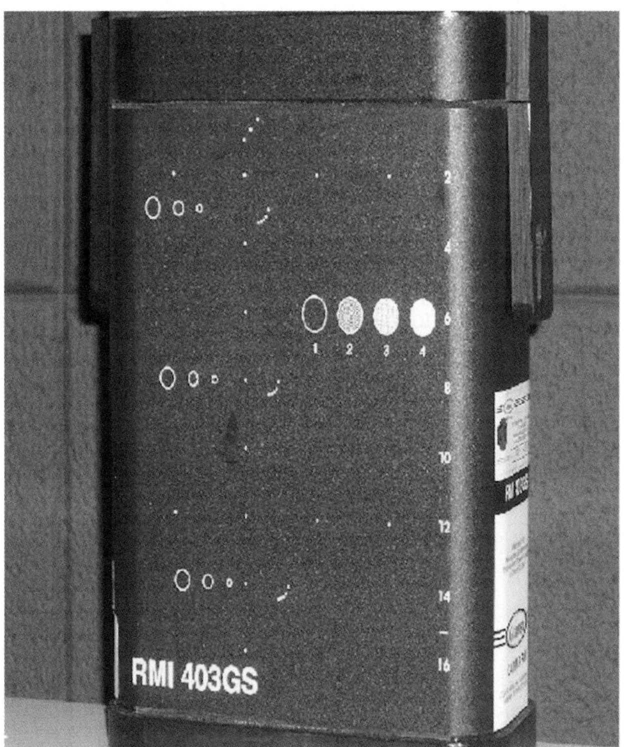

Figure 5-9 The tissue-equivalent phantom.

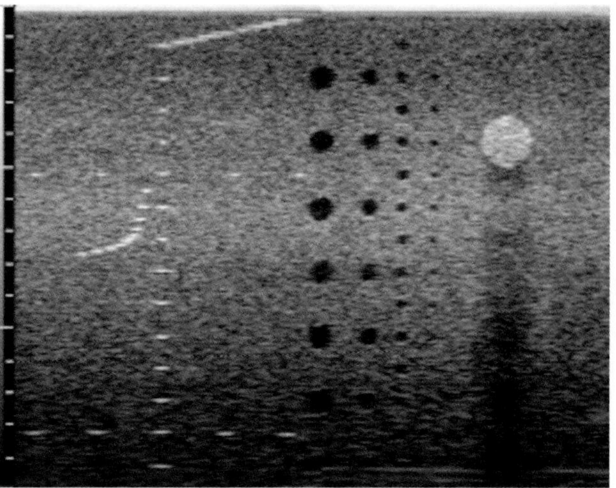

Figure 5-10 The sonographic appearance of one manufacturer's tissue-equivalent phantom.

The integrity of the tissue-equivalent phantom must be maintained, as the container must be airtight to avoid the degradation of the tissue properties inside the phantom. Also, the storage area temperature should be monitored to preserve the acoustic properties of the phantom. Sonographers should always check the manufacturer's instructions on proper care and maintenance of the phantom.

> **SOUND OFF**
> A slice-thickness phantom evaluates the elevational plane, the "third dimension" of the sound beam, perpendicular to the imaging plane.

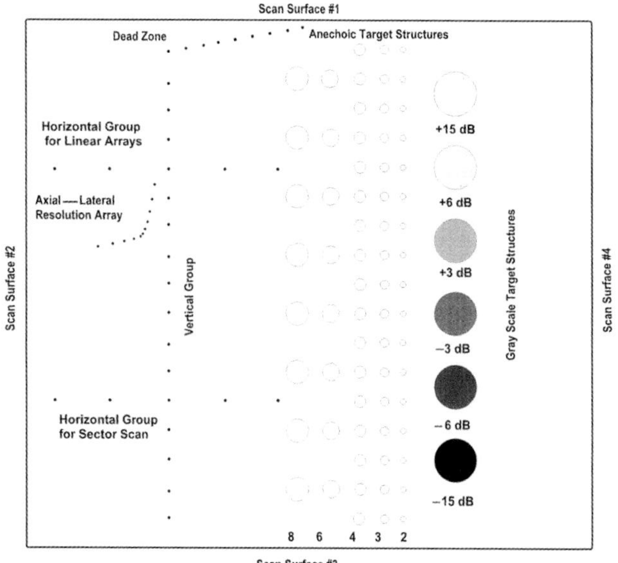

Figure 5-11 One company's schematic of a tissue-equivalent phantom.

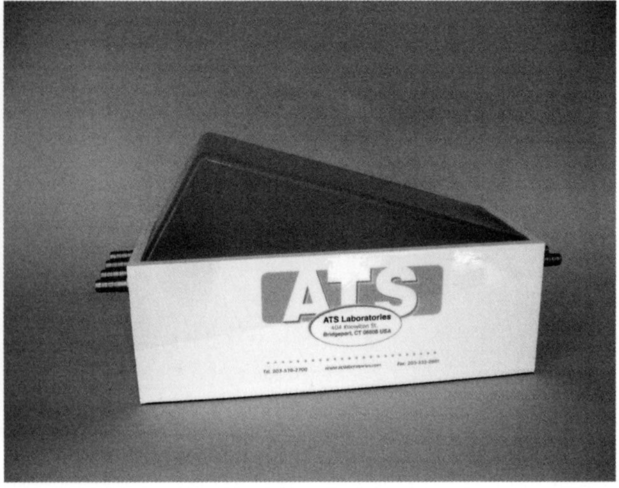

Figure 5-12 A Doppler testing phantom.

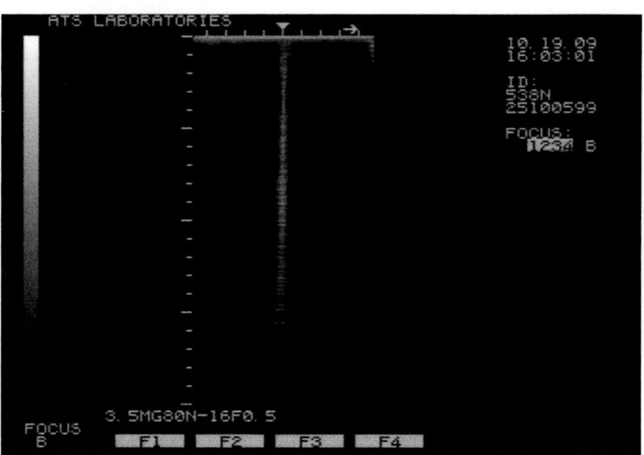

Figure 5-14 The sonographic appearance of the slice-thickness phantom.

Doppler Testing Phantom

The Doppler testing phantom evaluates the Doppler capabilities of imaging systems. These phantoms utilize a physically moving structure, such as a vibrating string or moving belt, or a circulation pump that moves blood-simulating fluid through the phantom. Thus, Doppler sensitivity, depth resolution, volume flow, and velocity accuracy can all be evaluated using a Doppler phantom (Figure 5-12).

Slice-Thickness Phantom

A **slice-thickness phantom** evaluates the **elevational plane**, the "third dimension," of the sound beam perpendicular to the imaging plane. If the sound beam is too thick, echoes appear inside cystic or fluid-filled structures (Figures 5-13 and 5-14).

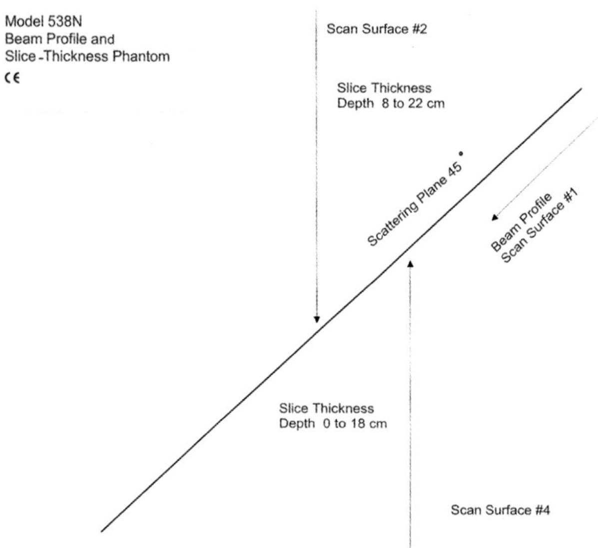

Figure 5-13 The anatomy of the slice-thickness phantom.

LAB ACCREDITATION AND CREDENTIALING

Reputable organizations that recognize ultrasound labs for their compliance with national performance standards exist. Lab accreditation procedures mandate that the lab meet specific, comprehensive guidelines governing departmental administration and policies, patient care, scanning protocols, and procedures.

Accrediting Agencies

Accrediting agencies in the field of sonography include the AIUM, the Intersocietal Accreditation Commission (IAC), and ACR. The AIUM is an organization that provides accreditation for ultrasound labs in the abdominal, musculoskeletal, contrast studies, high resolution studies, gynecology and obstetrics, and vascular sonography specialties. The IAC offers accreditation for vascular and echocardiographic labs, and the ACR provides opportunities for accreditation in general, vascular, pediatric, and ob/gyn ultrasound. Each accreditation agency plays a vital role in maintaining the standards of care that all patients expect and deserve (Table 5-4).

TABLE 5-4 Accrediting agencies and their websites

Accrediting Agency	Website
American College of Radiology (ACR)	http://www.acr.org/
American Institute of Ultrasound in Medicine (AIUM)	http://www.aium.org/
Intersocietal Accreditation Commission (IAC)	http://www.intersocietal.org

TABLE 5-5 Credential granting organizations and their websites

Credential Granting Organization	Website
American Registry for Diagnostic Medical Sonography (ARDMS)	http://www.ardms.org
American Registry of Radiologic Technologists (ARRT)	https://www.arrt.org/
Cardiovascular Credential International (CCI)	http://www.cci-online.org/

Professional Credentialing

Professional credentialing of sonographers and interpreting physicians is recommended for healthcare professionals practicing sonography. Lab accrediting organizations require professional certification(s) for practicing sonographers. Currently, the three main credentialing organizations that exist are the American Registry for Diagnostic Medical Sonography (ARDMS), Cardiovascular Credential International (CCI), and the American Registry of Radiologic Technologists (ARRT). Other organizations that test for specific areas (neurovascular and phlebology, for example) also exist for credentialing purposes.

The ARDMS represents tens of thousands of certified sonographers throughout the world. Certification exams are offered in several modalities. CCI offers certification exams in cardiac and vascular testing. The ARRT offers multiple certification exams in many areas of diagnostic imaging, including specialties in sonography (Table 5-5).

REVIEW QUESTIONS

1. Comprehensive preventative maintenance must be performed at least:
   a. Daily
   b. Semiannually
   c. Annually
   d. When a problem occurs

2. Which test object uses a moving belt, vibrating string, or a fluid pump?
   a. Contrast resolution phantom
   b. tissue-mimicking phantom
   c. Slice-thickness phantom
   d. Doppler phantom

3. Which of the following tests the ability of reflectors to be accurately imaged within the first centimeter of the sound beam?
   a. Sensitivity
   b. Dead zone
   c. Fresnel zone
   d. Axial resolution

4. The test used to evaluate the depth of reflectors from a transducer is called:
   a. Horizontal depth calibration
   b. Vertical depth calibration
   c. Dead zone
   d. Lateral resolution

5. All of the following are goals for a quality assurance program except:
   a. Document proper equipment performance
   b. Optimize image quality consistently
   c. Keep detailed results from quality assurance testing
   d. Report equipment malfunctions annually

6. The only certifying agency in this list that offers credentialing exams for cardiac and vascular testing is:
   a. ACR
   b. AIUM
   c. IAC
   d. CCI

7. Which of the following is a voluntary process that acknowledges an organization's competency and credibility according to standards and essentials set forth by a reliable source?
   a. Credentialing
   b. Accreditation
   c. Licensure
   d. Registration

8. Which of the following is the system's ability to detect echoes from weak reflectors?
   a. Uniformity
   b. Registration
   c. Sensitivity
   d. Dead zone

9. What type of errors will cause artificial echoes to appear within a cystic structure?
   a. Slice thickness
   b. Vertical depth calibration
   c. Registration
   d. Contrast resolution

10. Which of the following indicates the maximum depth of visualization?
   a. Vertical distance
   b. Horizontal distance
   c. Lateral resolution
   d. Sensitivity

11. Which of the following is a methodical way of evaluating equipment's performance on a routine basis to ensure proper and accurate equipment function?
   a. Accreditation
   b. Quality assurance
   c. Preventative maintenance
   d. Credentialing

12. Who among the following is responsible for ensuring an effective quality assurance program in the sonography lab?
   a. Physician
   b. Engineer
   c. Biomedical specialist
   d. Sonography staff

13. Which of the following is the ability to accurately identify reflectors that are arranged front to back and parallel to the ultrasound beam?
   a. Registration
   b. Axial resolution
   c. Vertical distance
   d. Lateral resolution

14. What is another term used for range accuracy?
   a. Lateral resolution
   b. Contrast resolution
   c. Depth calibration
   d. Focal filtering

15. Which of the following is the test object that evaluates the elevation resolution of the sound beam, which is perpendicular to the imaging plane?
   a. Test object
   b. Doppler testing phantom
   c. Tissue-equivalent phantom
   d. Slice-thickness phantom

16. What describes the system's ability to place echoes in the proper location horizontally and perpendicular to the sound beam?
   a. Horizontal calibration
   b. Azimuthal resolution
   c. Lateral determination
   d. Depth resolution

17. The test object that mimics the acoustic properties of human tissue and is used to ensure proper equipment performance is:
   a. Schlieren imaging phantom
   b. Doppler testing phantom
   c. Tissue-equivalent phantom
   d. Slice-thickness phantom

18. Which of the following is NOT likely to be evaluated by a Doppler phantom?
   a. Flow direction
   b. Subtle tissue differences
   c. Velocity measurement accuracy
   d. Accuracy of sample volume location

19. Which of the following is NOT an accrediting agency of sonography labs?
   a. American Institute of Ultrasound in Medicine
   b. American Registry of Diagnostic Medical Sonography
   c. Intersocietal Accreditation Commission
   d. American College of Radiology

20. Which of the following is NOT a credential granting body for sonographers?
   a. American Registry of Diagnostic Medical Sonography
   b. Cardiovascular Credential International
   c. American Registry of Radiographic Technologists
   d. American Institute of Ultrasound in Medicine

21. A new ultrasound (US) study is performed and compared to a gold standard. 200 patients were imaged. If the gold standard said that it found 100 studies were positive, and the US said that 90 studies were positive, how many studies are true positive?
   a. 100
   b. 90
   c. 10
   d. 1.11

22. Which of the following is defined as "how well a test can find that disease is present?"
    a. Positive predictive value
    b. Negative predictive value
    c. Accuracy
    d. Sensitivity

23. A new ultrasound (US) study is performed and compared to a gold standard. 200 patients were imaged. The gold standard found that 100 studies were positive, and of that 100, US found that 90 were positive. The gold standard said that 100 studies were negative, and of those 100, US found that 80 were negative. Which of the following represents the specificity of the US test?
    a. 80/20
    b. 80/100
    c. 100/80
    d. 110/20

24. What is the benefit of a quality improvement (QI) program in an ultrasound lab?
    a. Ensures equipment is functioning correctly
    b. Guarantees equipment is repaired properly
    c. Ensures staff are trained and evaluated routinely
    d. Provides for biomedical engineers to service machine

25. Negative predictive value is defined as:
    a. The number of negative (normal) exams an imaging test correctly identifies as negative compared to a gold standard
    b. If a test is good at finding positive and negative results compared to a gold standard
    c. The number of positive exams an imaging test correctly identifies as positive compared to a gold standard
    d. How good a test is at deciding if an exam is normal compared to a gold standard

SUGGESTED READINGS

AIUM.org Transducer Testing and Repair. Accessed November 11, 2023. https://www.aium.org/resources/official-statements/view/transducer-testing-and-repair, 2019.

Bushberg JT, Seibert JA, Leidholdt EM Jr, Boone JM. *The Essential Physics of Medical Imaging*. 4th ed. Wolters Kluwer; 2021.

Edelman SK. *Understanding Ultrasound Physics*. 4th ed. ESP Inc.; 2012.

Gaiser R, Fox TB. *Vascular Technology Examination PREP*. 2nd ed. McGraw Hill; 2021.

Grazhdani H, David E, Ventura Spagnolo O, et al. Quality assurance of ultrasound systems: Current status and review of literature. *J Ultrasound*. 2018;21:173–182.

Hedrick WR. *Technology for Diagnostic Sonography*. Mosby; 2013.

Kremkau FW. *Diagnostic Ultrasound: Principles and Instruments*. 10th ed. Saunders; 2020.

Kupinski A. *The Vascular System* (Diagnostic Medical Sonography Series). 3rd ed. Wolters Kluwer; 2022.

Miele F. *Ultrasound Physics and Instrumentation*. 6th ed. Miele Enterprises; 2022.

Zagzebski JA. *Essentials of Ultrasound Physics*. Mosby; 1996.

6

Patient Care and New Technologies

Outline

Introduction

This brief chapter will be used to discuss the role of a sonographer in patient care and the possible bioeffects of diagnostic ultrasound. Infection control, the practice of universal precautions, the sterile technique, and new technologies will be examined as well. Note that not everything in this section is on the current (as of this writing) ARDMS Sonography Principles and Instrumentation (SPI) content outlines. However, this book may be used for more than just the ARDMS SPI exam, and the content outlines change over time, necessitating the inclusion of additional materials. At the time of this writing, the September 2023 content outlines are current. Notations will be made where appropriate if a particular section is not included in the September 2023 content outlines.

Key Terms

- Items marked with an asterisk (*) are not specifically mentioned on the September 2023 ARDMS SPI content outline but may be on other credentialing examinations. Be sure to check the content of whatever exam you are taking.

acoustic cavitation—the production of bubbles in a liquid medium

acoustic radiation force impulse (ARFI) imaging—uses acoustic radiation force to compress the soft tissue and provides a qualitative measurement of stiffness without requiring pressure input from the sonographer

ALARA—stands for "as low as reasonably achievable" that is used to remind professionals to keep patient exposure to ultrasound at a minimum

automatic external defibrillator*—a portable device that is used to detect and treat abnormal heart rhythms with electrical defibrillation

contrast-enhanced ultrasound (CEUS)—type of imaging in which an ultrasound contrast agent containing microscopic gas bubbles is used to improve the visualization of structures or blood flow

diabetes mellitus*—a group of metabolic diseases that result from a chronic disorder of carbohydrates metabolism

diabetic ketoacidosis (DKA)*—a complication of diabetes that results from the severe lack of insulin

dwell time—the length of time the ultrasound transducer remains stationary over a volume of tissue

elastography—a sonographic technique used to evaluate the stiffness of a mass or tissue

ergonomics—the scientific study of creating tools and using equipment effectively in order to help the human body adjust to the work environment

fusion imaging*—technology that provides the ability to view alternate imaging modality (eg, CT or MRI) during real-time sonography; also referred to as hybrid imaging

Health Insurance Portability and Accountability Act (HIPAA)—US law that, among many goals, upholds patient confidentiality and requires the use of electronic medical records

Hepatitis*—inflammation of the liver

hypoglycemia*—a lower-than-normal blood sugar level

intravascular ultrasound—the technique that uses a miniature ultrasound transducer placed on a catheter and inserted into a circulatory system

mechanical index (MI)—the calculation used to identify the likelihood that cavitation could occur

nosocomial infection*—a hospital-acquired infection

radiation forces—forces exerted by a sound beam on an absorber or reflector that can alter structures

shear-wave elastography (SWE)*—the elastography technique that uses shear-wave information to analyze the stiffness of tissue

shear waves—the transverse waves that emanate within the tissue perpendicular to the beam

shock*—the body's pathologic response to illness, trauma, or severe physiologic or emotional stress

stable cavitation—nonthermal bioeffect in which bubbles are created in the tissue

strain elastography (SE)*—operator dependent type of elastography that measures the change in tissue as a result of compression

streaming—when acoustic fields cause motion of fluids

tachycardia*—rapid heart rate; a rate that exceeds the normal rate for the person's age

thermal index (TI)—the calculation used to predict the maximum temperature elevation in tissues

transient cavitation—nonthermal bioeffect in which bubbles are created in the tissue but collapse violently potentially causing cell damage

PATIENT CARE, SAFETY, AND COMMUNICATION

Patient Identification, Documentation, and Verification of Requested Examinations

The correct identification of patients who require sonographic procedures is a fundamental and yet crucial part of patient care. Sonographers should not limit the identification of a patient to simply asking the patient his or her last name. Verifying the patient's wristband information for identifying markers, which includes the patient's name, medical record number, and date of birth, is an essential part of patient care. All of this information should match with the requesting physician's information and relevant examination information. In some facilities, wristbands may have explicit colors that identify the patient as an outpatient or inpatient. Additionally, wristbands can indicate special precautions that should be taken for both the safety of the patient and healthcare workers.

In 2003, the HIPAA became effective in the United States. These HIPAA privacy rules influence many aspects of patient care and ensure that patient records are kept private by establishing certain standards or safeguards (Table 6-1). HIPAA also included a special provision to ensure that electronic transactions are securely performed.

Sonographers can play a key role in the protection of sensitive patient information. Computer monitors

TABLE 6-1 HIPAA goals

HIPAA Attempts To:
• Establish new standards for the release of health records • Protect health records by establishing new standards for healthcare professionals to follow • Apply strict penalties for those who violate patient confidentiality and patient rights • Provide more patient education

should be out of the viewing area of patients. Images should be viewed in a private locale, away from high-traffic areas. If viewing of images takes place outside of the healthcare facility, as in the case of publication and in the educational setting, patient identification and all distinctive markers should be omitted from the images. The discussion of sonographic studies and patient history should take place in a private area. Patient confidentiality must never be compromised, outside of the allowances afforded by HIPAA.

SOUND OFF
Proper documentation, both on the images obtained and of the procedure performed, is also crucial in the sequence of proper patient care.

Proper documentation, both on the images obtained and of the procedure performed, is also crucial in the sequence of proper patient care. According to the American Institute of Ultrasound in Medicine (AIUM), the documentation of sonographic images should include the patient's name and other identifying information, including facility information, date of the sonographic examination, and image orientation. The postexamination sonographic worksheet should include, but not be limited to, the patient's name, the date and type of examination, relevant clinical information and/or the International Classification of Diseases, 10th Revision (ICD-10) code, the name of patient's healthcare provider, and any other appropriate contact information.

SOUND OFF
If a patient does not speak English, or the national language, the sonographer should obtain an interpreter utilizing a translation phone or employee interpreter.

Patient Interaction, Effective Communication, and Obtaining a Clinical History

The role of a sonographer in patient care is critical. The sonographer should understand the physics of sound and should be able to relate the basic information about the use of ultrasound in medicine to patients. Therefore, sonographers should not only be capable of performing sonographic examinations but also be proficient in effectively communicating with their patients. An awareness of cultural diversity is essential, and sonographers should provide reasonable accommodations for those who have varying cultural or religious backgrounds.

Communication is the transfer of information from one person to another. It can be described as verbal or nonverbal. Verbal communication deals with spoken words. Picking the correct words to communicate with the patient is imperative. For example, the use of technical jargon may confuse the patient and result in the establishment of communication barriers. The details and explanation of the sonographic examination should be provided for the patient in clear, concise language and should always allow the opportunity for the patient to ask questions.

If a patient does not fluently speak English (or whatever the national language is), the sonographer should obtain an interpreter prior to the study taking place. Interpreters can be obtained via dedicated translation phone lines. Translation phones have two handsets, with the patient using one and the sonographer using the other. A translator on the line will inform the patient of what is said. In lieu of a translation phone, the sonographer may use an employee who speaks the same language. For medicolegal reasons, a patient's family member should not be used for translation purposes. Using a translator will ensure that the patient is completely informed about the procedure prior to the procedure being performed. Nonverbal communication can aid as an effective means of communication, and includes signs, hand gestures, facial expressions, and other body motions. Nevertheless, nonverbal gestures should never completely take the place of proper verbal communication. The reality is that the risk of litigation increases if a patient is not thoroughly informed of the procedure prior to its initiation.

Obtaining a thorough patient history is also a significant step toward proper patient care. Clinical history should be discussed with the patient before the sonographic examination begins. One goal of the sonographer should be to perform clinical correlation with the sonographic images acquired throughout the examination. There are several general questions that can be asked to start a conversation with patients who present with pain and those without noticeable pain (Tables 6-2 and 6-3). These questions should be followed by more in-depth questions that are not necessarily leading questions, but rather open-ended, to obtain further information. If performed rationally, and in sequence, a

TABLE 6-2 Clinical history questions for the patient who is complaining of pain

Universal Clinical History Question for the Symptomatic Patient
• Where is the problem or area of pain? • When did the pain start? • How severe is the pain? • What relieves the pain or causes it to increase? • What else happens when the pain begins?

TABLE 6-3 Clinical history questions for the patient who is not complaining of pain

Universal Clinical History Questions for the Asymptomatic Patient
• Are you a diabetic? • Do you have high blood pressure? • Do you smoke? • Do you take any medications? • Have you had any surgeries (related to the examination area)?

clinical enquiry can often lead to the discovery of previously undisclosed clinical concerns of the patient. Other sources of clinical history exist, including archived images, other diagnostic studies, laboratory findings, and family history. Especially useful to many sonographic studies is an analysis of other imaging examination reports, such as those created after computed tomography, magnetic resonance imaging, and radiographic studies. Sonographers should investigate these reports for relevant anatomic variants and pathology, so that the correlation between imaging modalities can increase accuracy in the diagnostic process. Sonographers should learn the aspects of obtaining basic vital signs. In some studies, obtaining a blood pressure is a part of the study, but it is also useful to be able to document vital signs in an emergency. Table 6-4 lists normal vital values for common vital signs, including heart rate, blood pressure, and temperature.

Consent is an important part of the patient care process. For noninvasive studies like transabdominal or transthoracic ultrasound, verbal consent is all that is required. You explain the examination to the patient, and they let you perform it. Endorectal ultrasound typically does not require written consent unless a procedure is to be performed, like oocyte retrieval or abscess drainage. For invasive studies, like biopsies, or studies requiring sedation, like transesophageal echocardiography, written consent is required. The examination must be explained to the patient along with the benefits and risks, and the patient and physician (or the nonphysician practitioner) must sign the form. If the patient does not speak English or the country's primary language fluently an interpreter must be used. Implied consent is when the patient is unable to provide consent, but services must be rendered immediately. For example, if an outpatient walks into the department and falls to the floor with no heartbeat, it is implied that they would want to be saved by any means necessary. Patients may have "do not resuscitate" orders, in which case the healthcare provider is not permitted to render life-saving aid unless otherwise specified in the chart. Patients have the right to refuse any examination, at any time, for any reason, even if having that procedure or examination would provide a better outcome. The healthcare provider can offer the patient information on the benefit of the examination, but the patient cannot be forced to have any study performed if they refuse.

TABLE 6-4 Vital signs

Vital Sign	Normal Values (Adult)
Heart rate	60-100 beats per minute (bpm)
Blood pressure	<120/80 Elevated 120-129/<80 Hypertension ≥130/≥80
Respirations	12 to 20 breaths per minute
Temperature (oral)	98.6 °F (37 °C)
Pulse oximetry	95%-100%
Skin color	Pale (pallor), blue (cyanotic), red (rubor), yellow (jaundice) may be abnormal

SOUND OFF
When emergency situations arise, sonographers must be prepared.

Emergency Situations

When emergency situations arise, sonographers must be prepared. Certification by the American Heart Association in Basic Life Support (BLS) should be maintained. Cardiopulmonary resuscitation (CPR) is most often used to counteract the effects of suspected cardiac arrest or heart attack. The classic presentation of cardiac arrest includes loss of consciousness, loss of blood pressure, dilation of the pupils, and possibly seizures. There are specific actions that the sonographer should be prepared to make in the event of cardiac arrest (Table 6-5).

TABLE 6-5 Sonographer's response to cardiac arrest

Sonographer's Response to Cardiac Arrest
1. In the presence of an unresponsive patient, shake the patient and ask, "Are you okay?" 2. If there is no response, call a "code." (In a nonhospital environment, call 911.) 3. If no one is near, shout for help. 4. Do not leave the patient. 5. Check the carotid pulse of an adult patient. 6. If there is no pulse, place the patient in the supine position and begin performing CPR.

If available, an **automatic external defibrillator** may be used to assess the patient's heart rhythm and administer a therapeutic shock, if necessary, to return the heart to normal rhythm.

SOUND OFF
Shock is the body's pathologic response to illness, trauma, or severe physiologic or emotional stress.

Sonographers should also be prepared to efficiently react to patients who may experience **shock**. Shock is the body's pathologic response to illness, trauma, or severe physiologic or emotional stress. There are several different classifications of shock (Table 6-6). The initial clinical manifestation of shock may not be obvious. However, as the body responds to the effects of shock, clinical observations can be made. The compensatory patient will experience cold and clammy skin, decreased urine output, increased respiration, reduced bowel sounds, and increased anxiety. If shock is allowed to progress, the patient's blood pressure will drop; their respirations will decrease; and they will experience **tachycardia**, chest pain, and possibly have a loss of mental alertness. In the irreparable stage of shock, vital organs such as the kidneys and liver shut down, and death is nearly unavoidable. The sonographer should immediately call for emergency assistance when any form of shock is suspected. For any emergency, the sonographer should know the procedures for calling for a "code blue" or other response that might require the rapid response team. Sonographers should also be prepared to perform CPR until the code team arrives and assist with patient care, if needed.

SOUND OFF
Although a "code" is commonly shorthand for "code blue," which includes cardiac/respiratory arrest or any other medical emergency, sonographers should know the other codes at their institutions. For example, "code red" is commonly used to signify a fire. What other codes do you know?

Some sonographic procedures require the patient to fast as part of preparation for the examination. Diabetic patients can be distinctly affected when they have not had anything to eat for an extended period. The sonographer should be aware if the patient is a diabetic because these emergency situations may be treated differently. Patients with **diabetes mellitus** may suffer from

TABLE 6-6 The classifications and explanation of shock

Classification of Shock	Explanation
Anaphylactic shock	A subcategory of distributive shock that results from an exaggerated allergic reaction, leading to vasodilation and pooling in the peripheral blood vessels. It can be caused by medications, iodinated contrast agents that are often used in x-ray procedures, and insect venoms.
Cardiogenic shock	Failure of the heart to pump the proper amount of blood to the vital organs. It can be caused by myocardial infarction, cardiac tamponade, dysrhythmias, or other cardiac pathology.
Distributive shock	When the blood vessels lack the ability to constrict and assist in the return of blood to the heart, leading to a pooling of peripheral blood. There are three types of distributive shock: neurogenic, septic, and anaphylactic.
Hypovolemic shock	When the amount of intravascular fluid decreases by 15% to 25%. It can be caused by internal or external hemorrhage, loss of plasma from burns, or fluid loss from vomiting, diarrhea, or medications.
Neurogenic shock	A subcategory of distributive shock in which there is a loss of the sympathetic tone causing vasodilation of the peripheral blood vessels. It can be caused by spinal cord injuries, severe pain, neurogenic damage, medications, lack of glucose, and adverse effects of anesthesia.
Obstructive shock	Results from pathologic conditions that interfere with the normal pumping action of the heart. It can be caused by pulmonary embolism, pulmonary hypertension, arterial stenosis, and possibly tumors that obstruct normal blood flow to the heart.
Septic shock	A subcategory of distributive shock in which there is an immune response of the body that leads to capillary permeability and vasodilation. It can be caused by invasive organisms, such as bacteria.

TABLE 6-7 Diabetic emergencies

Acute Complication of Diabetes Mellitus	Explanation
Hypoglycemia	Occurs when a patient has an excess amount of insulin or oral hypoglycemic medication in their system. This may be seen in the diabetic patient who has had nothing to eat for several hours.
Diabetic ketoacidosis (DKA)	A type of hyperglycemia more common in Type-I diabetics, DKA occurs when a patient has insufficient insulin, resulting in excess glucose production by the liver. DKA is an emergency that can lead to coma and death.
Hyperglycemic hyperosmolar nonketotic syndrome (HHNS)	Like DKA, but more common in Type-II diabetics, HHNS is seen in patients who are dehydrated and/or have an infection. HHNS is an emergency that can lead to coma and death.

three complications that the sonographer may have to recognize: **hypoglycemia**, **diabetic ketoacidosis (DKA)**, and hyperglycemic hyperosmolar nonketotic syndrome (HHNS, Table 6-7). Complications of diabetes include tachycardia, headache, blurred vision, extreme thirst, polyuria, or a sweet odor to the breath (in DKA). The sonographer should immediately notify the interpreting physician of the examination or emergency department physician and be prepared to monitor the patient's vital signs or assist the rapid response team in patient care procedures.

Infection Control and Universal Precautions

Healthcare workers can be exposed to various viruses during their daily practice. **Hepatitis** B and C viruses, human immunodeficiency virus (HIV), tuberculosis (TB), and methicillin-resistant *Staphylococcus aureus* (MRSA) are among the list of communicable diseases that may be transmitted in the hospital from a patient to a healthcare worker.

Toxins, certain drugs, some diseases, heavy alcohol use, and bacterial and viral infections can all cause hepatitis. Hepatitis B and C are transmitted via contact with infectious blood, semen, and other body fluids, from having sex with an infected person, sharing contaminated needles to inject drugs, or from an infected mother to her newborn. Hepatitis B vaccination is typically provided to all healthcare workers who may be exposed. It is a simple set of three injections. There is no present vaccine for hepatitis C, though medical treatments now exist.

Healthcare workers can also be the source of infections. A healthcare-associated infection (HAI) is also known as a **nosocomial infection**. These are discussed later in this section. If a living creature or person gives a patient a disease, it is called a **vector**. For example, rats were vectors of disease during the bubonic plague spread in Europe. If a patient gets infection from an object, it's called a **fomite**. For example, if a sonographer does not properly disinfect a transducer, a patient may get infection from the transducer, which in this case is a fomite. An **iatrogenic** injury is one that is caused (usually inadvertently) by a healthcare provider. For example, if a physician perforates the bowel during a colonoscopy, then that injury is considered iatrogenic. A summary of infection terminology is shown in Table 6-8.

SOUND OFF
MRSA is a type of *Staphylococcus* or "staph" bacteria that is resistant to many antibiotics.

HIV is the virus that leads to acquired immune deficiency syndrome (AIDS). It is spread by sexual contact with an infected person, by sharing needles with someone who is infected, through transfusions of infected blood or blood-clotting factors, or through childbirth or breast milk. In the healthcare setting, workers have been infected with HIV after being stuck with needles that are contaminated with HIV-infected blood and body fluids, although the risk is minimal.

TABLE 6-8 Infection terminology

Term	Definition
Vector	Living creature that spreads infection, including humans
Fomite	Nonliving object that spreads infection, like a dirty instrument
Iatrogenic	Inadvertent injury from a procedure performed in the healthcare setting. For example, accidental perforation of something that was not the target during an invasive procedure
Nosocomial	Healthcare-associated infection that manifests within 48 hours after admission to the institution

Patient Care and New Technologies

TB is an airborne disease found in the lungs, and possibly other organs, of an infected person. The TB bacteria are released from an infected individual most often when that person coughs, sneezes, speaks, or sings. People nearby, such as sonographers and other patients, may breathe in these bacteria and become infected. The TB skin test, the Mantoux tuberculin skin test, is performed to detect whether an individual is infected with TB. This test has been a mainstay in the detection and prevention of spread of TB in the healthcare setting. There is also a blood test for TB that does not require the individual to return to the lab to have the skin examined.

Multidrug-resistant organisms (MDROs) are pathogens, usually bacteria, that do not respond to conventional drugs formerly used to treat patients infected with those pathogens. MRSA is a type of *Staphylococcus* or "staph" bacteria that is resistant to many antibiotics. MRSA has become a rampant malady spread through close personal contact in the healthcare setting. Unfortunately, it is the healthcare worker who may be the means of transmission of this destructive organism. Most staph infections manifest as an infected area on the skin. There are other resistant strains of bacteria, like Vancomycin-resistant *enterococci* and drug-resistant TB, plus many more in a hospital environment.

Infection control, and consequently the reduction in the spread of infection, should be a priority in all sonography departments. The chain of infection begins with a pathogenic organism (Table 6-9) (Figure 6-1). Pathogens include viruses, fungi, and parasites. Pathogens need a reservoir to stay alive. The reservoir provides an environment in which the pathogen can grow or multiply. A reservoir could be found anywhere in the clinical setting, including on our hands, the ultrasound machine, and the examination table. Pathogens are also found in body fluids such as blood and urine, in the nose, and in the mouth. A portal of exit from the reservoir must be available for the pathogen to be transmitted to another individual. The mode of transmission by the hands is a common occurrence in the clinical environment.

TABLE 6-9 Chain of infection

Chain of Infection
1. Infectious agent
2. Reservoir
3. Portal of exit
4. Mode of transmission
5. Portal of entry
6. Susceptible host

SOUND OFF
The single most vital daily task that a sonographer can perform to prevent the spread of infection is the practice of regular hand hygiene.

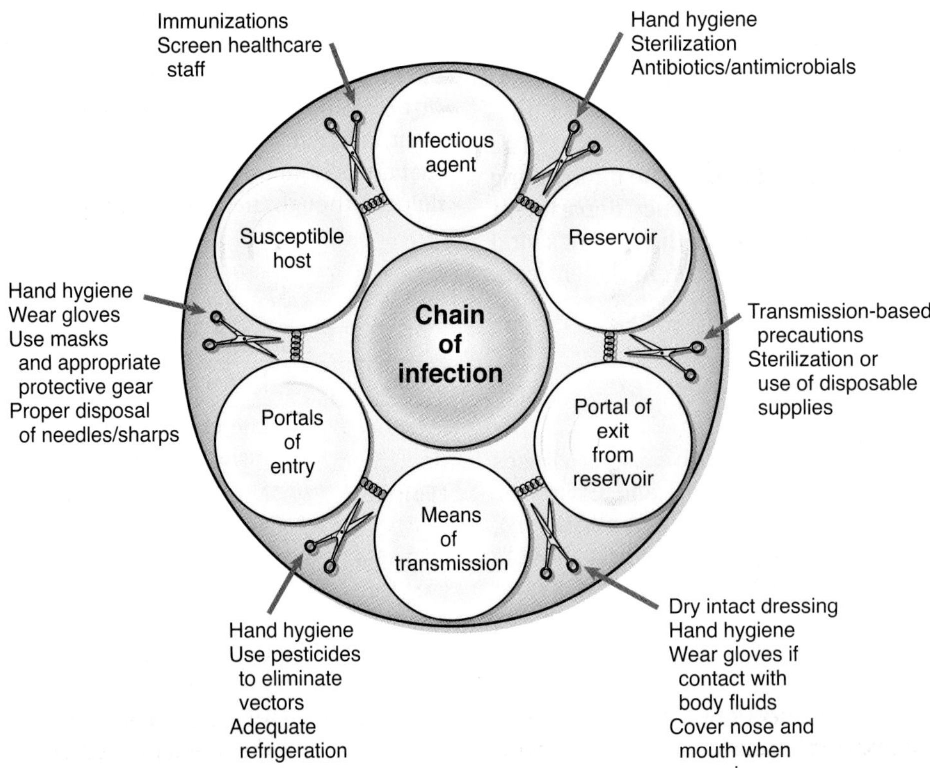

Figure 6-1 The infection cycle is demonstrated as a chain. The goal is to break the links of the chain to end the cycle.

Although the use of gloves should be a routine part of patient care, the single most vital daily task that a sonographer can perform to prevent the spread of infection is the practice of regular hand hygiene. Hand washing, when performed accurately, can reduce the spread of infection between patients significantly. Although alcohol-based hand rubs may be easily accessible, they should never take the place of hand washing in the presence of visibly soiled hands. Hand hygiene should take place before and after any contact with patients.

The use of other personal protective equipment (PPE) such as gowns and masks are also an effective means of reducing the spread of infection. PPEs are transmission barriers. They help prevent the transportation of pathogens from the infected person to the general environment (Figure 6-2).

The Occupational Safety and Health Administration and the Centers for Disease Control have established Standard Precautions that were previously referred to as Universal Precautions. These precautions deal with the safety measures that should apply to blood, all body fluids, secretions, excretions, nonintact skin, and mucous membranes. They not only encourage safe practices when dealing with patients but also promote cleanliness in the healthcare setting.

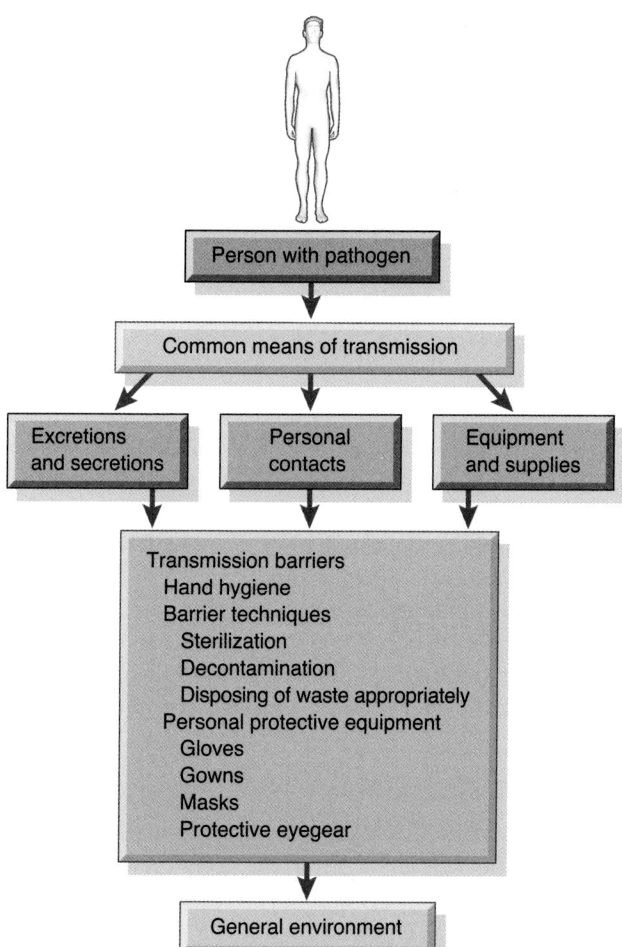

Figure 6-2 Transmission barriers help prevent the transporting of pathogens from the infected person to the general environment. Transmission barriers include hand hygiene, barrier techniques, and PPE.

> **SOUND OFF**
> One of the most widespread nosocomial infections is the urinary tract infection, caused by the incorrect use and placement of a Foley catheter bag.

Sonographers should try to prevent nosocomial infections. A nosocomial infection is a hospital-acquired infection. One of the most widespread nosocomial infections is the urinary tract infection, caused by the incorrect use and placement of a Foley catheter bag. The bag, when placed above or at the level of the urinary bladder, could allow the retrograde flow of urine into the bladder from the catheter bag. To minimize the potential impact from a urinary tract infection, the patient's catheter bag should be placed below the level of the urinary bladder. As mentioned earlier, the spread of MRSA is also a rapidly growing problem in hospitals and patient care facilities.

Appropriate disinfection of ultrasound equipment should be ensured. Various materials may be used to clean the ultrasound equipment daily between patients. The transducer, the transducer cord, and the control panel should all be cleaned with a manufacturer-approved disinfectant chemical. All gel should be wiped off the transducer prior to applying any disinfecting wipes or sprays, and the transducer should sit for the manufacturer-recommended time for disinfection. The use of wipes or sprays on a touch screen or the display may cause damage to the equipment, so be sure to correlate with manufacturer recommendations.

Some procedures require the use of a transducer probe cover and high-level disinfection after each examination. For example, endocavity transducers, such as transvaginal, transrectal, and transesophageal probes, may be soaked in a glutaraldehyde-based solution or some other form of cold high-level disinfection solution for the manufacturers' suggested submersion time. Some facilities may instead use a hydrogen-peroxide-based solution that is formulated for use within a specialized probe disinfection tabletop unit (see Chapter 1). Chemicals used for probe disinfection can be exceedingly hazardous to the sonographer's health. Thus, PPE and proper disposal techniques must be employed regardless of the method used. The disinfection of endocavity transducers should be documented in a log of some type. Regardless of the method used, transducers should be cleaned of all gel and dried prior to high-level disinfection.

TABLE 6-10 Several notable rules of surgical asepsis

1. Always be aware of what is considered sterile.
2. If an object's sterility is questionable, one must assume that the object is nonsterile.
3. Never reach or lean across a sterile field.
4. To be considered sterile, a person must don sterile gloves and a sterile gown.
5. The cuffs of a sterile gown are not considered sterile.
6. The edges of a sterile wrapper are not sterile.
7. Never leave a sterile tray unattended.
8. If you recognize that a sterile item has become contaminated, remedy the issue immediately.

Sterile Technique

Sterile technique, which may also be referred to as surgical asepsis, is the complete removal of microorganisms and their spores from an object or surface. Because sonographers are involved in procedures that require the sterile technique, they should have a fundamental understanding of the principles of maintaining a sterile field. Invasive procedures, such as biopsies and fluid drainage, require the practice of the sterile technique. There are many rules of surgical asepsis, though Table 6-10 provides several important rules to keep in mind.

BIOEFFECTS

Although the principle of piezoelectricity was discovered by Jacques and Pierre Curie in 1880, it was not until 1915 that it found a use: in sound navigation and ranging. Paul Langevin found that while it was possible for sound waves to detect underwater objects, like boat hulls and submarines, at higher intensities, it caused harm to some aquatic life. These findings were substantiated with further research. Therefore, it has been known for some time that there is a potential risk that ultrasound can cause harm to living tissue, especially with increased use of lung ultrasound and ultrasound contrast agents. Ultrasound machines should display the standard indices for monitoring output, **mechanical index (MI)** and **thermal index (TI)**. These indices, established by the Output Display Standard of 1992, help guide the sonographer in practicing ALARA, the "as low as reasonably achievable" principle that ensures sonographers are causing the least amount of harm related to putting sound energy into the body. The AIUM has several official statements on its website to guide practitioners of ultrasound on appropriate and safe use of ultrasound. The AIUM statements presented in this text can be found in the Suggested Readings section at the end of this chapter.

ALARA

Imaging a patient with ultrasound requires applying energy to living tissue. People who perform ultrasound are responsible for using the least amount of ultrasound exposure needed to obtain an acceptable diagnostic study. The principle of ALARA, which stands for "as low as reasonably achievable," tasks the sonographer/sonologist with utilizing ultrasound in as responsible and safe way as possible. Although the risk of harmful biologic effects is minimal when ultrasound is used on human tissue for diagnostic purposes, the ALARA maxim encourages the appropriate use of ultrasound for diagnostic purposes using the least time and least power possible. ALARA is an acknowledgment and reminder that although there has never been a documented adverse event related to diagnostic ultrasound alone, potential risks do exist and therefore exposure to ultrasound, especially at higher intensities, should be curtailed. The introduction to the AIUM official statement on ALARA reads as follows: The potential benefits and risks of each examination should be considered. The ALARA principle should be observed when adjusting controls that affect the acoustic output and by considering both the transducer dwell time and overall scanning time (AIUM, 2020). The AIUM official statement on ALARA can be found at: https://www.aium.org/resources/official-statements/view/as-low-as-reasonably-achievable-(alara)-principle.

Sound waves are attenuated in body tissues primarily through the creation of heat (absorption), and sound can have thermal and nonthermal effects on human tissues at certain intensities. The use of ultrasound contrast agents has shown adverse bioeffects in research settings in living creatures, so extra care should be taken to reduce power and minimize the dwell time, especially when using ultrasound contrast. There are two recognized types of potential bioeffects that may occur with ultrasound: thermal and nonthermal (aka mechanical).

Thermal Mechanism and Thermal Index

As sound travels through the body, attenuation occurs primarily through absorption, the conversion of sound to heat. Sound energy is converted to heat typically because of an increase in intensity and frequency. Elevation in the temperature of certain tissues has the potential to cause damage. For example, neonatal, embryonic, and fetal tissues are more sensitive to elevated temperatures, especially in tissues adjacent to bone. The TI is a calculation used to predict the

TABLE 6-11 Factors that affect thermal bioeffects

Factor	Effect on Thermal Bioeffects
Power output	Lower power output (aka output power or acoustic power) reduces the risk for bioeffects. Higher power output increases the risk for bioeffects.
Scanned vs. unscanned modes	In scanned modes, the beam is swept across the scanned volume, giving the tissue some cool down time before being insonated again. Scanned methods include B-mode and color Doppler. Unscanned modes send the sound wave down one scan line and deposit energy into the tissue with little time for cooling down. Unscanned modes include spectral Doppler and M-mode.
Perfusion	Increased tissue perfusion allows the heat to be dissipated more quickly. Poor perfusion permits heat to accumulate, increasing the risk for bioeffects.
Time	Dwell time: The longer the transducer stays over one area, the more heat has a chance to accumulate, which increases the risk for bioeffects. Keep the transducer moving, especially in areas where bone is in the scanned area. Overall time: The shorter the exam, the less exposure to the sound beam.

maximum temperature elevation in tissues because of the attenuation of sound. Although it is not possible to predict the exact temperature or increase in temperature at a given point in the body, sonographers should be aware that there is a possibility of a temperature increase given different parameters.

There are three subcategories for the TI:

- TIS—for use in soft tissue (fetus < 10 weeks, before bone calcifies)
- TIB—for use when bone is near the focal zone (fetus ≥ 10 weeks)
- TIC—for use when cranial bone is near the surface

The temperature in tissue increases with frequency because the rate of attenuation (attenuation coefficient) increases with frequency. The temperature increases with intensity because either more power is being applied or it is being applied over a smaller area (remember: intensity = power/area).

In addition to power output, the factors that affect thermal bioeffects include whether the mode is scanned or unscanned, tissue perfusion, overall scanning time, and the dwell time (Table 6-11). The maximum heating of tissue is related to the sound beam's spatial peak temporal average. The AIUM states that a beam that causes a temperature increase of less than 1.5 °C above the normal body temperature of 37 °C may be used without adverse effect. It is important to remember that absorption is greater in bone than in soft tissue, so the dwell time should be minimized, especially when scanning around bone. Given that fetal tissue is more sensitive to thermal bioeffects, and the fetal brain is encased in bone, especially later in pregnancy, it is important to minimize the dwell time when imaging the fetal brain. In other words, if the image is not easily obtainable, move the probe and then come back after a moment to allow the tissue to cool. In general, according to the AIUM's Recommended Maximum Scanning Times for Displayed Thermal Index (TI) Values (2022), if the TI is ≤0.7, then there is no time limit for scanning. At thermal indices >0.7, time limits have been published and are available at https://www.aium.org/resources/official-statements/view/recommended-maximum-scanning-times-for-displayed-thermal-index-(ti)-values.

SOUND OFF

In order, from the least risk of thermal bioeffects to the highest risk for bioeffects:

B-mode < color Doppler < M-mode < spectral Doppler

Nonthermal Mechanism and Mechanical Index

Nonthermal mechanisms for bioeffects include **radiation forces**, **streaming**, and **acoustic cavitation**, with the last being the most worrisome. Nonthermal mechanisms may also be referred to as mechanical mechanisms. Radiation force is the "push" force of ultrasound (remember—sound waves are mechanical in nature). Do not conflate "radiation force" with "ionizing radiation." Sound waves are not on the electromagnetic spectrum like ionizing radiation and are not harmful like ionizing radiation. However, there is a push force to the tissue, which has the potential to cause streaming in fluids in the tissue, which has the potential to cause stress and cell death. (Flashback to Chapter 1: sound is a pressure wave created by a mechanical action.)

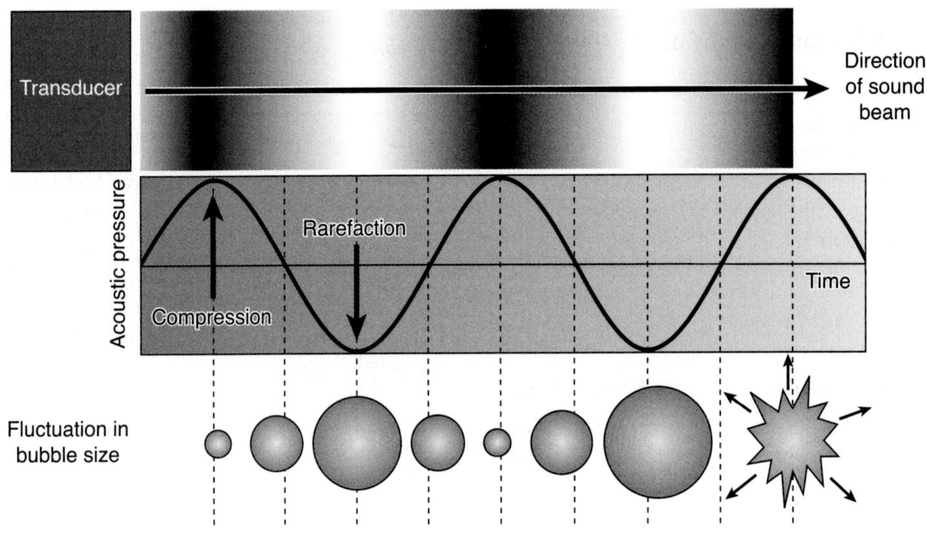

Figure 6-3 Cavitation. As ultrasound travels through tissue **(top)**, it causes alternating compression and rarefaction **(middle)**. Gas is drawn out of a solution during rarefaction, creating bubbles. These bubbles can fluctuate in size in a stable fashion with the changing tissue pressure. However, they may collapse. This collapse can result in local energy release and a focal increase in temperature at the microscopic level **(bottom)**.

Acoustic cavitation is the action of an acoustic field within a medium to generate bubbles (Figure 6-3). There are two types of cavitation: stable and inertial (or transient). **Stable cavitation** produces bubbles that oscillate, or fluctuate, in size but do not rupture. **Transient (aka inertial) cavitation** has the potential of causing the most biologic damage caused by the collapse of the bubble. With transient cavitation, larger bubbles are produced and subsequently they violently rupture (collapse). The risk is highest at low frequencies and where the bubbles are the largest, which is observed during the peak rarefactional pressure (ie, at the lowest pressure). The rupture of these bubbles produces a shock wave and an increase in tissue temperature in that area. This sudden increase in temperature has been associated with biologic effects, although only an area consisting of several cells is affected.

SOUND OFF
The three types of nonthermal (mechanical) bioeffects are radiation force, streaming, and acoustic cavitation.

The MI was developed to assist in evaluating the likelihood of cavitation occurring, especially transient (inertial) cavitation. The MI is directly related to the pressure (in MPa) and inversely related to the frequency of the transducer (in MHz). The FDA maximum (for diagnostic scanners) for MI is 1.9, and there are no observed adverse effects in tissues without existing gas bodies below an MI of 1.9. In ophthalmic ultrasound, the maximum MI is 0.23. In tissues with existing gas bodies, including contrast agents, the MI should be <0.4. Table 6-12 sums up the important numbers for bioeffects.

SOUND OFF
What is an "existing gas body?" Tissues in the body containing air or gas are called "existing gas bodies." They include the GI tract (intestines), lungs, and any tissue with ultrasound contrast agents.

TABLE 6-12 Summary of important numbers in bioeffects

Thermal or Mechanical	Description
Thermal	Ultrasound can be used without any concern for thermal bioeffects if the tissue's temperature increase is less than 1.5 °C and greater than the normal body temperature of 37 °C
Thermal	TI ≤ 0.7 has no time limit for scanning
Mechanical	FDA maximum MI: 1.9
Mechanical	MI maximum without existing gas bodies: 1.9
Mechanical	MI maximum with existing gas bodies: 0.4
Mechanical	MI maximum in contrast agents: 0.4

TABLE 6-13 How to minimize the risk of all bioeffects

1. Reduce the output power when able
2. Minimize overall scanning time
3. Minimize the dwell time—keep the probe moving when possible, especially if over bone and/or scanning an embryo or fetus
4. Minimize the use of Doppler and avoid the use of Doppler in the first trimester except when indicated
5. Use ultrasound only for medical diagnostic purposes
6. Avoid scanning over the eye, bone, and bowel/lung when able
7. Use shortened, evidence-based protocols to reduce exam time

SOUND OFF
The thermal indices relate to the beam's spatial peak temporal average intensity, whereas the MI relates to the beam's peak rarefactional (negative) pressure, which is related to the spatial peak pulse average intensity.

Although the manufacturers of ultrasound equipment display the mechanical and thermal indices and set up presets to ensure that the output is decreased for certain examinations, ultimately it is up to the sonographer to ensure that ALARA is practiced. Table 6-13 provides suggestions on how to minimize bioeffects when scanning.

ADVANCED TECHNOLOGIES IN SONOGRAPHY

Elastography

SOUND OFF
Elastography and fusion imaging are not listed on the September 2023 content outlines for the ARDMS SPI examination but may be on other credentialing examinations or future versions of the ARDMS SPI examination.

One of the mainstays of the clinical exam has always been manual palpation. Feeling the hardness or softness of a breast lesion, for example, is a standard part of a breast sonogram, with the sonographer having the knowledge that cancers tend to be hard and benign lesions tend to be soft. As with most clinical findings, palpation is subjective and potentially misleading, as many benign lesions may feel firm on palpation. **Elastography** uses sound waves to virtually palpate lesions in the body to evaluate stiffness. On most machines, elastograms are presented in dual-screen mode, with the B-mode image on one side of the screen and the elastogram on the other side. The elastogram presents a change in shades of gray or colors indicating variations of stiffness. Elastography is also being used most recently in determining the presence of liver fibrosis in patient with known liver disease. The literature is mixed concerning the efficacy of elastography, and its use varies by institution.

SOUND OFF
SE measures the tissue strain or change in tissue length as a result of compression. It is qualitative and only provides a color-coded scale for evaluating tissue stiffness.

There are two general methods for performing elastography: **strain elastography** and **shear-wave elastography (SWE)**. SE measures the tissue strain or change in tissue length as a result of compression. SE is operator dependent because it requires the operator to manually apply compression to the tissue. The operator must apply steady, repeated compressions, which consequently lead to high interoperator variability. Some machines use the patient's breathing or cardiovascular pulsations to apply the needed compressions, but there is still variability in the degree of compression applied to the tissue. SE is qualitative and only provides a color-coded scale (soft→hard) for evaluating tissue stiffness (Figure 6-4). **Acoustic radiation force impulse (ARFI) elastography** is like SE but uses the acoustic radiation force, the mechanical push force of ultrasound, to compress the soft tissue. SWE provides a qualitative (ie, numerical value) measurement of stiffness without requiring pressure input from the sonographer.

SOUND OFF
The speed of the shear waves is measured as they travel through tissue, providing the quantitative result.

SWE, also referred to as transient elastography, uses ARFI to produce the push pulse but measures the speed of the **shear waves** to analyze the stiffness of the tissue. A longitudinal sound wave generated from the transducer applies pressure to the tissue, resulting in transverse wave generation 90° to the point of impact (Figure 6-5). The analogy would be like dropping a stone onto a pond—the rock is the push force, and ripples emanate laterally from where the stone hit. With SWE, not only the compression is applied by the sound

Patient Care and New Technologies

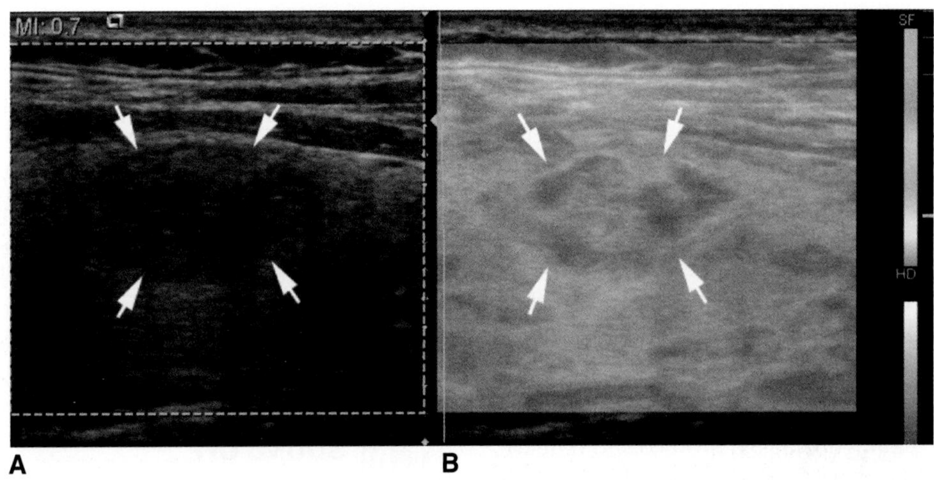

Figure 6-4 Elastogram of a thyroid nodule (*arrows*). **A.** Representative grayscale image of a hypoechoic thyroid nodule (*arrows*). **B.** Color depiction of the strain results. Correlation with the color scale on the right reveals that this nodule is stiffer than the rest of the thyroid gland, which theoretically increases the risk of malignancy.

pulse itself, but also a quantitative result is produced in the form of pressure, in kilopascals (kPa) or velocity in m/s. The speed of the shear waves is measured as they travel through tissue, providing the quantitative result. Specialized ultrafast ultrasound machines are required to produce SWE data. Figure 6-6 is a shear-wave elastogram showing the pressure of the lesion in m/s. A growing use of SWE in general sonography is measuring liver stiffness in patients with chronic liver disease. The aim of liver SWE is to reduce the number of liver biopsies that need to be performed in patients with chronic liver disease.

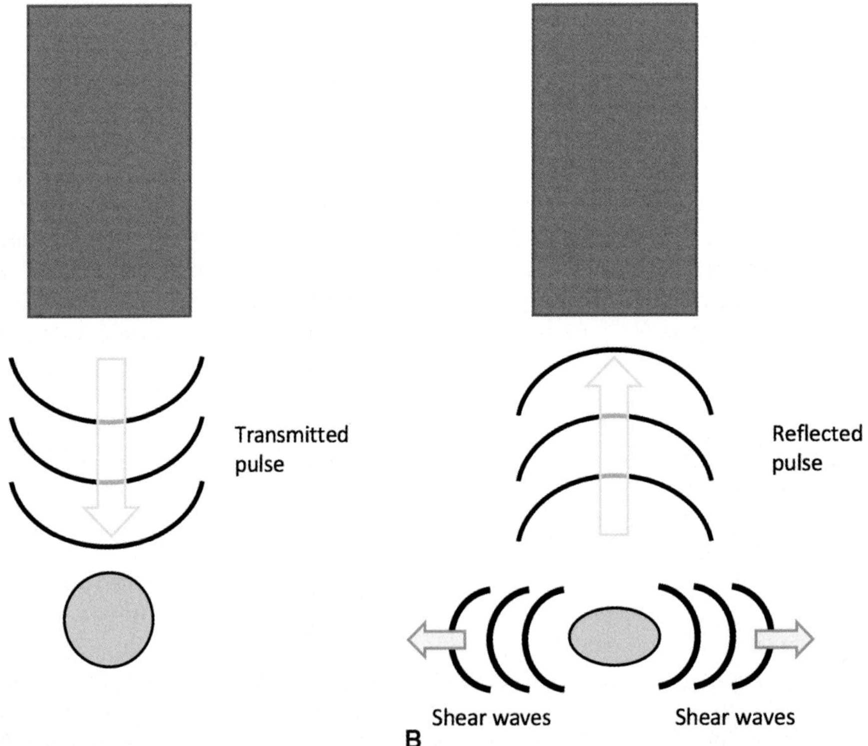

Figure 6-5 Shear-wave elastography. **A.** The pulse is sent out. **B.** Vertical waves (*single vertical arrow*) are generated where the pulse hits the object, but transverse waves (*short arrows*) are generated 90° to the point of impact, emanating from where the object is located.

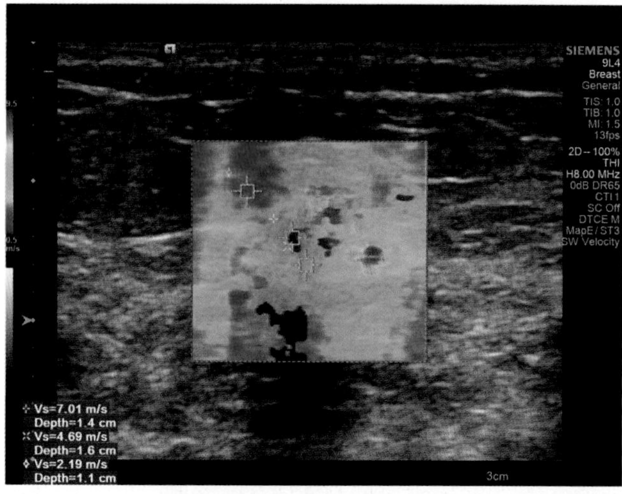

Figure 6-6 A shear-wave elastogram of a breast lesion.

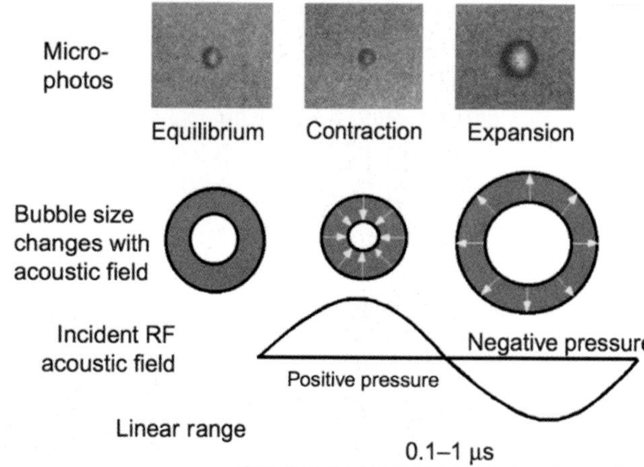

Figure 6-7 This image depicts microbubbles under high and low pressure. Under low pressure, a harmonic signal is produced.

Contrast-Enhanced Ultrasound

Although the Food and Drug Administration (FDA) did not approve ultrasound contrast outside of the heart until 2016, **contrast-enhanced ultrasound (CEUS)** has been utilized for decades as part of research applications within the United States. Like contrast agents used in other imaging disciplines, ultrasound contrast agents help in the visualization of blood vessels and in the identification of neoplasms. There are many studies demonstrating the use of CEUS in imaging the liver, kidneys, genitourinary tracts, and many other applications, albeit as part of research protocols or off label. Although the FDA granted approval for CEUS, it was for limited use and for only one contrast agent, Lumason. However, there is potential for other approved applications in the future.

Ultrasound contrast agents are different from those used in MRI and CT. The typical CEUS agent is a microbubble, usually smaller than 10 μm. These contrast agents are designed to survive passage through the lungs, liver, or kidneys. The bubble shell may be albumin, a phospholipid, a surfactant, a cyanoacrylate, or possibly another type of substance. The gas inside the bubble can be sulfur hexafluoride, perfluorocarbon, or air. Because of the substantial impedance mismatch between soft tissue and air/gas, contrast increases the reflectivity of sound, and therefore these contrast agents are designed to increase reflection approximately 300-fold, enabling better visualization of small blood vessels.

SOUND OFF
The typical CEUS agent is a microbubble composed of a shell and an inert gas.

When ultrasound strikes the microbubble, it causes the bubble to resonate, creating a harmonic signal that is detected by the transducer (Figure 6-7). The harmonic signal that it produces is similar to the principles discussed in the "Tissue Harmonic Imaging" section of this book (see Chapter 3). CEUS enables the visualization of very small blood vessels and isoechoic tumors that would have otherwise been missed during routine sonographic imaging. Figure 6-8 demonstrates the superior visualization of a liver neoplasm with the use of CEUS.

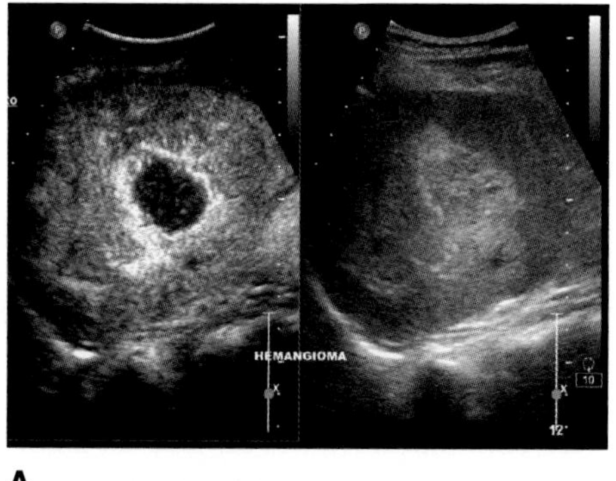

A

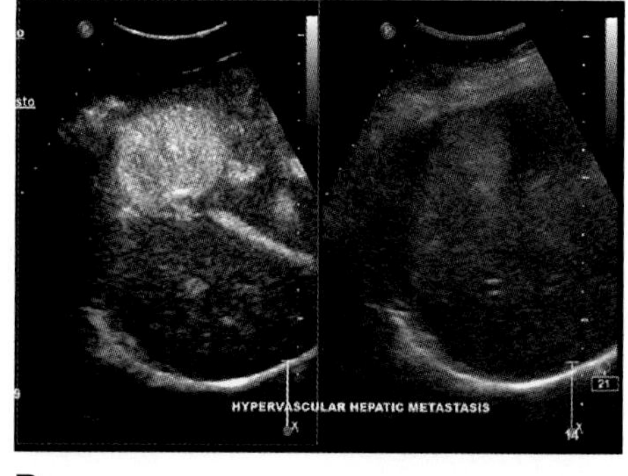

B

Figure 6-8 Contrast-enhanced ultrasound. **A.** Contrast-enhanced sonogram of the liver demonstrates a benign tumor. **B.** Contrast-enhanced sonogram of the liver in another patient demonstrates a hypervascular malignant tumor.

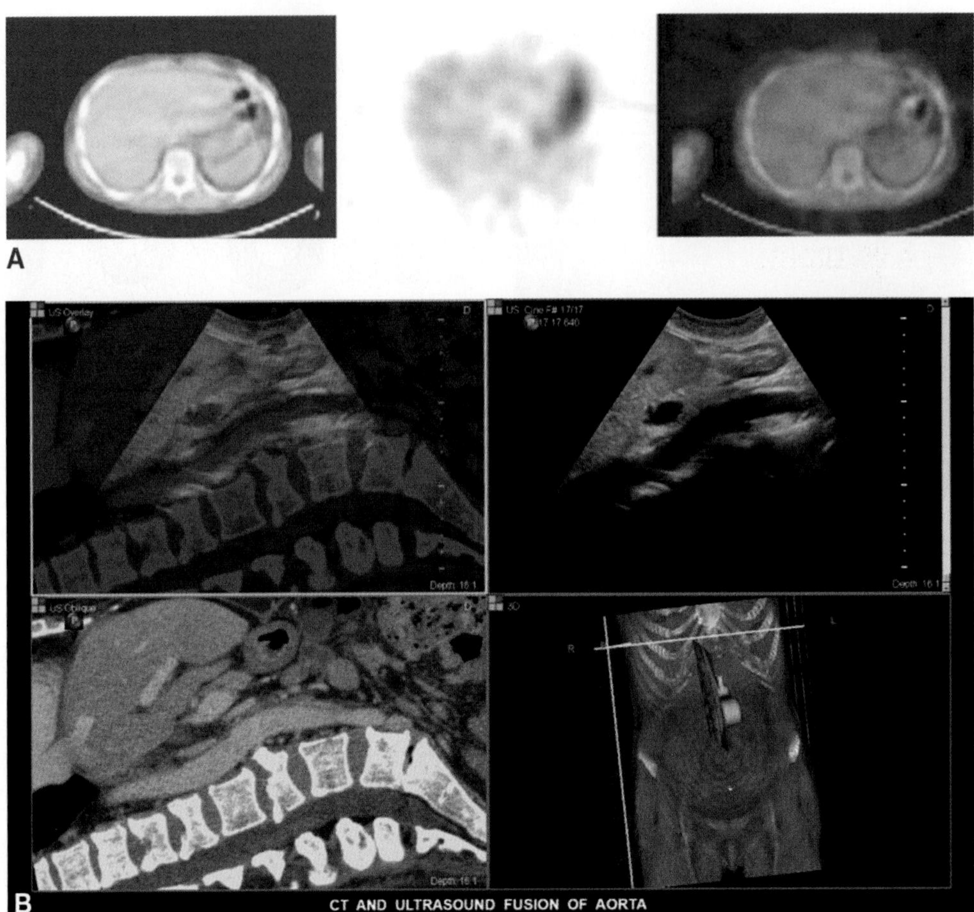

Figure 6-9 Fusion or hybrid imaging. **A.** An example of hybrid or fusion imaging. This study combined single-photon emission computed tomography and CT. **B.** These images combine CT and ultrasound. With permission from Philips Ultrasound.

Other (research-based) uses of CEUS include targeted delivery of drugs through a specialized outer shell and medication inside the bubble. After the microbubbles reach the area of interest, high-intensity sound waves can be used to pop the bubbles, releasing the medication contained within. CEUS is also used in subharmonic imaging (SHI), which is a technique that uses the signal information produced at one-half the fundamental frequency to suppress the tissue information to better display the microvasculature. SHI is also being used for noninvasive pressure measurements in the heart and liver.

Fusion Imaging

One innovation that several ultrasound manufacturers use is called **fusion imaging**, also referred to as hybrid imaging. Fusion imaging enables the simultaneous display of real-time sonography and a stored CT or MRI. Using a tracking system, the machine knows where the transducer is placed on the patient and automatically moves the CT or MRI image to correspond with the plane of the sonographic image. The advantage of fusion imaging is that although certain lesions are better seen with CT or MRI, real-time sonography offers improved needle guidance and the ability to assess relevant anatomy during procedures such as tissue ablation (Figure 6-9).

Intravascular Ultrasound

Intravascular ultrasound (IVUS) is a procedure that pairs a miniature ultrasound transducer and a vascular catheter (Figure 6-10). The IVUS probe is placed in the circulatory system and the transducer is used to analyze the vessel wall. IVUS has a role in evaluating plaque morphology and arterial and venous intervention. In arterial stenosis and occlusion intervention, IVUS may be used preprocedure, during the procedure, and postprocedure. There is a growing list of functions for IVUS, beyond the 2D assessment of plaque within vessels. The combination of IVUS and 3D sonography is being utilized in hopes of providing improved diagnosis and enhanced treatment of otherwise difficult to evaluate vascular conditions.

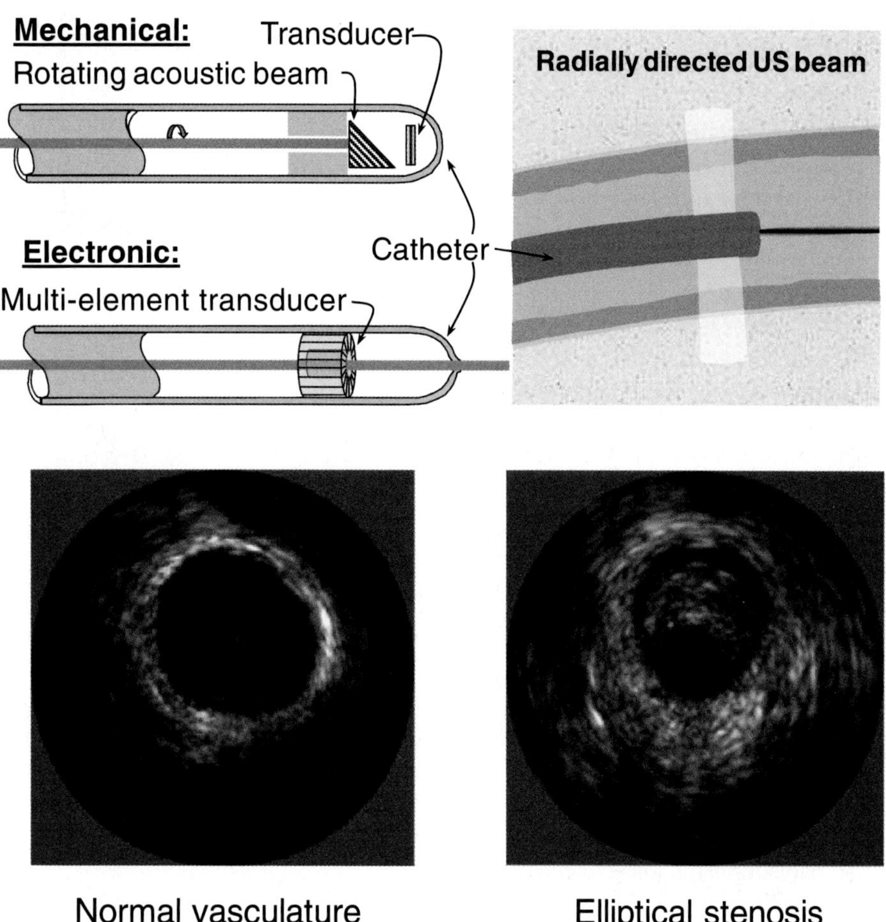

Figure 6-10 Intravascular ultrasound. A transducer is mounted on a catheter and placed into a blood vessel for the assessment of stenosis. Images from within the vessel demonstrate normal vasculature **(lower left)** and a vessel with a stenosis **(lower right)**.

SOUND OFF
Elastography and fusion imaging are not listed on the September 2023 content outlines for the ARDMS SPI examination but may be on other credentialing examinations or future versions of the ARDMS SPI examination.

SOUND OFF
MLA is an advanced type of beamforming that provides better frame rates, better lateral resolution, and improved signal-to-noise ratio compared to single-line acquisition.

Multiline Acquisition

Throughout most of this text, ultrasound imaging has relied on the pulse-echo method in which a pulse of sound is transmitted, and the returning echoes create one scan line of information. When the scan lines are placed next to each other, a single image, or frame, is produced. Single-line acquisition only requires one piezoelectric element to send and receive sound and minimal amounts of memory to process hundreds of shades of gray. **Multiline acquisition** is a more recent type of beamforming with array transducers in which a wide beam is transmitted and received, and parallel processing is performed by a graphic processing unit that sorts out all echo information to produce the image. MLA is a technique similar to other techniques such as plane-wave imaging and synthetic aperture in which the beamformer is virtual. All these techniques, sometimes referred to as "the new physics," allow for ultrafast imaging with very high frame rates (in the thousands for grayscale imaging and hundreds for color Doppler).

A similar imaging methodology that removes some of the limitations of the wide beam used in MLA (namely worse lateral resolution) is zone imaging. Zone imaging receives multiple beams simultaneously with dynamic receive focusing, which eliminates the need for transmit focal zones. This method creates very narrow beams that are focused in all planes.

ERGONOMICS

Work-Related Musculoskeletal Disorders

A fundamental appreciation of **ergonomics** is vital for a sonographer to have a long and satisfying career. Ergonomics is the scientific study of creating tools and using equipment effectively to help the human body adjust to the work environment. For a sonographer, ergonomics is geared toward recognizing the potential for, and thus preventing, work-related musculoskeletal disorders (WRMSDs).

Preventing WRMSDs can be accomplished by combining the use of proper body mechanics, creating a practical work environment with room design, and by using equipment that is functionally supportive for the occupation of the sonographer. The use of proper body mechanics ensures that the spine is always in appropriate alignment, including movements that require sitting, standing, and lifting. Room design should offer proper lighting, seating, and good air quality. Equipment design, such as high-definition, adjustable exam tables and monitors, lightweight transducers, foam pads, and cable braces can also avert strain to specific, overworked muscle groups. Stretching during the day can help prevent injury and should be factored into the daily schedule.

The symptoms of WRMSDs include those associated with inflammation, such as swelling, numbness, burning, muscle spasm, stabbing pains, tingling, loss of sensation, and perhaps a "pins and needles" feeling in the affected region. The recognition of these symptoms is critical for a sonographer, and they should not be ignored. The damage from WRMSDs is cumulative, and thus the devastation of the affected area occurs over time. For a sonographer, these types of injuries result from repetitive strain and are thus referred to as repetitive strain disorders or injuries.

SOUND OFF
The shoulder is the most common source of pain for a sonographer.

Tendinitis, tenosynovitis, epicondylitis, bursitis, and pinched nerves are all examples of repetitive strain disorders. The neck, back, feet, elbows, wrists, and hands are common locations of pain for sonographers. However, the shoulder is the most common source of pain for them. To prevent shoulder discomfort and repetitive damage, sonographers should decrease shoulder abduction while performing sonograms. The suggested position of the scanning arm is no more than a 30° angle of abduction (Figure 6-11). A sonographer should place the patient as near to oneself as practical because this situation will reduce the amount of reach needed to perform most examinations. To ease neck and shoulder strain, the display should be positioned so that it is closer to the patient, although never over the patient's head, reducing the awkward position of aiming the body toward the patient and the head away from the patient. On the website https://healthysonographer.com/, the "magic triangle" is described, which demonstrates how the machine, display, and sonographer are positioned to minimize strain (Figure 6-12).

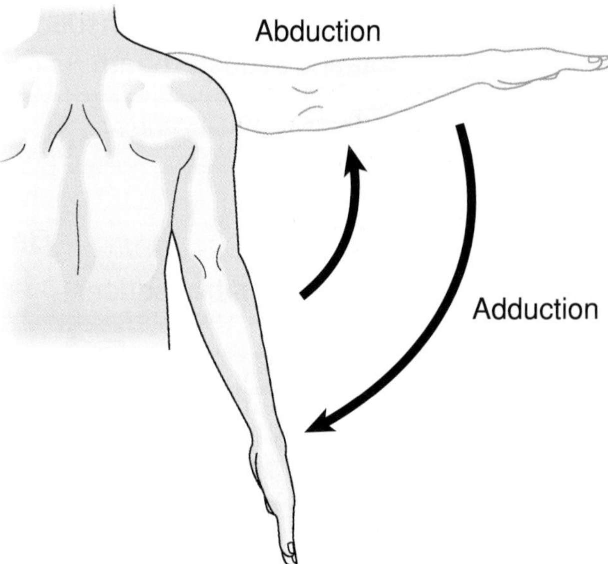

Figure 6-11 Abduction and adduction of the arm. The sonographer should work to decrease arm abduction.

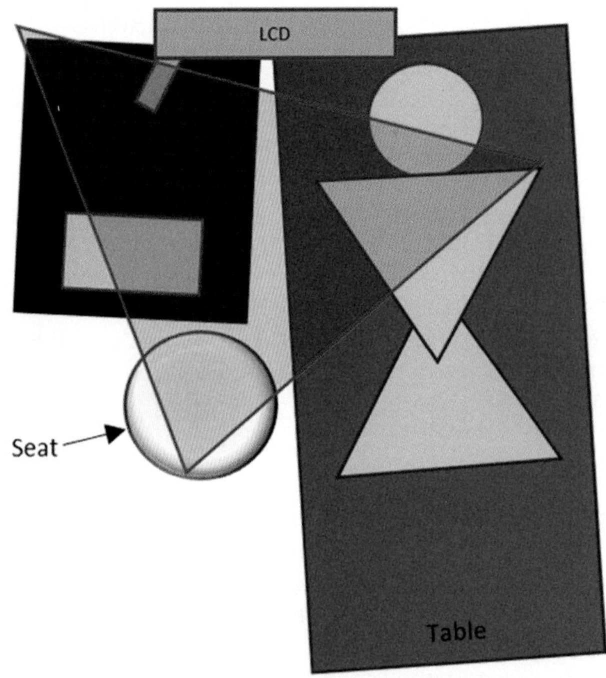

Figure 6-12 The "magic triangle." The "magic triangle," in pink, is adapted from Canon Medical Systems USA website healthysonographer.com. The "magic triangle" approach describes how the US panel, the display, the patient, and the sonographer are positioned to make the patient the focus, not the machine. This positioning can reduce strain from poor sonographer positioning.

REVIEW QUESTIONS

1. What term and philosophy relates the amount of exposure time for the patient during a sonographic examination?
   a. Nonthermal mechanisms
   b. Mechanical mechanism
   c. As low as reasonably achievable
   d. Health Insurance Portability and Accountability Act

2. Sonographers should verify the patient's wristband information for identifying markers. Identifying markers include which of the following?
   a. Patient's race
   b. Medical record number
   c. Date of registration
   d. Birth place

3. If a patient does not speak English, or the national language, the sonographer should:
   a. Use picture cards
   b. Cancel the examination
   c. Provide an interpreter
   d. Offer the patient paper and use hand gestures

4. Which of the following is true regarding thermal bioeffects?
   a. The highest intensity is at the surface in a focused transducer
   b. Lower frequencies result in higher attenuation of sound
   c. Scanned modes are higher risk than unscanned modes
   d. The dwell time should be minimized when over bone

5. What is the name of the clinical finding when a patient's face is too pale?
   a. pallor
   b. rubor
   c. cyanosis
   d. jaundice

6. What technology permits the imaging of blood vessels with contrast-enhanced ultrasound?
   a. Tissue harmonic imaging
   b. Shear-wave elastography
   c. Fusion imaging
   d. A-mode imaging

7. What is defined as the action of an acoustic field within a fluid to generate bubbles?
   a. Thermal index
   b. Cavitation
   c. Dehydration
   d. Streaming

8. What is it called when an acoustic field causes motion of fluids?
   a. Streaming
   b. Cavitation
   c. Hydrostatic pressure
   d. Radiation forces

9. The calculation used to predict the maximum temperature elevation in tissues because of the attenuation of sound is the:
   a. Spatial temporal index
   b. Nonmechanical index
   c. Mechanical index
   d. Thermal index

10. The maximum heating of tissue is related to the sound beams:
    a. Spatial average peak average
    b. Spatial peak temporal average
    c. Spatial average temporal average
    d. Spatial average

11. The Health Insurance Portability and Accountability Act attempts to do everything below except:
    a. Establish new standards for the release of health records.
    b. Protect health records by establishing new standards for healthcare professionals to follow.
    c. Apply strict penalties for those who violate patient confidentiality and patient rights.
    d. Promote high-quality cleanliness in the healthcare setting.

12. Which of the following is defined as forces exerted by a sound beam on an absorber or reflector that can alter structures?
    a. Cavitation
    b. Radioactive mechanism
    c. Radiation forces
    d. Nonmechanical strengths

13. Which of the following forms of cavitation has the most potential for inducing biologic damage?
    a. Acute
    b. Chronic
    c. Transient
    d. Stable

14. The calculation used to assist in evaluating the likelihood of cavitation to occur is referred to as the:
    a. Inertial index
    b. Mechanical index
    c. Nonmechanical index
    d. Thermal index

15. Which of the following would be the best described as the failure of the heart to pump the proper amount of blood to the vital organs?
    a. Distributive shock
    b. Neurogenic shock
    c. Hypovolemic shock
    d. Cardiogenic shock

16. A nosocomial infection is best described as a:
    a. Hospital-acquired infection
    b. Infection caused by mosquito bite
    c. Injury caused by malpractice
    d. An airborne disease found in infected persons' lungs that is spread by coughing

17. Which of the following could be a cause of anaphylactic shock?
    a. Cardiac tamponade
    b. Diarrhea
    c. Contrast agents
    d. Lack of glucose

18. Which of the following would be considered one of the most common nosocomial infections?
    a. AIDS
    b. Hepatitis B
    c. Urinary tract infections
    d. Tuberculosis

19. An infectious agent needs to initially have which of the following to grow and survive?
    a. Means of transmission
    b. Portal of entry
    c. Portal of exit
    d. Reservoir

20. The thermal index most appropriate for use at 20 week is the
    a. TIB
    b. TIC
    c. TIS
    d. TIA

21. When viewing sonographic images outside of the clinical arena, all the following pieces of information are required to be removed except:
    a. Patient's name
    b. Facility
    c. Date
    d. Image orientation

22. Which of the following is best described as an airborne disease that is spread by bacteria released from an infected individual when that person coughs, sneezes, speaks, or sings?
    a. Methicillin-resistant *Staphylococcus aureus*
    b. Hepatitis B
    c. Tuberculosis
    d. Hepatitis C

23. What is the FDA maximum for mechanical index?
    a. 0.4
    b. 1.0
    c. 1.4
    d. 1.9

24. Assuming there is no attenuation, the highest intensity of the beam is located where?
    a. At the surface
    b. At the focal point
    c. 2- to 3-cm deep from the surface
    d. Between 10- and 15-cm deep

25. Which technique measures the stiffness of the tissue?
    a. Fusion imaging
    b. IVUS
    c. Elastography
    d. Contrast-enhanced ultrasound

26. For optimal ergonomics, which of the following is true?
    a. The ultrasound machine's LCD should be placed over the patient's head
    b. The machine should be greater than 3 feet away from the table
    c. The machine and table should be positioned to minimize the reach of the sonographer
    d. Pads and cable braces should be used in people with previous injury only

27. Hepatitis is a form of:
    a. Liver inflammation
    b. Urinary tract disorders
    c. Respiratory infection
    d. Biliary inflammation

28. All the following are considered to be part of non-thermal mechanisms of biologic effects except:
    a. Radiation forces
    b. Streaming
    c. Acoustic cavitation
    d. Tissue heating

29. What is the primary reason why the intensity of sound decreases as sound moves through soft tissue?
    a. Reflection
    b. Enhancement
    c. Cavitation
    d. Absorption

30. From a bioeffects standpoint, below what peak temperature can soft tissue be insonated indefinitely?
    a. 0.5 °C
    b. 1.5 °C
    c. 2.5 °C
    d. 3.5 °C

31. Which of the following does not qualify as "an existing gas body?"
    a. Liver cells
    b. Lungs
    c. Intestines
    d. Contrast agents

32. Which of the following would be described as a complication of diabetes that results from a severe lack of insulin, in which case the patient's breath may have a sweet smell?
    a. Hypoglycemia
    b. Diabetic ketoacidosis
    c. Hypovolemic shock
    d. Neurogenic shock

33. In tissues that contain well-defined gas bodies, no effects have been observed for in situ peak rarefactional pressures below a mechanical index value less than approximately:
    a. 0.4
    b. 0.8
    c. 2
    d. 100

34. Regarding the prevention of work-related musculoskeletal disorders, the sonographer's scanning arm should be in a position that is no more than a:
    a. 20° angle of adduction
    b. 20° angle of abduction
    c. 30° angle of adduction
    d. 30° angle of abduction

35. Which ultrasound contrast agent is currently FDA approved for use in adult livers?
    a. Viewsonic
    b. Lumason
    c. Levovist
    d. Definity

36. Which of the following is a violation of HIPAA?
    a. Asking a coworker for help lifting a patient
    b. Asking the radiologist to review your study after completion
    c. Telling your spouse that a certain famous person was in your department that day
    d. Calling the patient's nurse with the patient's results after the ultrasound

37. Which of these is true regarding the sterile technique?
    a. Never reach across a sterile field
    b. The edges of a sterile wrapper are considered sterile
    c. If sterile gloves become contaminated, wash with soap and water to decontaminate them
    d. Sterile trays do not need to be covered if left unattended

38. Human immunodeficiency virus may be spread by all the following means except:
    a. Sexual contact
    b. Handshake
    c. Needle stick
    d. Blood transfusion

39. A heart rate above normal is called
    a. Bradycardia
    b. Brachycephaly
    c. Tachypnea
    d. Tachycardia

40. Which of the following statements is true regarding handwashing?
    a. Alcohol-based hand rubs can be used to take the place of handwashing in all circumstances.
    b. Handwashing should occur before and after any contact with patients.
    c. Handwashing is not an effective means to prevent the spread of infection.
    d. Alcohol-based hand rubs should never be used in conjunction with handwashing.

41. In the presence of a nonresponsive adult patient, which pulse should be evaluated?
    a. Radial
    b. Tibial
    c. Carotid
    d. Temporal

42. Personal protective equipment includes all of the following except:
    a. Gloves
    b. Glutaraldehyde-soaking solution
    c. Gowns
    d. Face masks

43. Which of these uses high-frequency ultrasound mounted on a catheter to view the endoluminal lining of vessels?
    a. Contrast-enhanced ultrasound
    b. Elastography
    c. Fusion imaging
    d. Intravascular ultrasound

44. What would be the most likely means of transmission of the human immunodeficiency virus from a patient to a sonographer?
    a. Exposure to fecal material
    b. Holding the patient's hand without a glove
    c. Needle stick
    d. Coughing

45. What would be the most likely means of transmission of tuberculosis from a patient to a sonographer?
    a. Exposure to fecal material
    b. Holding the patient's hand without a glove
    c. Needle stick
    d. Coughing

46. Nonthermal mechanisms for bioeffects may also be referred to as:
    a. Thermal mechanisms
    b. Mechanical mechanisms
    c. Thermal indices
    d. Absorption influence

47. What is the type of injury that occurs when a patient hemorrhages after an invasive medical procedure?
    a. portal of entry
    b. hospital acquired infection
    c. iatrogenic
    d. fomite

48. Which of the following statements is true concerning the biologic effects of diagnostic sonography?
    a. The risk of harm to the patient is minimal when performing diagnostic ultrasound without contrast agents
    b. Ultrasound causes dangerous bioeffects and should only be used in an emergency
    c. Ultrasound has no potential to cause bioeffects to the tissue
    d. The only biologic effect of diagnostic ultrasound exposure is cavitation

49. All of the following are true statements about the use of gloves except:
    a. Gloves should be used when there is any expected contact with infected materials
    b. Gloves can be used to replace handwashing
    c. Gloves should be changed between patients
    d. Gloves are considered personal protective equipment

50. Which of the following best describes transient (inertial) cavitation?
    a. The type of cavitation in which there is a production of cavernous spaces within tissue
    b. The type of cavitation that produces bubbles that oscillate, or fluctuate, in size but do not rupture
    c. The type of cavitation in which bubbles do not exist
    d. The type of cavitation in which larger bubbles are produced and rupture violently

SUGGESTED READINGS

AIUM. *Medical Ultrasound Safety*. 3rd ed. American Institute of Ultrasound in Medicine; 2014.

AIUM ALARA Principle. As Low as Reasonably Achievable (ALARA) Principle. Accessed November 26, 2023 from https://www.aium.org/resources/official-statements/view/as-low-as-reasonably-achievable-(alara)-principle, 2020.

AIUM Guidelines for Cleaning and Preparing External- and Internal-Use Ultrasound Transducers and Equipment Between Patients as Well as Safe Handling and Use of Ultrasound Coupling Gel. Accessed November 26, 2023 from https://www.aium.org/resources/official-statements/view/guidelines-for-cleaning-and-preparing-external--and-internal-use-ultrasound-transducers-and-equipment-between-patients-as-well-as-safe-handling-and-use-of-ultrasound-coupling-gel, 2022.

AIUM Prudent Use and Clinical Safety. Accessed November 26, 2023 from https://www.aium.org/resources/official-statements/view/prudent-clinical-use-and-safety-of-diagnostic-ultrasound, 2019.

AIUM Statement and Recommendations for Safety Assurance in Lung Ultrasound. Accessed December 21, 2023 from https://www.aium.org/resources/official-statements/view/statement-and-recommendations-for-safety-assurance-in-lung-ultrasound

AIUM Statement on Biological Effects of Ultrasound in Vivo. Accessed November 26, 2023 from https://www.aium.org/resources/official-statements/view/statement-on-biological-effects-in-tissues-with-ultrasound-contrast-agents-2, 2022.

AIUM Statement on Mammalian Biological Effects of Ultrasound in Vivo. Accessed June 25, 2017 from http://www.aium.org/officialStatements/9, 2021.

American Institute of Ultrasound in Medicine Web site. Available at: https://www.aium.org/resources/official-statements

Canon Medical Systems USA. Healthy sonographer. Accessed December 24, 2023 from https://healthysonographer.com/

Carlsen JF. Strain elastography ultrasound: An overview with emphasis on breast cancer diagnosis. *Diagnostics*. 2013;3(1):117–125.

Centers for Disease Control and Prevention. Available at: http://www.cdc.gov/

Craig M. *Essentials of Sonography and Patient Care*. 2nd ed. Saunders; 2006.

Edelman SK. *Understanding Ultrasound Physics*. 4th ed. ESP Inc.; 2012.
Harvey CJ, Blomley MJ, Eckersley RJ, Cosgrove DO. Developments in ultrasound contrast media. *Eur Radiol.* 2011;11(4):675–769.
Kremkau FW. *Diagnostic Ultrasound: Principles and Instruments*. 9th ed. Saunders; 2016.
Lee MW. Fusion imaging of real-time ultrasonography with CT or MRI for hepatic intervention. *Ultrasonography.* 2014;33(4):227–239.
OSHA. Available at: https://www.osha.gov/dte/grant_materials/fy10/sh-20839-10/hand_hygiene.pdf, 2016.
Penny S. *Introduction to Sonography and Patient Care.* Wolters Kluwer; 2016.
Rumack C, Wilson S, Charboneau J. *Diagnostic Ultrasound.* 4th ed. Mosby; 2011.
Secemsky EA, Mosarla RC, Rosenfield K, et al. Appropriate use of intravascular ultrasound during arterial and venous lower extremity interventions. *Cardiovasc Interv.* 2022;15(15):1558–1568.
Sikora A, Zahra F. Nosocomial infections. Accessed November 26, 2023 from https://www.ncbi.nlm.nih.gov/books/NBK559312/, 2023.
Szabo TL. *Diagnostic Ultrasound Imaging: Inside Out.* Elsevier; 2014.
Torres L, Dutton A, Linn-Watson T. *Patient Care in Imaging Technology.* 7th ed. Wolters Kluwer; 2010.

Appendix

TABLE A-1 Parts of the ultrasound system and important points to remember

Parts of the Ultrasound System	Important Points to Remember
Transmit beam former	• Responsible for generating voltage pulses that determine PRF and PRP • Responsible for shaping and steering of the beam and apodization • Consists of many of the components listed in this table

Pulser (aka Transmitter)	• Part of a transmit beam former
	  • Generates the voltage that drives the transducer
	  • Pulser sends signal to many channels, each of which consists of a delay and its piezoelectric element
	• Directly controls the amount of power entering the patient

Receiver	• Processes the return echo coming back from the patient in this order:
	  • Amplification: Increases or decreases all echo amplitudes equally
	  • Compensation: Adjusts the brightness of echoes to correct for attenuation with depth
	  • Compression: Decreases the range of amplitudes present within the system (opposite of dynamic range)
	  • Demodulation: Makes the signal easier for the system to process; includes rectification and smoothing
	  • Rejection: Eliminates (suppresses) low-level echoes that do not contribute to useful information on the image

Analog-to-digital converter	• Converts analog information from the transducer to the digital (binary) form required by the scan converter and computer • Also called the digitizer
Transmit/receive switch	• Ensures the electrical signals travel in the correct direction • Ensures that the pulser voltages go to the transducer, and the received voltages from the transducer go to the amplifier

Scan converter/image memory	• Part of the image processor
	• The summer is part of the machine responsible for creating the scan lines
	  • Digital memory: Uses computer memory (which uses binary language) to store the image information on an image matrix that corresponds to pixels on the display
	  • Digital-to-analog (D-to-A) converter: Converts the binary back to the analog form to get the signal ready for video output
	• Settings that can be adjusted after the image has been stored in memory are called "postprocessing" functions

Display	• LCD: Liquid crystal display, also called a flat-panel display. Two polarized filters in front of a light source. Sandwiched between the filters are liquid crystals that twist/untwist with the application of electricity to determine if the backlighting gets through or not
Recording and storage	• PACS: Picture archiving and communication system. Uses a computer network to store images and videos. Can transmit images to remote locations. Backed up by RAID array • Film: Obsolete. Replaced by PACS. Thermal paper may also be used to print images. • CD/DVD: Optical disk storage • USB flash drives: Portable, removable storage device

TABLE A-2 Binary conversion

To convert TO binary:
Converting to binary is not difficult: just remember the number **1**.

- Create a table of columns
- Starting with the right-hand column, write the number 1

Populate the remaining columns (working right to left) by doubling the number

16	8	4	2	1

How far to the left do you need to go? Depends on what you want to convert. For example, to convert the number 30 to binary, you go no higher than the number 30. Try it: Fill out the grid below by doubling, starting with the number 1:

32	16	8	4	2	1

Look at the leftmost column—notice it is a 32. That is higher than 30, so ignore it or do not write it. You do not need it. The highest column we need is 16. How many times does 16 go into 32? The answer can *only* be a 0 or a 1. Sixteen goes into 30 one time, so we put a 1 under the "16" column as follows:

16	8	4	2	1
1				

- You have to subtract 16 from the original 30 now, because you just used it up
  - 30 – 16 = 14. Move down the column. How many times does 8 go into 14?

Once; so add the "1" under the "8"

16	8	4	2	1
1	1			

- Now subtract 8 from 14

14 – 8 = 6. How many times does 4 go into 6? Once; so add it under the "4"

16	8	4	2	1
1	1	1		

6 – 4 = 2. How many times does 2 go into 2? Once; so add it under the "2"

16	8	4	2	1
1	1	1	1	

2 – 2 = 0. How many times does 1 go into 0? None; so add a 0 under the "1"

16	8	4	2	1
1	1	1	1	0

- There you have it! The binary of 30 is 11110

To convert FROM binary:
To convert from binary, look at how many digits there are in the number. For example, 11110 has five digits. Draw a grid, with as many columns as there are digits.

16	8	4	2	1

Five digits, five columns. Now, populate the columns with the binary number

16	8	4	2	1
1	1	1	1	0

All of the columns that have a "1" in it, add those up.

16 + 8 + 4 + 2 = <u>30</u>

Image Optimization Review Questions

*NOTE: Color versions of applicable figures are available in the Image Bank at thePoint.lww.com/penny_spi2e

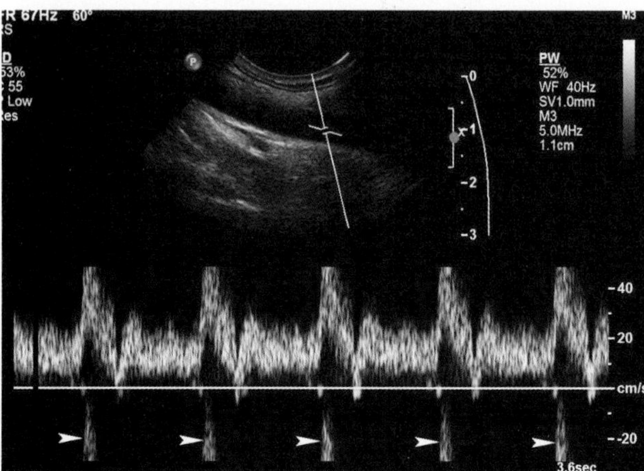

Figure ic.1

1. Spectral Doppler waveform (Figure ic.1) could be corrected by:
   a. Increasing the wall filter
   b. Decreasing the 2D gain
   c. Increasing the spectral gain
   d. Lowering the baseline

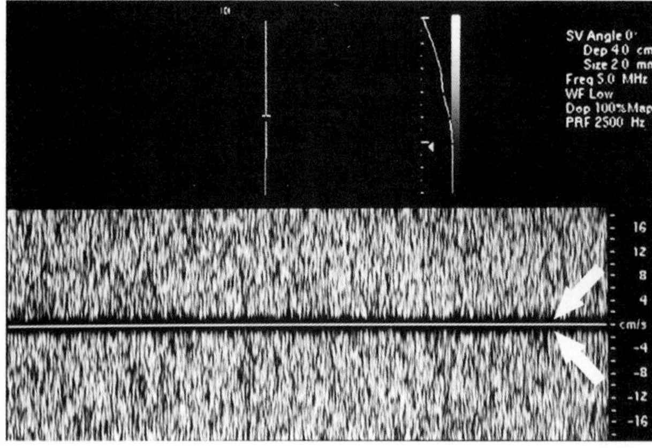

Figure ic.2

2. The arrows in this image (Figure ic.2) indicate:
   a. The signals removed by the wall filter
   b. The signals removed by decreasing the dynamic range
   c. The increased depth of the reflector
   d. The decreased pulse repetition frequency

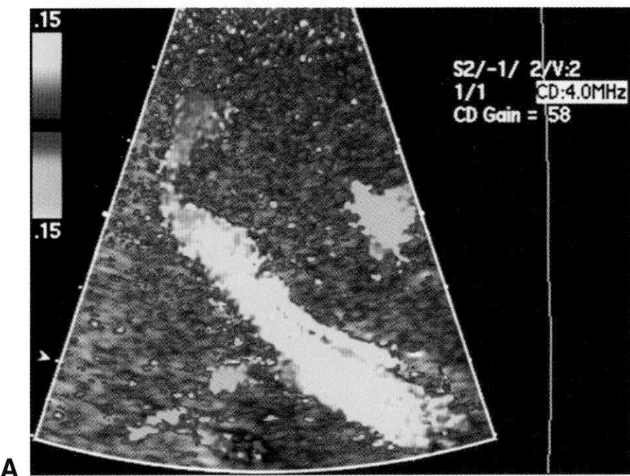

A

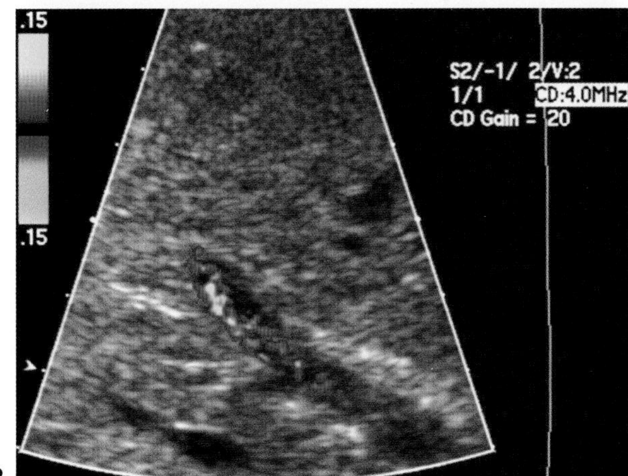

B

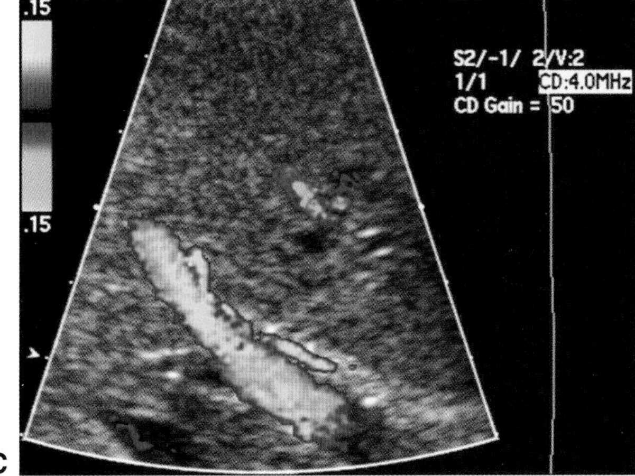

C

***Figure ic.3**

3. The color gain settings in image "A" (Figure ic.3) is:
   a. Too high
   b. Too low
   c. Correct

4. The color gain setting in image "B" (Figure ic.3) is:
   a. Too high
   b. Too low
   c. Correct

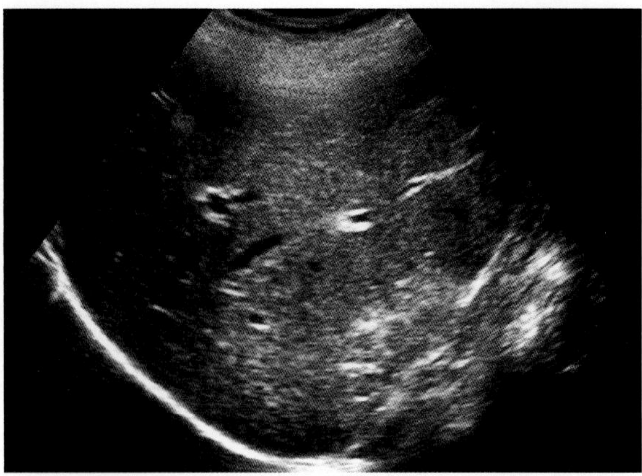

Figure ic.4

5. How could a sonographer adjust the following image of a liver (Figure ic.4) to obtain a more diagnostic representation of the anatomy?
   a. Increase the operating frequency
   b. Increase the near-field time-gain compensation
   c. Decrease the spatial pulse length
   d. Decrease the overall gain

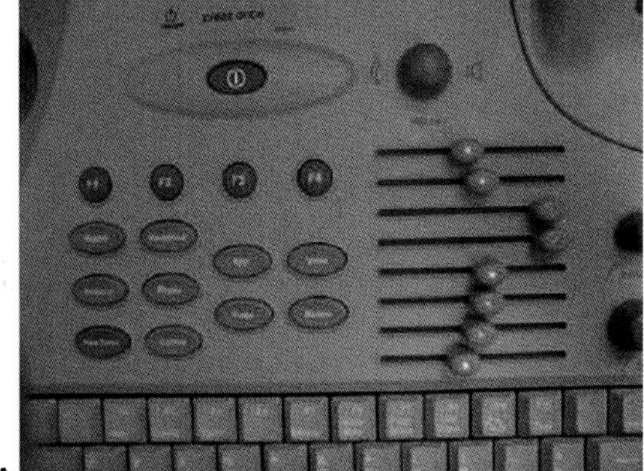

A

B

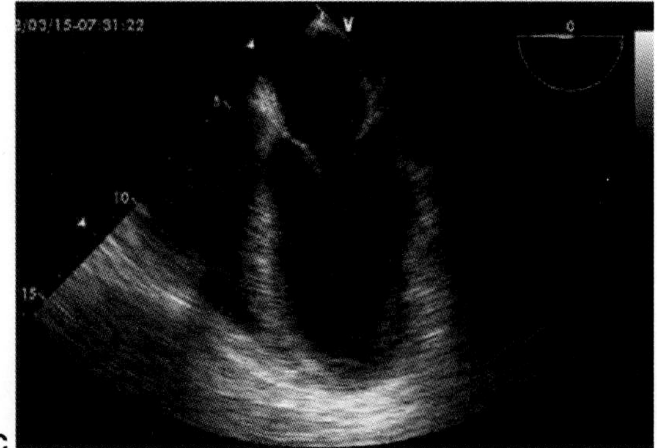

C

Figure ic.5

6. What control did a sonographer most likely adjust to obtain the bottom image in this image series (Figure ic.5)?
   a. Depth
   b. Time-gain compensation
   c. Wall filter
   d. Pulse repetition frequency

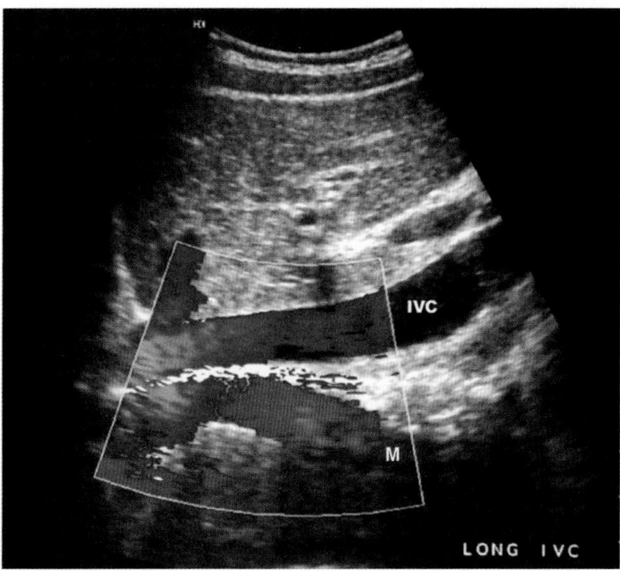

***Figure ic.6**

7. What can the sonographer do to reduce the likelihood of this artifact (Figure ic.6)?
   a. Decrease the gain and/or angle
   b. Increase the gain and decrease the angle
   c. Decrease the depth and increase the frequency
   d. Increase the depth and the overall gain

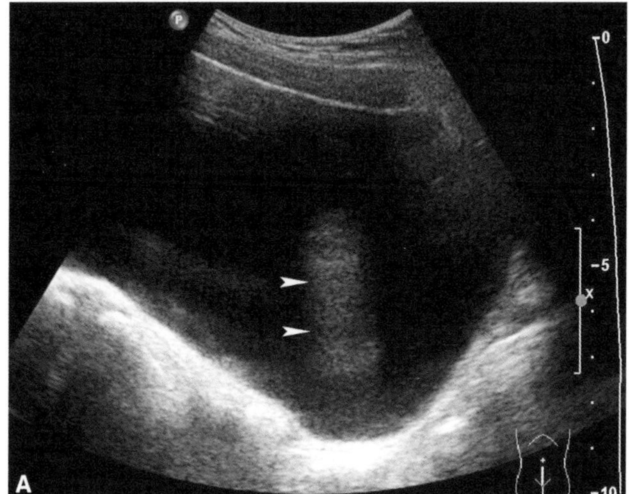

B

Figure ic.7

8. The artifact in the following image (Figure ic.7) on the left (*arrows*) was corrected by increasing the:
   a. Frequency
   b. Depth
   c. Overall gain
   d. Time-gain compensation

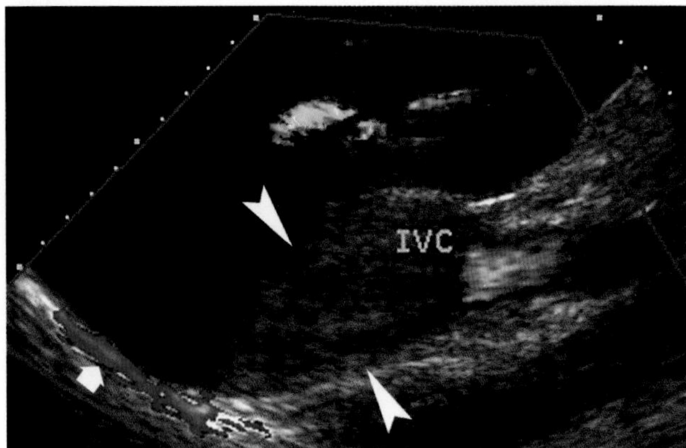

*Figure ic.8

9. The artifact identified by the short arrow in this image (Figure ic.8) can be eliminated by:
   a. Increasing the gain
   b. Decreasing the pulse repetition frequency
   c. Having the patient hold his or her breath
   d. Increasing the output power

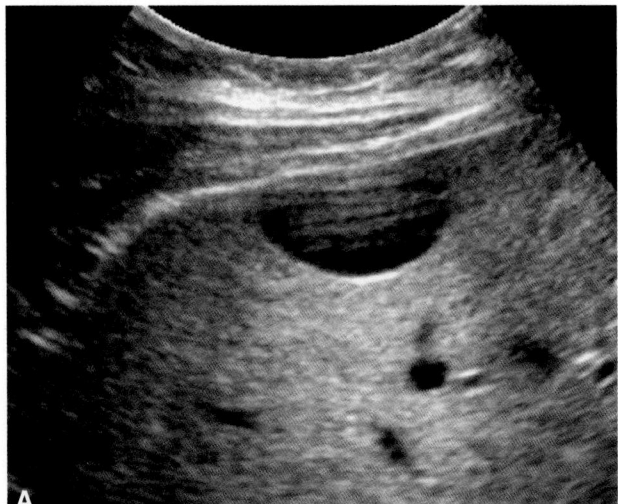

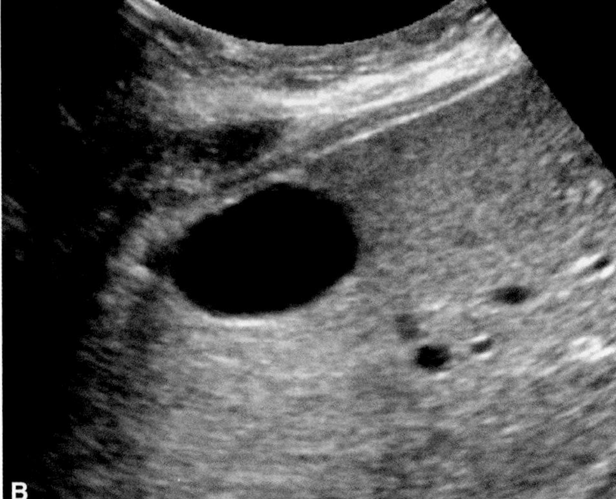

Figure ic.9

10. How did the sonographer correct for the artifact noted in image "A" in this figure (Figure ic.9)?
    a. Reducing the number of transmit zones
    b. Increasing the overall gain
    c. Repositioning the transducer
    d. Deactivating tissue harmonics

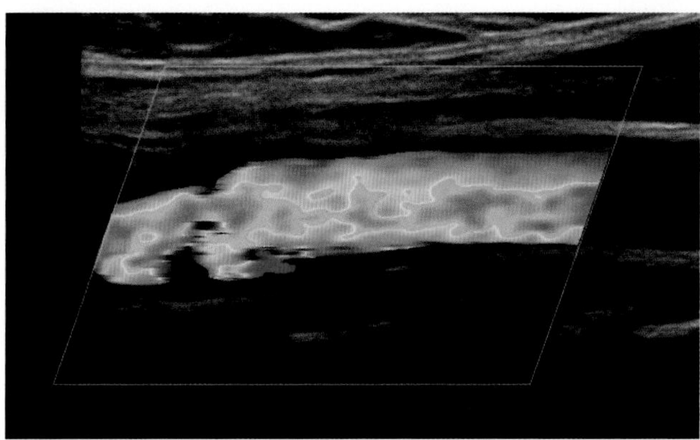

*Figure ic.10

11. What is the appropriate correction to fix this image (Figure ic.10)?
    a. Increase the pulse repetition frequency
    b. Increase the color gain
    c. Increase the frequency
    d. Increase the wall filter

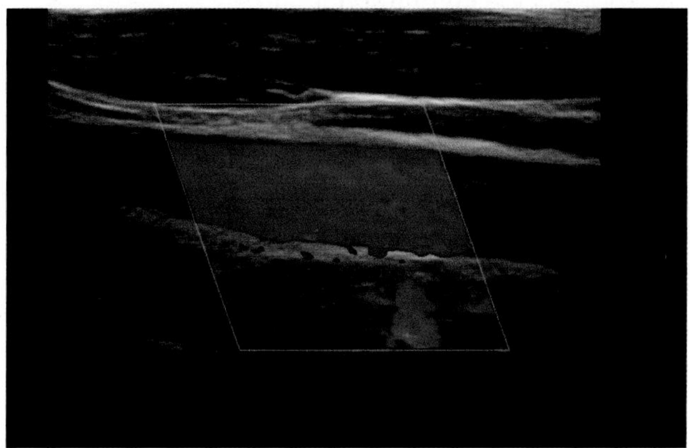

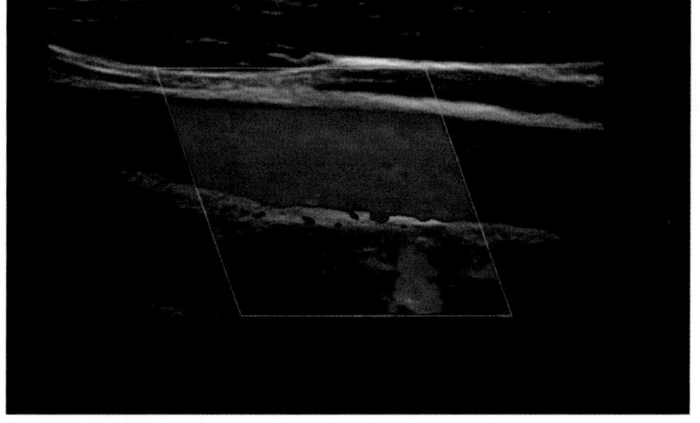

*Figure ic.11

12. In this image (Figure ic.11), what appears to be wrong?
    a. The color gain is too low
    b. The color gain is too high
    c. The scale is too low
    d. The scale is too high

*Figure ic.12

13. What is the best way to make this vessel fill better (Figure ic.12)?
    a. Decrease the scale
    b. Increase the color gain
    c. Decrease the baseline
    d. Change the color steer

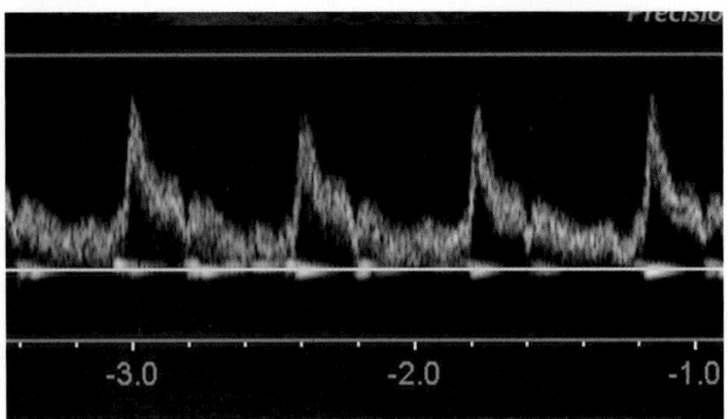

Figure ic.13

14. What is the control that will optimize this spectral waveform (Figure ic.13)?
    a. Scale
    b. Sweep speed
    c. Wall filter
    d. Baseline

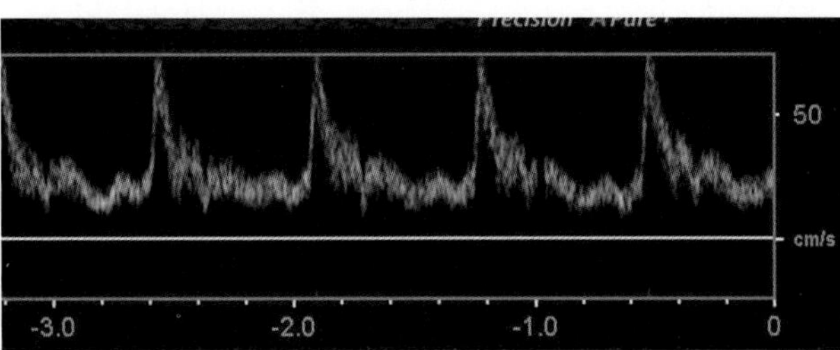

Figure ic.14

15. What is the proper action to improve this spectral waveform (Figure ic.14)?
    a. Increase the baseline
    b. Increase the pulse repetition frequency
    c. Increase the wall filter
    d. Increase the sweep speed

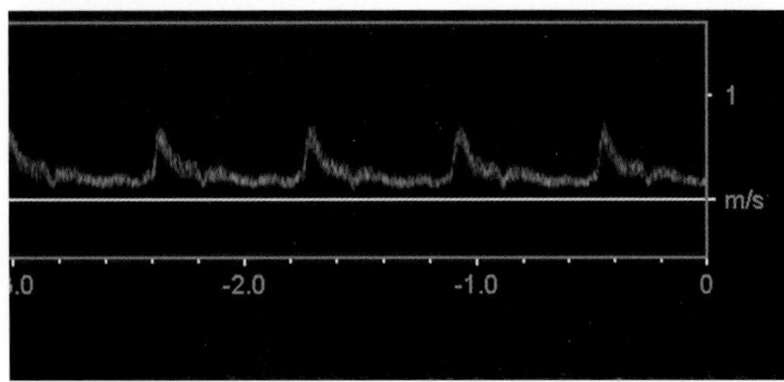

Figure ic.15

16. What is wrong with this image (Figure ic.15)?
    a. Too much spectral broadening
    b. There is aliasing
    c. The waveform is the wrong size
    d. The spectral gain is too high

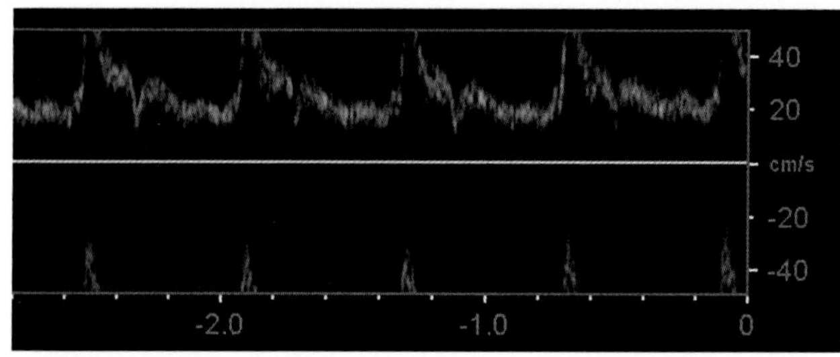

Figure ic.16

17. Which of the following will fix this image (Figure ic.16)?
    a. Decrease the pulse repetition frequency/scale
    b. Raise the baseline
    c. Decreasing the Doppler angle
    d. Decrease the operating frequency

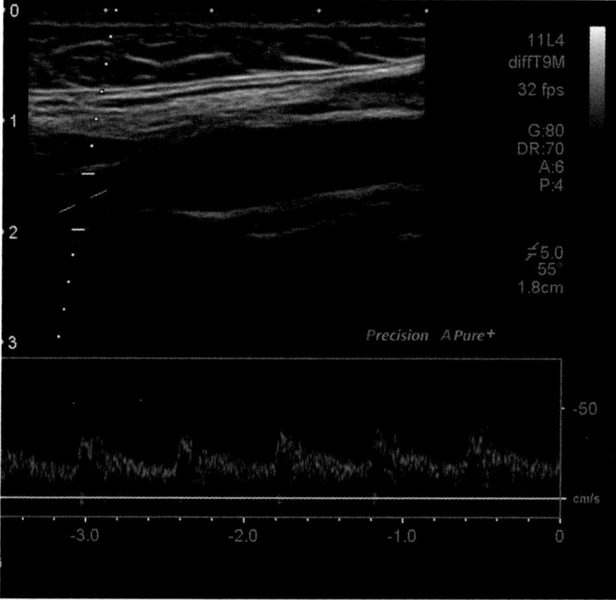
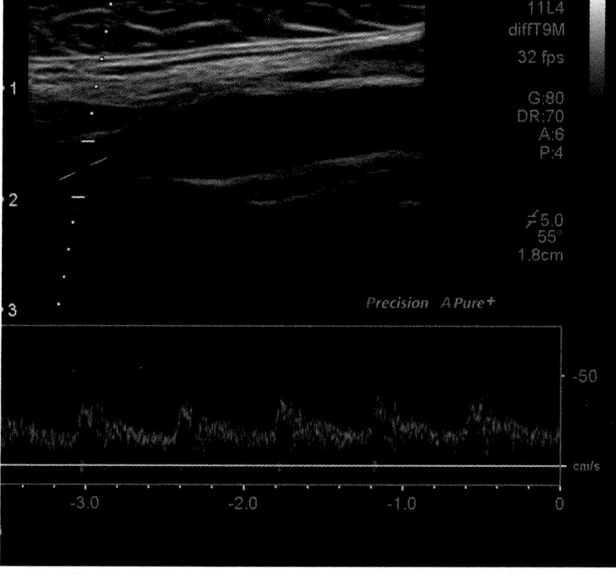

Figure ic.17

18. The spectral broadening seen in this image can be corrected by what means (Figure ic.17)?
    a. Use continuous wave
    b. Decrease the sample volume size
    c. Increase the spectral gain
    d. Increase the pulse repetition frequency

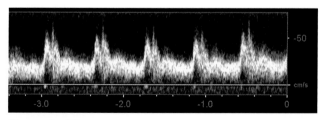

Figure ic.18

19. The problem with this image is (Figure ic.18):
    a. Aliasing makes it impossible to accurately measure velocities
    b. The wall filter is too high, obscuring low velocity flow
    c. The spectral gain is too high, causing the overmeasurement of velocities
    d. The scale is too high, causing the waveform to appear too small

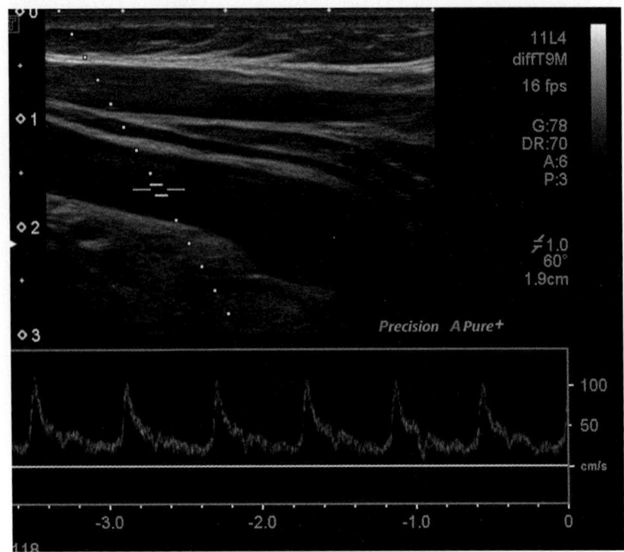

Figure ic.19

20. What is wrong with this image (Figure ic.19)?
    a. The angle correction is incorrect
    b. The spectral gain is too high
    c. The baseline is too high
    d. The spectral cursor steer is incorrect

Registry Review Exam

1. Which of the following is true about sound?
   a. The molecules in the medium propagate perpendicular to the direction of the beam
   b. Sound is a mechanical wave
   c. Sound is a form of ionizing radiation
   d. Sound is able to propagate through a vacuum

2. The frequency ranges for ultrasound are:
   a. <20 Hz
   b. 20 to 20,000 Hz
   c. >20 kHz
   d. >2000 Hz

3. The speed of sound in soft tissue is:
   a. 1.54 mm/s
   b. 1540 m/s
   c. 1540 km/s
   d. 1.54 m/μs

4. Which of the following transducers fires the elements in sequence and in groups?
   a. Linear sequenced array
   b. Phased array
   c. Continuous-wave transducer
   d. Single-element transducer

5. Which of the following is an appropriate unit for wavelength?
   a. Millimeters
   b. Hertz
   c. Microseconds
   d. Milliliters

6. Enhancement is caused by:
   a. Structures with high levels of attenuation
   b. Propagation speed errors
   c. Snell's law
   d. Weakly attenuating structures

7. The wavelength in a material having a propagation speed of 1.5 mm/μs employing a transducer frequency of 5.0 MHz is:
   a. 0.3 mm
   b. 0.3 cm
   c. 0.6 mm
   d. 3.0 mm

8. A piezoelectric element has the ability to transform
   a. Electrical energy into light and heat
   b. Electrical energy into mechanical energy
   c. Mechanical energy into radiation
   d. Audible sound into ultrasound

9. Arrange the following media in correct order from the lowest attenuation to the highest:
   a. Air, fat, muscle, bone
   b. Muscle, fat, air, blood
   c. Urine, fat, bone, air
   d. Muscle, air, fat, bone

10. Arrange the following media in terms of propagation speed from the lowest to the highest:
    a. Air, fat, muscle, bone
    b. Bone, fat, air, muscle
    c. Bone, muscle, fat, air
    d. Muscle, air, fat, bone

11. If the frequency doubles, what happens to the wavelength?
    a. It quadruples
    b. It doubles
    c. It is halved
    d. Frequency has no relationship to wavelength

12. What happens to intensity if the amplitude of a signal is halved?
    a. Quartered
    b. Quadrupled
    c. Halved
    d. No change

13. Which of the following describes the percentage of time that sound is being transmitted?
    a. Intensity
    b. Amplitude
    c. Pulse repetition period
    d. Duty factor

14. A 3-dB gain would indicate an increase in intensity by:
    a. 2 times
    b. 4 times
    c. 8 times
    d. 10 times

15. Ignoring the effects of attenuation, the intensity of the ultrasound beam is usually greater at the focal zone because of:
    a. Decreased attenuation
    b. The smaller beam area
    c. Bernoulli's principle
    d. A shorter duty factor

16. Attenuation can be defined as:
    a. Progressive weakening of the sound beam with propagation
    b. Product of the density of tissue and the speed of sound in the tissues
    c. The reflection of the ultrasound back to the transducer
    d. Redirection of the transmitted wave after crossing an interface

17. Which of the following is the lowest intensity listed, assuming PW operation?
    a. SPTP
    b. SATP
    c. SPTA
    d. SATA

18. What is the definition of the beam uniformity ratio?
    a. The spatial peak intensity divided by the temporal average intensity
    b. The spatial peak intensity divided by the spatial average intensity
    c. The temporal average intensity divided by the spatial average intensity
    d. The temporal peak intensity divided by the spatial peak intensity

19. Continuous-wave Doppler has a duty factor of:
    a. <1%
    b. 100%
    c. >100%
    d. 50%

20. The spatial pulse length is defined as the product of the ____________ and the number of ____________ in a pulse.
    a. cycles, frequency
    b. frequency, velocity
    c. wavelength, cycles
    d. frequency, wavelength

21. With phased array transducers, the transmitted sound beam is steered by:
    a. Steering the piezoelectric elements via a motor
    b. A lens attached to the face of the transducer
    c. Varying the timing of pulses to the individual piezoelectric elements
    d. Varying the amplitude of pulses to the individual piezoelectric elements

22. If the gain of an amplifier is 18 dB, what is the new gain (in dB) if the power is reduced by half?
    a. 15 dB
    b. 9.0 dB
    c. 36 dB
    d. 0.5 dB

23. Which of the following statements is true?
    a. With PW operation, temporal peak equals the pulse average
    b. With CW operation, the temporal average equals the pulse average
    c. The spatial average is usually the same as the spatial peak
    d. The spatial peak is typically highest near the transducer's edge

24. Which of the following best describes specificity?
    a. The ability of a test to predict a negative result
    b. The ability of a test to determine that a patient has a disease
    c. The ability of a test to predict positive and negative results
    d. The ability of a test to say who had a false positive result

25. Ultrasound undergoes an attenuation of an average of ________ dB/cm for each megahertz of frequency.
    a. 1
    b. 0.7
    c. 0.33
    d. 0.25

26. Sound strikes an interface and 74% of the sound is reflected at the interface. What is intensity transmission coefficient in this case?
    a. 1.06
    b. 6.00
    c. 0.26
    d. 0.04

27. Acoustic impedance is defined as the product of:
    a. The density mismatch between two interfaces
    b. A change in velocity that occurs at an oblique incidence
    c. The product of the speed of sound and density of the tissue
    d. The wavelength and frequency

28. Rayleigh scattering occurs when
    a. A reflector is significantly smaller than the wavelength
    b. There is a 100% reflection at an interface
    c. There is a specular reflection
    d. Side lobes are present in the beam

29. Assuming normal incidence, if medium 2 impedance is equal to medium 1 impedance:
    a. 100% of the intensity will be reflected
    b. 100% of the intensity will be transmitted
    c. The reflection and transmission coefficients will be equal
    d. The answer cannot be determined without knowing the impedances

30. What is the total amount of attenuation of a 3.5-MHz pulse after passing through 2 cm of soft tissue?
    a. 7 dB
    b. 3.5 dB
    c. 17 dB
    d. 1.75 dB

31. The thinner the piezoelectric element:
    a. The lower the impedance
    b. The higher the operating frequency
    c. The higher the amplitude
    d. The lower the Doppler frequency shift

32. The unit for impedance is:
    a. dB
    b. mW/cm^2
    c. Rayls
    d. No units

33. A sound beam encounters an interface at a 90° angle. If the speed of sound in the first tissue is 1540 m/s and the speed of sound in the second tissue is 1450 m/s, which of the following numbers most closely approximates the angle of beam transmission?
    a. <90°
    b. 90°
    c. >90°
    d. Need the impedance to compute angle of transmission

34. 1000 patients are examined by a new ultrasound test and the results are compared to the gold standard, which is in this case is computed tomography (CT). CT found that 700 of the 1000 studies were negative, but ultrasound only found 500 were negative. Of the 300 studies positive by CT, ultrasound determined that 250 were positive. What is the negative predictive value (NPV) of this test?
    a. 500/550
    b. 500/700
    c. 750/1000
    d. 250/450

35. Ensuring that ultrasound labs are practicing according to a set of established standards and maintaining an acceptable level of quality is known as
    a. Credentialing
    b. Quality correction
    c. Bioeffects
    d. Accreditation

36. The correct equation for Snell's law is:
    a. $R = (Z_2 - Z_1)^2/(Z_2 + Z_1)^2$
    b. $Z = pc$
    c. $\sin \theta_t = (C_2/C_1) \times \sin \theta_i$
    d. $Fd = 2\ f\nu \cos \theta / c$

37. The attenuation coefficient of sound in soft tissue can be defined by which of the following equations?
    a. One half the frequency times the path length
    b. Frequency/6
    c. Frequency/2
    d. Frequency × 2

38. The intensity transmission coefficient is equal to:
    a. 100% + intensity reflection coefficient
    b. 100% − intensity reflection coefficient
    c. The square of the angle of transmission
    d. (Intensity transmission coefficient)/2

39. The range equation explains:
    a. Side lobes
    b. Distance to reflector
    c. Attenuation
    d. Calibration

40. The value for attenuation coefficient for 6-MHz ultrasound in soft tissue is:
    a. 3 dB/cm
    b. 1 dB/cm/Hz
    c. 3 dB/cm^2
    d. 2 dB

41. What must be known in order to calculate distance to a reflector?
    a. Attenuation, propagation speed, density
    b. Attenuation, impedance
    c. Travel time, propagation speed
    d. Density, propagation speed

42. Specular reflections:
    a. Are not dependent on the angle of incidence
    b. Occur when the interface is smaller than the wavelength
    c. Arise from interfaces smaller than 3 mm
    d. Occur when the interface is larger than the wavelength

43. What is the reflected intensity from a boundary between two materials if the incident intensity is 1 mW/cm^2 and the impedance of medium 1 is 25 and the impedance of medium 2 is 75?
    a. 0.25 mW/cm^2
    b. 0.33 mW/cm^2
    c. 0.50 mW/cm^2
    d. 1.0 mW/cm^2

44. The layers of material within the transducer which have an intermediate impedance between the transducer element and human tissue are known as the:
    a. Filler medium
    b. Damping medium
    c. Acoustic medium
    d. Matching layers

45. Which of the following relates bandwidth to operating frequency?
    a. Near zone
    b. Piezoelectric crystal
    c. Quality factor
    d. Far zone

46. The piezoelectric effect can best be described as:
    a. Density of tissue and the speed of sound in the tissues
    b. Mechanical deformation that results from a high voltage applied to the face of the crystal that in turn generates a pressure wave
    c. The increase in intensity that occurs as the beam area decreases in tissue
    d. The decrease in intensity that results from the application of a damping material

47. Which of the following materials is most commonly used in ultrasound transducers?
    a. Lead zirconate titanate
    b. Barium sulfate
    c. Epoxy loaded with tungsten
    d. Quartz

48. Divergence refers to:
    a. Bending of the sound beam crossing a boundary
    b. Conversion of sound to heat
    c. Reflection of the beam at an interface
    d. Spreading out of the ultrasound beam

49. The preferred method for high level disinfection of endocavity ultrasound transducers is:
    a. Soap and water
    b. Steam
    c. Cold disinfection
    d. Autoclave

50. A transducer with which frequency would have the thickest element(s)?
    a. 2 MHz
    b. 3.5 MHz
    c. 5 MHz
    d. 7.5 MHz

51. Which of the following is best defined as the ability to discriminate between two closely spaced reflectors?
    a. Temporal resolution
    b. Range accuracy
    c. Spatial resolution
    d. Amplification

52. Which of the following is an effect of focusing?
    a. Improved lateral resolution
    b. Improved axial resolution in the near zone
    c. Increased beam divergence in the near zone
    d. Higher frequency

53. Bandwidth is:
    a. A source of artifacts
    b. A potential shade of gray
    c. The range of frequencies produced by the transducer
    d. Undesirable interference or noise

54. The part of the transducer that is most likely to be embedded with tungsten is:
    a. The matching layer
    b. The backing material
    c. The piezoelectric element
    d. The electrical shielding

55. The acoustic impedance of the transducer's matching layer:
    a. Is chosen to improve the efficiency of transmission of sound into the body
    b. Is chosen to have increased internal reflections
    c. Determines the operating frequency
    d. Varies with frequency of the transducer

56. When building a transducer, adding has more damping has what effect on the bandwidth?
    a. Stays the same
    b. Increases
    c. Decreases
    d. Damping and bandwidth are unrelated

57. The region where the sound beam diameter is the smallest is referred to as the:
    a. Fresnel spot
    b. Focal point
    c. Near field
    d. Far field

58. The near-zone length is determined by:
    a. Propagation speed
    b. Frame rate
    c. Pulse repetition frequency
    d. Transducer frequency

59. A two-element continuous-wave transducer:
    a. Is able to determine the depth of the reflectors
    b. Has an adjustable focal zone
    c. Is only used for spectral Doppler
    d. Has better color Doppler sensitivity

60. A wave's initial intensity is 2 mW/cm^2. There is an increase of 10 dB. What is the final intensity?
    a. 4 mW/cm^3
    b. 8 mW/cm^2
    c. 12 mW/cm^2
    d. 20 mW/cm^2

61. Which of the following is described best as a transducer that has multiple elements in a curved shape?
    a. Continuous-wave transducer
    b. Mechanical sector
    c. Curvilinear array
    d. Linear array

62. What is the name of the control that compensates for attenuation related to path length?
    a. Near gain
    b. Dynamic range
    c. Time-gain compensation
    d. Reject

63. What part of the machine creates the scan lines in the pulse-echo system of ultrasound?
    a. Receiver
    b. Scan converter
    c. Demodulator
    d. Transducer

64. What portion of the ultrasound system provides the electrical impulses to the transducer?
    a. Pulser
    b. Receiver
    c. Scan converter
    d. Time-gain compensation controls

65. What Doppler mode uses the amplitude of the Doppler shift in order to produce an image demonstrating flow in a vessel?
    a. Power Doppler
    b. Color Doppler
    c. Pulsed-wave spectral Doppler
    d. Continuous-wave spectral Doppler

66. Identifying tissues with similar shades of gray equates most to which of the following?
    a. Axial resolution
    b. Lateral resolution
    c. Temporal resolution
    d. Contrast resolution

67. Most current ultrasound systems have ______ shades of gray available.
    a. 256
    b. 64
    c. 32
    d. 4

68. How many bits per pixel can be displayed with 4 bits of memory?
    a. 2
    b. 4
    c. 8
    d. 16

69. The spatial resolution capabilities of the system are primarily functions of the:
    a. Pulser
    b. Transducer
    c. Receiver
    d. Display

70. What is the change to operating frequency if the depth is doubled?
    a. There is no change to operating frequency
    b. The operating frequency is doubled
    c. The operating frequency is only increased if the depth decreases
    d. The frequency is halved and the pulse repetition frequency is doubled

71. Preprocessing of the information that is fed to the scan converter:
    a. Enlarges each pixel to provide a magnified image
    b. Determines the display brightness assigned to stored grayscale levels
    c. Determines the assignment of echoes to predetermined gray levels
    d. Determines the frame rate of the image

72. Which of the following do grayscale systems typically use as a means of signal dynamic range reduction?
    a. Rejection
    b. Compression
    c. Relaxation
    d. Edge enhancement

73. Area is expressed by which of the following units?
    a. m/s
    b. cm
    c. cm^2
    d. cm^3

74. If the frequency of a transducer is increased, which of the following will undergo a decrease in numerical value?
    a. Axial resolution
    b. Propagation speed
    c. Temporal resolution
    d. Pulse repetition period

75. With tissue harmonic imaging,
    a. The propagating pressure wave causes the image to be distorted
    b. There is worse lateral resolution
    c. There is a higher risk for bioeffects
    d. There are decreased artifacts near the surface

76. Which of the following is in the range of infrasound?
    a. 1.5 kHz
    b. 15 Hz
    c. 25 Hz
    d. 1 MHz

77. Which of the following is in the range of audible sound?
    a. 15 Hz
    b. 25,000 Hz
    c. 18 kHz
    d. 2 Hz

78. Which of the following can be changed by the operator?
    a. Frequency
    b. Wavelength
    c. Propagation speed
    d. Pulse repetition frequency

79. Which of the following is the time it takes for one cycle to occur?
    a. Period
    b. Frequency
    c. Wavelength
    d. Pulse repetition period

80. The length of the pulse is the:
    a. Period
    b. Wavelength
    c. Pulse repetition frequency
    d. Spatial pulse length

81. Assuming oblique angle of incidence, if the propagation speed of medium 1 is greater than the propagation speed of medium 2, what will the angle of transmission be?
    a. Greater than the angle of incidence
    b. Less than the angle of incidence
    c. Equal to the angle of incidence
    d. Propagation speed does not influence the angle of transmission

82. A 5-MHz wave travels through 5 cm of soft tissue. If a 3.5-MHz transducer is selected instead, what happens to the propagation speed of the medium?
    a. Increases
    b. Decreases
    c. No change
    d. Not enough information given

83. The slowest propagation speed is found in which medium?
    a. Bone
    b. Air
    c. Muscle
    d. Liver

84. Which of the following represents the strength of the beam?
    a. Frequency
    b. Intensity
    c. Q-factor
    d. Duty factor

85. Which of the following is the unit of pressure amplitude?
    a. W/cm^2
    b. mm
    c. mW
    d. Pascal

86. Which of the following is the unit of intensity?
    a. W/cm^2
    b. mW
    c. Pascal
    d. dB/cm

87. What else changes with a change in amplitude?
 a. Resonating frequency
 b. Output power
 c. Wavelength
 d. Spatial pulse length

88. Which of the following will increase the acoustic exposure to the patient?
 a. Increased receiver amplification
 b. Increased time-gain compensation
 c. Decreased pulse repetition frequency
 d. Increased acoustic output

89. Which operator control adjusts the intensity of the transmitted pulse?
 a. Receiver gain
 b. Depth of scanning
 c. Power
 d. Time-gain compensation

90. What happens to the intensity if the power is doubled?
 a. No change
 b. It doubles
 c. It quadruples
 d. It is halved

91. The number of pulses that occur in 1 second is the:
 a. Pulse repetition frequency
 b. Pulse repetition period
 c. Pulse duration
 d. Duty factor

92. What is along the *x*-axis on a spectral Doppler waveform?
 a. Depth
 b. Amplitude
 c. Time
 d. Velocity

93. What is are the units of spatial pulse length?
 a. μs
 b. m
 c. m/s
 d. m/s^2

94. What testing device is used to measure acoustic output (intensity) level?
 a. Tissue phantom
 b. AIUM test phantom
 c. Doppler flow phantom
 d. Hydrophone

95. What is the principle that states sound waves are the result of the interference of many wavelets produced at the face of the transducer?
 a. Doppler's principle
 b. Bernoulli's principle
 c. Huygen's principle
 d. Poiseuille's principle

96. When using tissue harmonic imaging, the frequency used is
 a. Four times the fundamental frequency
 b. Double the fundamental frequency
 c. Equal to the fundamental frequency
 d. One half the fundamental frequency

97. In B-mode imaging, amplitude is located on the __ -axis of the image
 a. *x*
 b. *y*
 c. *c*
 d. *z*

98. Which of the following determines the radial resolution of a system?
 a. Pulse repetition frequency
 b. Impedance
 c. Spatial pulse length
 d. Duty factor

99. The axial resolution can be improved by decreasing the ______________ or increasing the ______________.
 a. Impedance, pulse duration
 b. Wavelength, number of cycles in a pulse
 c. Propagation speed, spatial pulse length
 d. Number of cycles in a pulse, frequency

100. Two reflectors are 1.3 mm apart in a plane that is parallel to the beam. The spatial pulse length of the transducer is 2.6 mm. These two reflectors:
 a. Will show up as one dot on the screen
 b. Will show up as two dots on the screen
 c. Will not show up on the image at all
 d. Will have poor lateral resolution

101. In what zone does beam divergence occur?
 a. At the face of the transducer
 b. Focal zone
 c. Fraunhofer zone
 d. Fresnel zone

102. The larger the aperture of a single element transducer,
 a. The shorter the near zone
 b. The longer the near zone
 c. The more divergence there is in far field
 d. The shorter the Fresnel zone

103. The ability to resolve two reflectors that lie parallel to the beam is the _______ resolution of a system
   a. Axial
   b. Lateral
   c. Elevational
   d. Temporal

104. The more focal zones used,
   a. The worse the azimuthal resolution
   b. The worse the temporal resolution
   c. The better the axial resolution
   d. The shorter the spatial pulse length

105. In a 1D array transducer, the slice-thickness plane is focused:
   a. Using 2D technology
   b. Using a matrix array
   c. Electronically
   d. Using a lens

106. If sound encounters a reflector in water, the reflector will appear to be _______ on the ultrasound image compared to where it is actually located:
   a. Too far away
   b. Too close
   c. In the correct location
   d. Not enough information to tell

107. What is the maximum temperature increase below which there should be no thermally induced biologic effects for an indefinite time period?
   a. 95 °C
   b. 10 °C
   c. 4 °C
   d. 1.5 °C

108. Two sound beams with different frequencies are traveling through soft tissue. Which beam will travel faster?
   a. The higher frequency sound
   b. The lower frequency sound
   c. Both will travel at the same speed
   d. Cannot be determined

109. There is a higher potential for work-related musculoskeletal disorders beyond what angle of arm abduction?
   a. 15°
   b. 30°
   c. 45°
   d. 60°

110. What is the name for the smallest amount of digital storage in a computer?
   a. The bit
   b. The pixel
   c. The byte
   d. The megabyte

111. In the Fresnel zone of a single element focused transducer,
   a. The beam diameter is a constant
   b. The beam diameter diverges
   c. The beam area varies with the amount of damping
   d. The beam area decreases with distance from the transducer

112. Signals from the transducer to the scan converter are in what format?
   a. Analog
   b. Digital
   c. Binary
   d. Hexadecimal

113. Which of the following is true about color Doppler?
   a. Each pixel can be both color and grayscale at the same time
   b. Each pixel can either be grayscale or color
   c. Pixels cannot be colorized
   d. The gain determines the color priority of the pixels

114. Which of the following preserves the pixel density when enlarging the image?
   a. Read zoom
   b. Write magnification
   c. Max zoom
   d. Postprocessing magnification

115. What is the relationship between the amplitude of sound and its frequency?
   a. Directly related
   b. Inversely related
   c. No relation
   d. Sometimes they are related, sometimes not

116. Which Doppler setting determines the preference for the display of color pixels versus grayscale pixels?
   a. Priority
   b. Gain
   c. High pass filter
   d. Sweep speed

117. Which of the following is true about axial resolution?
    a. It decreases with depth
    b. It increases with depth
    c. It does not vary with depth
    d. It is best at the focal zone

118. If the ______________ is increased, the flow increases.
    a. Pressure differential
    b. Resistance
    c. Length of vessel
    d. Viscosity of blood

119. Bernoulli's principle states that velocity and _______ have an inverse relationship to each other with no change in the net energy of the system
    a. Propagation speed
    b. Pressure
    c. Frequency
    d. Volume flow

120. The most common type of flow found in the body is:
    a. Plug
    b. Turbulent
    c. Laminar
    d. Chaotic

Answer Key for Registry Review Exam

1. **B.** Sound is a mechanical, longitudinal wave and not part of the electromagnetic spectrum like ionizing radiation.
2. **C.** Ultrasound, which is defined as sound that is above the range of human hearing, is described as sound with a frequency >20,000 Hz (20 kHz).
3. **B.** Sound travels through soft tissue at 1540 m/s.
4. **A.** The linear sequenced array fires the elements in groups and in sequence.
5. **A.** Wavelength is a distance, therefore the unit must be a unit of distance such as millimeters.
6. **D.** Enhancement occurs when sound passes through a weakly attenuating structure, such as a fluid-filled structure, although enhancement is not limited to fluid-filled structures.
7. **A.** Wavelength = c/f. Therefore, 1.5 mm/μs ÷ 5 MHz = 0.3 mm.
8. **B.** Ultrasound transducers convert mechanical energy into electrical energy and vice versa.
9. **C.** The order of attenuation in the list provided is: urine, fat, bone, air. Air is the highest attenuator of ultrasound.
10. **A.** Note that this order is for propagation speed, not attenuation. Air has the slowest propagation speed and bone has the highest.
11. **C.** Frequency and wavelength are inversely related. If frequency doubles, wavelength is halved.
12. **A.** Intensity is proportional to the amplitude squared, so if the amplitude is halved, the resulting intensity is one-fourth the original intensity.
13. **D.** Duty factor is the percentage of time the sound is being transmitted.
14. **A.** A gain of 3 dB results in doubling of intensity (or power).
15. **B.** Intensity equals power divided by area. The area is smallest in the focal zone; therefore, the intensity is the highest (assuming no losses due to attenuation).
16. **A.** Attenuation is the weakening of the strength of the beam, typically from absorption, reflection, or scattering.
17. **D.** SATA is the lowest of the intensities.
18. **B.** The beam uniformity ratio, also known as the beam uniformity coefficient or "SP/SA factor" equals spatial peak divided by spatial average.
19. **B.** Continuous-wave Doppler is transmitting 100% of the time, therefore the DF = 100%.
20. **C.** SPL = λn, or wavelength times the number of cycles in the pulse.
21. **C.** Phased array transducers operate by shocking the elements with minute time differences in between.
22. **A.** If the power is reduced by half it is the same as a change of −3 dB. Therefore, 18 dB − 3 dB = 15 dB. Note that the answer is in dB, not units for power or intensity (W or W/cm^2).
23. **B.** The duty factor is 1 (100%) with CW, so if TA = PA × DF, with CW the TA = PA.
24. **A.** Specificity is the ability of a test to predict someone will be free of disease. On the Chi square it is True Negative divided by the sum of the True Negative and False Positive.
25. **B.** The average rate of attenuation in soft tissue is 0.7 dB/cm/MHz. Some authors use 0.5 dB/cm/MHz.
26. **C.** The percent reflected at an interface (IRC) and the percent transmitted at an interface (ITC) must total 1 if using decimals (or 100%, if using percentages). If the ITC = 0.74 (74%), the IRC must equal 0.26 (26%) because 1 − 0.74 = 0.26.
27. **C.** $Z = \rho c$, or impedance equals density times propagation speed.
28. **A.** Rayleigh scattering occurs from reflectors that are significantly smaller than the wavelength of the incident beam, such as red blood cells.
29. **B.** If the impedances of two media are identical, there cannot be reflection and there will be 100% transmission of sound.

30. **B.** Total attenuation (dB) = ½f × path length. Therefore (0.5 × 3.5 MHz) × 2 cm = 3.5 dB.

31. **B.** The thinner the piezoelectric element, the higher the operating (a.k.a. resonating, or center) frequency.

32. **C.** The unit for impedance is Rayls, named after Lord Rayleigh.

33. **B.** There can be no refraction, or change in the angle of transmission, when sound strikes a reflector at 90° to the interface, regardless of propagation speeds.

34. **A.** Negative predictive value describes the patients who receive a negative test result and do not have the disease. It is calculated by using True Negative divided by True Negative + False Negative [D/(C + D)]. In this case, the True Negative value is 500 and the False Negative value is 50. NPV = 500/550.

35. **D.** Accreditation is the process by which an ultrasound lab applies to an organization to show that it meets the standards as determined by this organization.

36. **C.** Snell's law describes refraction at an interface. The equation has angles and propagation speeds, which are a clue.

37. **C.** The attenuation coefficient in soft tissue is equal to one half of the frequency and is in dB/cm.

38. **B.** ITC = 100% – IRC. The intensity transmission coefficient (ITC, % of transmitted sound at an interface) is 100% minus the IRC (% of reflected sound at an interface).

39. **B.** The range equation ($d = ct/2$) provides the distance to the reflector.

40. **A.** The attenuation coefficient (in dB/cm) in soft tissue is equal to one half of the frequency.

41. **C.** To calculate distance to the reflector, the travel time (specifically round-trip time) and propagation speed must be known.

42. **D.** Specular reflections occur when the interface (border) is larger than the incident wavelength.

43. **A.** First, solve for IRC (IRC = $[(Z_2 + Z_1)/(Z_2 + Z_1)]^2$). IRC = $(0.5)^2$ = 0.25 or 25%. This means that 25% of the sound coming from the transducer was reflected. To solve for the reflected intensity, solve for I_r. ($I_r = I_i \times$ IRC) → 1 mW/cm^2 × 0.25 = 0.25 mW/cm^2.

44. **D.** The matching layers have an impedance between that of the piezoelectric element and the skin in order to improve transmission of sound into the patient.

45. **C.** Quality factor (or Q-factor) = operating frequency/bandwidth.

46. **B.** The piezoelectric effect occurs when electricity is applied and a pressure wave is generated and vice versa.

47. **A.** The transducer element in modern-day transducers is commonly a ceramic made-up of lead zirconate titanate (PZT).

48. **D.** Divergence is a spreading of the wavefront and commonly occurs in the far zone of a sound beam. The more divergence present the worse the lateral resolution.

49. **C.** High level disinfection of endocavity ultrasound transducers must be performed with cold disinfection methods, like a soak in an approved disinfection liquid or a warmed peroxide misting unit.

50. **A.** The thicker the element, the lower the frequency, so the lowest frequency has the thickest element.

51. **C.** Spatial resolution is the ability to discern two closely spaced reflectors as individual reflectors.

52. **A.** Focusing improves lateral resolution and is unrelated to axial resolution.

53. **C.** Bandwidth is the range of frequencies produced by the transducer. These additional frequencies outside of the center frequency can be used for imaging and allow for "multifrequency" transducers.

54. **B.** The backing material is usually an epoxy containing tungsten and is needed to shorten the spatial pulse length.

55. **A.** The matching layer(s) impedance is chosen to improve the efficiency of transmission of sound into the body.

56. **B.** If the amount of damping increases, the bandwidth increases.

57. **B.** The beam is smallest at the focal point (a.k.a. focal zone or focus).

58. **D.** The near-zone length is determined by frequency and element diameter.

59. **C.** CW transducers, which utilize two elements, only produce a spectral waveform.

60. **D.** An increase of 10 dB is equal to a change of 10 times the initial intensity.

61. **C.** The curvilinear array (aka curved, convex) transducer has multiple elements on a curvature.

62. **C.** Compensation is the same as time gain compensation, or TGC.

63. **B.** The scan converter processes the received signals and creates the scan lines that are stored in memory until ready to be displayed.

64. **A.** The pulser is responsible for producing the voltage pulses that drive the transducer.

65. **A.** Power Doppler uses the amplitude of the Doppler shift (but not the shift itself) to produce an image of flow in a vessel.

66. **D.** Contrast resolution is the ability to distinguish different tissues by using varying shades of gray.

67. **A.** Most current ultrasound systems have 256 shades of gray (8 bits).

68. **D.** Shades of gray are 2^n, where n = the number of bits per pixel in memory. $2^4 = 16$.

69. **B.** The transducer determines primarily the spatial (axial, lateral) resolution of the system.

70. **A.** Depth does not affect the frequency as frequency is determined primarily by the thickness of the piezoelectric element, but the ability to penetrate, the depth of penetration, is determined by the frequency.

71. **C.** Preprocessing assigns received amplitudes to predetermined shades of gray.

72. **B.** Compression is the opposite of dynamic range. Increasing the compression reduces the dynamic range.

73. **C.** The unit for area is cm^2.

74. **A.** If the frequency is increased the wavelength is decreased, which decreases the spatial pulse length, which decreases the numerical value of the axial resolution. The lower the numerical value of the axial resolution, the better the axial resolution of the transducer.

75. **D.** With tissue harmonic imaging, there are decreased near-field artifacts.

76. **B.** Infrasound is sound with a frequency less than 20 Hz, and 15 Hz is less than 20 Hz.

77. **C.** Audible sound is in the frequency range of 20 to 20,000 Hz, and 18 kHz is 18,000 Hz, which is within that range.

78. **D.** Pulse repetition frequency is changed by adjusting the depth. The others cannot be changed by the operator.

79. **A.** Period (T) is the time it takes for one cycle to occur, in μs.

80. **D.** Spatial pulse length is the length of the pulse in mm, and is equal to the wavelength multiplied by the number of cycles in a pulse.

81. **B.** Since the propagation speed of medium 2 is less than the propagation speed of medium 1, the angle of transmission will be less than the angle of incidence ($\theta_2 < \theta_1$ if $C_2 < C_1$).

82. **C.** Propagation speed is only determined by the medium (specifically stiffness and density).

83. **B.** The slowest propagation speed of sound is through air. Remember: do not mix up the charts for attenuation and propagation speed.

84. **B.** Intensity is a parameter that represents the strength of the beam related to beam area.

85. **D.** Pascal (Pa) is the unit for pressure amplitude.

86. **A.** W/cm^2 is the unit of intensity.

87. **B.** Amplitude is a measure of the strength of the beam. A change in amplitude will change the output power.

88. **D.** Any term with "output" or "power" is a pulser function, so increasing the acoustic output increases exposure to the patient.

89. **C.** Increasing the power increases the intensity of the transmitted pulse. Intensity is directly related to power.

90. **B.** Intensity and power are directly proportional, so a doubling of the power causes a doubling of the intensity.

91. **A.** Pulse repetition frequency (PRF) is the number of pulses per second.

92. **C.** Time is represented along the *x*-axis of the spectral waveform.

93. **B.** The spatial pulse length is a distance, so meters (m) is the most correct answer.

94. **D.** The hydrophone is used by physicists or biomedical engineers to test output intensity.

95. **C.** Huygen's principle states that sound waves are the result of the interference of many wavelets produced as the face of the transducer.

96. **B.** Tissue harmonic imaging (THI) produces images using sound produced by the patient's tissue. THI produces images using the second harmonic, which is double the fundamental frequency.

97. **D.** In B-mode imaging amplitude is the brightness of the dot, which is considered the *z*-axis of the image.

98. **C.** Radial, or axial resolution, is determined by the spatial pulse length. Remember LARRD for the axial resolution synonyms: longitudinal, axial, radial, range, and depth.

99. **D.** Decreasing the number of cycles in a pulse (n) or increasing the frequency (f) will improve the axial resolution. The number of cycles in a pulse can be decreased by adding more damping during transducer construction.

100. **B.** The axial resolution is one half of the spatial pulse length. Therefore, the axial resolution is 1.3 mm. Since the distance between the reflectors is equal to (or greater than) the axial resolution, they will be resolved as two individual echoes.

101. **C.** Divergence occurs in the far zone, or Fraunhofer zone.

102. **B.** The larger the aperture, or element diameter, of a single element transducer, the longer the near zone.

103. **A.** Resolution of two echoes parallel to the beam is the axial resolution.

104. **B.** The more focal zones that are used, the worse the temporal resolution.

105. **D.** The slice-thickness plane is focused with a lens in 1D array transducers.

106. **A.** If sound travels through a medium with a propagation speed less than 1540 m/s, the reflectors will be displayed too far away on the image.

107. **D.** A maximum temperature increase of 1.5 °C appears to be safe for an indefinite time period according to AIUM guidelines.

108. **C.** Both frequencies will propagate at the same speed. Frequency and propagation speed are unrelated in a given medium as propagation speed is determined solely by the stiffness and density of the medium.

109. **B.** There is a higher risk of work related musculoskeletal disorders with arm abduction beyond 30 degree angle.

110. **A.** The bit, or binary digit, is the smallest unit of digital memory.

111. **D.** In the Fresnel zone, or near zone, the beam area decreases with distance from the transducer.

112. **A.** The signal from the transducer is an analog signal. This signal needs to be converted to digital via the A to D converter, or digitizer, before being transmitted to the scan converter and computer memory.

113. **B.** Pixels can either be color or grayscale; they cannot be both at the same time.

114. **B.** Write magnification enlarges the image before the image is stored in digital memory, thus preserving the pixel density. Write magnification is a preprocessing function and the image must be live, not frozen.

115. **C.** Amplitude and frequency are unrelated. Amplitude is the strength of the beam based on the strength of the voltage pulse, and the frequency is determined by the thickness of the element and the propagation speed of the element itself.

116. **A.** Priority, or color write priority, is a setting that lets the operator choose between preferentially displaying color information over grayscale information and vice versa.

117. **C.** Axial resolution does not vary with depth. Axial resolution is determined by the spatial pulse length, which does not vary with depth.

118. **A.** If the pressure differential is increased, there is an increase in flow. Poiseuille's Law states that the pressure difference (ΔP) is directly proportional to flow (Q).

119. **B.** Benoulli's principle states that if velocity increases there must be a corresponding decrease in pressure (and vice-versa) to preserve the net energy of the system. Bernoulli's principle describes why, in a nonhemodynamically significant stenosis, the velocity increases in the stenosis and undergoes a corresponding pressure drop.

120. **C.** Laminar flow, in which the center of the vessel has the fastest flow and the flow adjacent the vessels walls is the slowest, is the most common type of flow in the body.

Image Optimization Answers and Rationale

1. **D.** This image depicts aliasing (*arrowheads*), and in this case it can be corrected by lowering the baseline.
2. **A.** This image has resulted from excessive gain with resultant noise. The region on each side of the baseline represents signals that are removed by the wall filter.
3. **A.** Gain setting at 58 dB. Color Doppler image of the portal vein at a high gain setting demonstrates excessive color noise.
4. **B.** Gain setting at 20 dB. An image with a low color gain setting shows minimal detectable flow in the portal vein.
5. **D.** This image results from an overall gain that has been adjusted too high, resulting in an image that is too bright. The overall gain should be decreased.
6. **B.** The time-gain compensation (TGC) was adjusted.
7. **A.** This is Doppler mirror image artifact, and it can be minimized by decreasing color gain and/or using an angle that is less than 90°.
8. **B.** Range ambiguity artifact (*arrowheads*) within a bladder, resulting from the operation of concurrent beams (image A). The artifact disappears when the depth of display is increased (image B).
9. **C.** The blue color along the diaphragm (*short arrow*) is color flash artifact caused by motion of solid tissue. Having the patient hold his or her breath would hopefully eliminate this artifact, though the sonographer could also try decreasing the gain or increasing the pulse repetition frequency (PRF).
10. **C.** Reverberation artifact is noted in this hepatic cyst (A). By repositioning the transducer so that the cyst is deeper in the image, the reverberation artifacts are eliminated and the cyst is entirely anechoic (image B).
11. **A.** In this image, there is excessive color aliasing. That indicates that the PRF/scale setting is too low. If the PRF/scale setting is at a maximum and the aliasing persists, it is an indication of a high velocity that needs to be further interrogated with spectral Doppler.
12. **B.** There is "bleeding" of color pixels outside of the vessel, indicating a color gain setting that is too high.
13. **D.** The color gate is 90° to the vessel. Color Doppler cannot be performed at a 90° angle. The steering of the color gate should be adjusted.
14. **C.** There is clutter along the baseline indicating a wall filter that is too low. Increasing the wall filter will remove the artifact. Be careful not to set the wall filter too high, or important diastolic information may be erased.
15. **B.** In this image, the waveform is touching the top of the spectral window. The spectral waveform should occupy about two-thirds of the spectral window. Increasing the PRF/scale will make the waveform smaller.
16. **C.** In this image, the waveform is too small. The spectral waveform should occupy about two-thirds of the spectral window. Decreasing the PRF/scale will make the waveform larger and more optimized.
17. **D.** Aliasing occurs when the Doppler shift exceeds the Nyquist limit. If the PRF/scale is at a maximum, then lower the Doppler frequency, increase the Doppler angle, or use a continuous-wave (CW) probe. A better answer for this image would be to lower the baseline, but that option was not provided so you are required to find the next best option.
18. **B.** Spectral broadening may occur for several reasons, and it is not always pathologic. Using a smaller gate size, decreasing the spectral gain, or moving to the center of the vessel are all ways to help reduce spectral broadening. CW spectral waveforms will usually have spectral broadening because of the large and nonadjustable sample volume size.
19. **C.** The spectral gain is too high, which increases the risk of overmeasuring the velocities.
20. **A.** In this image, the angle correction is not parallel to the wall, yielding incorrect velocities. The angle correction should be parallel to the wall of the vessel. Note that in echocardiography a 0° angle is assumed, and no angle correction is used.

Answer Key for Chapter Review Questions

Chapter 1

1. **A.** Stiffness is the ability of an object to resist compression and relates to the hardness of a medium.
2. **A.** Duty factor is equal to pulse duration (PD) divided by pulse repetition period (PRP). PRP is inversely related to pulse repetition frequency (PRF), so an increase in PRF would lead to an increase in duty factor because they are directly related.
3. **B.** Bone, which has a propagation speed of 4080 m/s, has the highest propagation speed.
4. **D.** Lung tissue, which has a propagation speed of 660 m/s, has the lowest propagation speed. Do not confuse propagation speeds with attenuation values. Air has the highest relative attenuation, but the lowest propagation speed.
5. **C.** Depth and PRF are inversely related. As imaging depth increases, the PRF decreases.
6. **D.** Refraction is a redirection of the transmitted sound beam. Snell's law describes the angle of transmission at an interface based on the angle of incidence and the propagation speeds of the two media.
7. **B.** Pressure is typically expressed in pascals. You may also see kPa (kilopascals) or MPa (megapascals).
8. **B.** The typical range of frequency for diagnostic ultrasound is 2 to 15-20 MHz, although some transducers may go as low as 1 MHz and as high as 28 MHz. In this question, 2 to 20 MHz is the best answer.
9. **A.** The attenuation coefficient (in dB/cm) is the rate at which sound is attenuated per unit depth. It is equal to one half of the frequency (*f*/2) in soft tissue.
10. **A.** Micro- is a metric prefix that denotes one-millionth (10^{-6} or 0.000001).
11. **D.** Wavelength is the distance over which one cycle occurs, or the distance from the beginning of one cycle to the end of the same cycle.
12. **B.** For refraction to occur, there must be an oblique angle of incidence and different propagation speeds.
13. **A.** Areas of high pressure and density are referred to as compression. Areas of low pressure are referred to as rarefaction.
14. **C.** Spatial pulse length equals the number of cycles in the pulse multiplied by the wavelength.
15. **A.** Density is typically measured in kilograms per centimeter cubed.
16. **A.** Attenuation is a decrease in the amplitude and intensity of the sound beam as sound travels through tissue. There are three mechanisms of attenuation: absorption, reflection, and scattering.
17. **B.** Attenuation in soft tissue is equivalent to the attenuation coefficient (*f*/2, in dB/cm) multiplied by the path length (in cm). The total amount of attenuation that occurs if a 6.0-MHz sound beam travels through 4 cm of soft tissue is –12 dB (3 dB/cm × 4 cm).
18. **B.** Depth and PRP are directly related. Therefore, as imaging depth increases, the PRP increases.
19. **D.** Duty factor, the percentage of time that sound is being transmitted, has no units. It is a percentage.
20. **C.** The duty factor is the percentage of time the ultrasound system is producing a sound.
21. **A.** Density and propagation speed are inversely related. Propagation speed is directly related to stiffness.
22. **B.** Power is proportional to the amplitude squared, so power decreases as amplitude decreases. Power is measured in W or mW. Intensity and power are directly related.
23. **A.** Wavelength (λ) is determined by the sound source (frequency, determined by the transducer) and the medium (propagation speed). Wavelength is inversely related to frequency, not directly related.

24. **A.** Propagation speed is determined by the stiffness and density of the medium. Therefore, propagation speed is only determined by the medium.

25. **C.** Pulse repetition frequency is defined as the number of ultrasound pulses emitted in 1 second. PRF is determined by imaging depth.

26. **D.** Pulse duration is the time it takes for a pulse to occur, but only includes the "on," or transmitting time.

27. **D.** Intensity is proportional to the amplitude squared. If the amplitude is doubled, the intensity is quadrupled.

28. **A.** Frequency is determined by the sound source only. Specifically, it is the thickness of the element and the propagation speed of the element that determines frequency.

29. **B.** "Centi" denotes hundredths.

30. **B.** The angle of transmission is greater than 40° because the propagation speed of medium two is greater than the propagation speed of medium 1 ($\theta_2 > \theta_1$ if $c_2 > c_1$).

31. **C.** Refraction is the change in direction of the transmitted sound beam that occurs with oblique incidence and dissimilar propagation speeds.

32. **A.** Propagation speed can be measured in millimeters per microsecond or meters per second.

33. **B.** Absorption, the creation of heat in the tissue as sound travels, is a significant contributor to attenuation.

34. **D.** In clinical imaging, the wavelengths measure between 0.1 and 0.8 mm. Only one of these answers was in mm, and since wavelength is a distance (length) the units are mm.

35. **B.** Duty factor is the percentage of time that sound is being transmitted. With continuous-wave (CW) ultrasound, there is constant sound transmission. Therefore, the duty factor for CW is 100%, or 1

36. **B.** Amplitude, intensity, and power represent the strength of the beam. Wavelength is the length of the wave.

37. **B.** Intensity and power are directly related. If power is decreased by half, intensity is decreased by half.

38. **A.** Damping of the sound decreases the spatial pulse length by decreasing the number of cycles in a pulse (*n*).

39. **C.** Axial resolution (also known as radial, range, longitudinal, or depth resolution) is improved when the pulse is shorter, which occurs when damping is used in a pulsed-wave (PW) transducer.

40. **A.** The pulse repetition period is the time from the start of one pulse to the start of the next pulse, and therefore, it includes the "on" (or transmit) and "off" (or listening) times.

41. **B.** Pressure is measured in pascals (Pa) or pounds per square inch.

42. **C.** Intensity is essentially equal to the power of a wave divided by the area over which the power is distributed.

43. **C.** Although modern transducers may be made of a variety of materials, the ceramic commonly used is a combination of lead zirconate titanate (PZT).

44. **C.** Power is proportional to the amplitude squared. They do not have a one-to-one relationship. If amplitude doubles, then power increases by four times. If the amplitude is halved, the power is quartered.

45. **B.** Rarefaction is an area in the sound wave where the molecules are spread wider apart. This occurs in areas of low pressure and density. Be careful not to confuse "rarefaction" with "refraction."

46. **B.** Density and propagation speed are inversely related. If only the density of the medium is increased, then the propagation speed will decrease.

47. **D.** Sound is a mechanical and longitudinal wave. Sound waves are pressure waves, which are created by a mechanical action, like vocal cords or a vibrating piezoelectric element. Longitudinal waves are waves in which the molecules vibrate in a direction that is parallel to the direction of wave travel.

48. **D.** Amplitude is the maximum or minimum deviation of an acoustic variable from the average value of that variable (a.k.a. the baseline).

49. **C.** 0.5 MHz is 500,000 Hz, which is an ultrasonic frequency. The ultrasonic range is defined as "greater than 20,000 Hz."

50. **D.** The average speed of sound in all soft tissue is considered to be 1540 m/s or 1.54 mm/µs. This number is the average of all the propagation speeds found within the human body.

Chapter 2

1. **D.** The focus is the narrowest part of the ultrasound beam. The beam narrows in the near (Fresnel) zone and diverges in the far (Fraunhofer) zone.
2. **C.** The damping material, same as backing material, is the part of the transducer assembly that reduces the number of cycles produced in a pulse.
3. **C.** The frame rate is determined by the number of lines per frame/line density, number of focal zones, and the imaging depth (PRF).
4. **D.** Temporal resolution, also known as frame rate, is the ability to display moving structures in real time.
5. **B.** If the depth is increased, the frame rate would typically decrease. According to the question, it didn't. Therefore, something else decreased to cancel out frame rate. If the number of lines per frame is decreased, that would increase the frame rate, causing no change to the frame rate.
6. **A.** The sector phased array comes to a point at the top because all of the scan lines come from a common point of origin.
7. **B.** The bandwidth is the range of frequencies present with the beam. It is the highest available frequency minus the lowest available frequency. In this case, 7.5 MHz − 4.5 MHz = 3 MHz.
8. **B.** Frequency, along with crystal diameter (aperture), determines the divergence in the far field.
9. **A.** An increase in line density would decrease temporal resolution. The other choices would all improve temporal resolution (frame rate).
10. **D.** Decreasing the imaging depth, which is the same as increasing the PRF, would increase the frame rate.
11. **B.** The diameter of the beam in the near zone (Fresnel zone) decreases from the face of the transducer to the focal zone.
12. **A.** Most transducers usually have better axial resolution than lateral resolution. The synonyms for axial resolution are LARD: longitudinal, axial, radial, range, and depth. The synonyms for lateral resolution are LATA: lateral, angular, transverse, and azimuthal.
13. **C.** A large crystal diameter (aperture) and high frequency would increase the near-zone length the most compared to the other options listed.
14. **C.** A large crystal diameter (aperture) and high frequency would produce the least amount of beam divergence in the far field.
15. **A.** Imaging (pulsed-wave) transducers have low quality factors ("Q-factor") and wide bandwidths. Remember that "quality" in this sense means the "purity" of the beam, not image quality. Low Q-factor and wider bandwidths are due to damping, which is used to shorten the spatial pulse length, resulting in better axial resolution.
16. **B.** Damping material decreases the spatial pulse length by decreasing the number of cycles (*n*) in a pulse.
17. **A.** A curved firing pattern of the piezoelectric elements indicates focusing of the beam.
18. **C.** In an unfocused, single-element transducer, the focal point measures one half of the beam width at the face of the transducer.
19. **B.** The matching layer (technically plural: matching layers) is the component of the transducer that is used to minimize the impedance mismatch between that of the element and that of the patient's skin.
20. **B.** The bandwidth is the range of frequencies within the sound beam. All of today's PW transducers are considered broadband, which means they have a range of frequencies available for use.
21. **A.** Constructive interference occurs when in-phase waves meet and the amplitudes of the two waves are added to form one large wave.
22. **C.** The spatial pulse length has no effect on temporal resolution. The other choices listed all cause a change in temporal resolution, or frame rate.
23. **A.** The matching layer is composed of epoxy resin loaded with tungsten. Lead zirconate titanate is found in the piezoelectric material.
24. **D.** The linear sequenced array does not have elements arranged in a ring.
25. **A.** The width of the beam varies with depth, therefore the lateral resolution varies with depth.
26. **C.** Damping improves axial resolution by shortening the pulse. The pulse is shorter because damping decreases "*n*," the number of cycles in a pulse.
27. **B.** The vector image shape has a flat top and angled sides, which is the shape of a trapezoid.
28. **B.** Temporal resolution is another term for frame rate.

29. **C.** The far zone may also be referred to as the Fraunhofer zone.

30. **D.** Huygen's principle states that waves are the result of the interference of many wavelets produced at the face of the transducer.

31. **B.** Elevational resolution refers to the resolution in the third dimension of the beam, the slice-thickness plane.

32. **A.** In a single-element, unfocused transducer, the higher the frequency, the longer the near-zone length.

33. **C.** Phasing is a method of focusing and/or steering the beam by applying electrical impulses to the piezoelectric elements with small time differences between shocks.

34. **A.** Spatial resolution consists of axial, lateral, elevational, and contrast resolution.

35. **A.** Continuous-wave (CW) transducers do not time how long it takes pulses to travel so they have no range resolution. In other words, no image is produced.

36. **A.** CW transducers do not produce an image, only spectral Doppler.

37. **B.** The phased array transducer is also referred to as a sector or vector transducer.

38. **C.** The backing material, also known as the damping material of the transducer assembly, reduces the number of cycles produced in a pulse.

39. **B.** The phased array produces a pie-shaped, or sector image. Some phased array transducers produce a vector shape image, which is like a sector but has a flat top.

40. **B.** The matching layer, or face of the transducer, is the part of the transducer that comes in contact with the patient.

41. **D.** Heat sterilization will kill pathogens but will unfortunately destroy the transducer as well. Piezoelectric elements in a transducer can never be taken to the Curie point or beyond after they are created.

42. **A.** Range resolution, also referred to as axial resolution, is the ability to accurately identify reflectors that are arranged parallel to the ultrasound beam. Remember: LAARD.

43. **C.** Destructive interference occurs when out-of-phase waves meet. The amplitude of the resultant wave is smaller than either of the original waves.

44. **A.** A thinner piezoelectric element will yield a higher frequency. A thicker piezoelectric element will yield a lower frequency.

45. **B.** Since the SPL is 0.3 mm, the axial resolution is 0.15 mm. The distance to the reflectors (0.2 mm), which is greater than the axial resolution, so two reflectors will be imaged.

46. **C.** Of the choices listed, the curved sequence array would be best suited for imaging abdominal structures. Endocavitary probes tend to be high frequency and linear transducers have a limited depth and near field of view. Continuous-wave transducers do not produce an image.

47. **D.** Endocavity transducers are used internally but cannot image deep, linear sequenced arrays are also used more superficially. CW transducers do not produce an image. The curvilinear transducer is commonly used for abdominal scanning.

48. **B.** The frame rate is equal to the pulse repetition frequency divided by the lines per frame.

49. **A.** The higher the temporal resolution, or frame rate, the better the ability to represent structures in real time.

50. **B.** Ultrasound transducers are typically disinfected using a high-level disinfectant soaking solution, although transducers may be disinfected using a warmed hydrogen peroxide mist produced inside of a tabletop device.

Chapter 3

1. **B.** Output (a.k.a. power, acoustic output, etc) is a pulser function. Changing the output changes the intensity of the pulse and introduces more energy into the patient. Increasing the output also increases the potential risk for bioeffects.

2. **D.** Compensation (TGC) is the receiver function that changes the brightness of the echo amplitudes to compensate for attenuation with depth.

3. **C.** Rectification and smoothing are part of the "demodulation" component of the receiver.

4. **B.** The pixel, or picture element, is the smallest part of the image.

5. **A.** The pulser sends its signal to a pulse delay which sends the signal at the appropriate time to the piezoelectric elements. The pulse delay plus the element are called a transmit channel.

6. **B.** The transmit/receive switch directs the signals in the correct direction (to the transmit part of the transducer or the reception part of the transducer).

7. **A.** A bistable image (obsolete) is black and white with no other shades of gray.
8. **A.** LCD, or liquid crystal displays, use a backlight (fluorescent or light emitting diode) to produce an image.
9. **C.** In tissue harmonic imaging, sound is transmitted at the fundamental frequency (f_0), but received at two times the fundamental ($2f_0$).
10. **B.** A RAID array is a series of hard drives interconnected so that one drive backs up another drive. This creates a redundant backup system for the critical data stored on the PACS.
11. **D.** The number of shades of gray is equal to 2^n, where n = number of bits in memory ($2^6 = 64$ shades of gray).
12. **B.** The stronger the reflector, the brighter (whiter) the dot on the display.
13. **A.** The spatial detail of the display is improved with an increase in pixel density.
14. **A.** Slice thickness artifact is a result of a too wide elevational (slice thickness) plane.
15. **C.** Enhancement occurs behind a weak attenuator, most commonly from a structure containing a fluid (like a cyst). Enhancement can also occur deep to a weakly attenuating solid masses.
16. **A.** Output power is controlled by the pulser.
17. **D.** Reject (suppression; threshold) removes unwanted noise from the signal by eliminating echoes below a certain threshold.
18. **C.** Compression is the opposite of dynamic range, which is the range of echo amplitudes in a signal. Increasing the compression, decreases the dynamic range. Higher compression means fewer shades of gray.
19. **B.** Mirror-image artifact occurs because of sound refracting off of a strong reflector, causing a duplicate object to appear on the other side of the strong reflector.
20. **D.** $d = ct/2$. To compute the distance to the reflector, you need to know the round-trip time and the propagation speed of the medium. Assuming soft tissue, $d = 0.77t$ where "d" is the depth of the reflector and "t" represents the round-trip time of the pulse.
21. **A.** Contrast resolution is the ability to discern different shades of gray from each other.
22. **B.** Postprocessing of the signal occurs after the image has been frozen. Many functions on today's modern ultrasound machines can be adjusted after the freeze button has been pressed, although the exact functions will vary by manufacturer. Read zoom is a postprocessing function.
23. **B.** In B-mode, or brightness mode imaging, the brightness of the dot corresponds to the strength of the reflector.
24. **C.** M-mode, or motion mode imaging, displays movement of the reflectors as they occur along one scan line.
25. **D.** Time is along the x-axis of an M-mode image with depth along the y-axis.
26. **B.** The patient produces the harmonic signal that is received by the transducer.
27. **A.** In tissue harmonic imaging, the fundamental (transmitted) frequency is filtered out of the received signal and only the harmonic signal produced by the patient is displayed.
28. **D.** The range equation is $d = 0.77t$, where t is the round-trip time. Only the time to the reflector is given, not the round-trip time. Therefore, the given time must be doubled to 52 μs ($d = 0.77(52) = 40$ mm, or 4 cm). Another way to solve this problem is using the 13 μs rule: 26 μs is 2×13, which would be equal to 2 cm (20 mm) if the round-trip time had been provided. However, the one-way time was provided, so double 20 mm (20 mm × 2) to get the correct dept of 40 mm or 4 cm.
29. **C.** Rewrite the range equation to solve for round-trip time ($t = d/0.77$) ($t = 20/0.77 = 26$ μs). More practically, use the 13 μs rule: If it takes 13 μs for sound to travel 10 mm (1 cm), it takes 26 μs for sound to travel 20 mm (2 cm).
30. **B.** Apodization is a technique used by the beam former to reduce grating lobe artifact by minimizing the voltage strength on the elements closest to the edge of the transducer and higher voltages to the elements in the center of the transducer.
31. **A.** The beam former determines the strength, or amplitude, of the voltage pulses.
32. **C.** Coded excitation improves the signal-to-noise ratio of the image, in that there is less noise.
33. **B.** Optimizing the TGC is needed if only part of the image is too bright/dark, but if the image is underpenetrated, decreasing the frequency will allow for better visualization in the far field and no additional energy to the patient. Increasing the output (power) should be the last option.

34. **B.** Read zoom is a postprocessing function, whereas write zoom is a preprocessing function.

35. **C.** Write zoom is the higher-quality zoom because it preserves the pixel density. It is a preprocessing function, and therefore the image must be live.

36. **D.** Compensation, or TGC (time-gain compensation) is needed to brighten the echoes that are diminished because of attenuation.

37. **C.** The voxel, or volume element, is the smallest component of a 3D image.

38. **B.** Fill-in (or pixel) interpolation is needed when there are gaps between scan lines. The machine assumes what pixels should be placed in between the scan lines based on the shades of gray along the actual scan lines.

39. **D.** Digital Imaging and Communications in Medicine (DICOM) is the standard used in imaging for data exchange.

40. **A.** Reverberation occurs when sound bounces between two strong reflectors.

41. **D.** Grating lobes are an artifact that occurs with array transducers, and occur when sound energy is produced off of the main axis of the beam.

42. **A.** Muscle has a propagation speed greater than the soft-tissue average of 1540 m/s. When the actual propagation speed is greater than 1540 m/s, the reflector will be placed too close to the transducer.

43. **B.** Shadows are formed from sounds traveling through strongly attenuating areas.

44. **D.** Echo information goes from the memory to the digital-to-analog converter to be sent to an analog display or other output.

45. **A.** A-mode, or amplitude mode, may still used in ophthalmology imaging.

46. **A.** The receiver does not affect the amount of sound entering the patient.

47. **C.** $2^1 = 2$ shades of gray, or bistable (black and white).

48. **A.** Ring-down occurs from vibrating foci of air but may also be caused by small surgical clips, etc.

49. **B.** Frequency compounding improves contrast resolution and reduces speckle by imaging with multiple frequencies and averaging them out.

50. **D.** The machine always assumes 1540 m/s, which may be a cause of artifact.

Chapter 4

1. **C.** The heart provides the potential energy at the beginning of the cardiovascular system in the form of blood pressure.

2. **B.** A color without any other colors added to it is called a hue. If a color is pure red, blue, etc, that is its hue. Saturation is when white is added to a hue. The more white there is, the less saturated the hue is.

3. **A.** In plug flow, which occurs in large vessels (eg, aorta) and at the entrance of vessels, almost all the blood cells are traveling at the same velocity, giving it a flat or blunted profile.

4. **B.** When the scale (PRF) setting is increased, the Nyquist limit is increased, thereby decreasing the likelihood of aliasing.

5. **A.** The frequency of CW transducers is determined by the oscillator frequency. There is no user controllable range gate with CW, and no pulses as sound is driven continuously. Also with CW, there is no aliasing.

6. **C.** The Doppler shift is highest when the beam is parallel to flow (ie, at a 0° angle).

7. **B.** To eliminate aliasing the frequency shift needs to be decreased and the PRF needs to be increased. Increasing the PRF increases the Nyquist limit.

8. **A.** The frequency of the reflected sound increases as sound moves toward the transducer.

9. **A.** The higher the pressure difference, the greater the amount of flow. Poiseuille's Law describes the relationship between pressure (P) and volume flow (Q).

10. **C.** Amplitude is not part of the Doppler equation and therefore does not affect the frequency shift.

11. **A.** Voltage (pressure difference) = Current (flow) × Resistance ($V = IR$). Ohm's Law is analogous to Poiseuille's Law in which $Q = \Delta P/R$. Flow is directly related to the pressure difference and inversely related to resistance.

12. **C.** A Reynolds number >2000 indicates turbulence.

13. **B.** $Q = VA$. As the area increases, the velocity decreases to maintain volume flow as a constant.

14. **B.** Venous blood only flows from the abdomen and lower extremity during expiration. During inspiration or Valsalva maneuver, venous blood flow below the diaphragm ceases.

15. **A.** Gravity causes the highest hydrostatic pressure to be in the feet of a standing patient.

16. **B.** A 75% decrease in area is equivalent to a 50% decrease in diameter.

17. **D.** A multiphasic flow pattern is one where there is flow above and below the zero-flow baseline. This was formerly referred to as biphasic or triphasic flow.

18. **C.** If there is no reflector motion, the reflected frequency equals the incident frequency.

19. **B.** The higher the frequency, the greater the intensity of the scatter.

20. **A.** An increase in the Doppler angle causes a decrease in the frequency shift because the frequency shift is calculated based on the cosine of the angle, not the angle itself.

21. **D.** Phase quadrature is the part of the machine used to detect positive versus negative frequency shifts.

22. **B.** Two piezoelectric elements are needed for a CW device. One element continuously sends and the other continuously receives.

23. **C.** Aliasing occurs when the signal is not sampled often enough.

24. **D.** Fast Fourier transform (FFT) is the signal processing technique used for spectral Doppler.

25. **C.** The RI = (PSV – EDV)/PSV. One way to remember this is (A-B)/A where A is PSV and B is EDV.

26. **A.** The spectral amplitude is proportional to the number of red blood cells present within the signal.

27. **B.** Inertia is based on Newton's first law, which states that an object at rest stays at rest and an object in motion stays in motion unless acted on by an outside force.

28. **B.** The sweep speed adjusts the number of waveforms that appear on the spectral display at one time.

29. **C.** When the spectral gain is too high, the velocities may be overmeasured.

30. **D.** At a 90° angle to flow the Doppler shift is zero. Therefore, the Doppler shift is lowest at a 90° angle.

31. **C.** Autocorrelation is the signal processing technique used for color Doppler imaging.

32. **D.** Tissue Doppler imaging uses a low-pass filter to eliminate RBC signals and measure the movement of the walls of the heart. This is the opposite of the high-pass (or wall) filter that eliminates wall motion in favor of the moving RBCs.

33. **B.** Power Doppler uses the strength, or amplitude, of the frequency shift, which is equivalent to the number of RBCs present.

34. **B.** In triplex mode, the spectral waveform is displayed simultaneously with the color and 2D image.

35. **A.** The duty factor, or percentage of time the sound is being transmitted, of a CW beam is 1 or 100%.

36. **C.** CW beams have a large sample volume that may sample several vessels at once.

37. **B.** Color Doppler has very poor temporal resolution (slow frame rates) compared to 2D/grayscale imaging.

38. **A.** Color Doppler is a PW technique, and therefore has the same limitation as spectral Doppler regarding aliasing.

39. **C.** Aliasing occurs at a frequency shift greater than ½ PRF. If the PRF is 5000 Hz, then the Nyquist limit is 2500 Hz, or 2.5 kHz. Therefore, any frequency shift higher than 2.5 kHz would exhibit aliasing.

40. **D.** The frequency shift is typically 1/1000th of the operating frequency, which is in the audible range of sound (20 to 20,000 Hz).

41. **C.** The typical color Doppler ensemble length is 10 to 20 pulses per scan line, although it may be as low as 3 (also known as packet size).

42. **A.** Laminar flow has its highest velocities in the center of the vessel and slowest flow toward the walls. The slowest flow is at the boundary layer, where RBCs are stationary and move progressively faster toward the center of the vessel.

43. **D.** Color Doppler imaging cannot measure peak systolic or end diastolic velocities, but only mean velocities.

44. **B.** Power Doppler, a.k.a. color Doppler energy or amplitude Doppler, is obtained by measuring the amplitude of the Doppler shift, which is equivalent to the number of RBCs present. Power Doppler cannot measure velocity or identify direction of flow.

45. **C.** According to Bernoulli, in a region of narrowing in a nonhemodynamically significant stenosis, there is an increase in the velocity of the blood along with a corresponding decrease in pressure.

46. **D.** In the presence of turbulence, there is spectral broadening, a vertical thickening of the spectral envelope.

47. **C.** The pressure of the inside of a vessel compared to the outside pressure is its transmural pressure.

48. **B.** A delay in the upstroke of an arterial waveform, or dampened (tardus parvus) waveform, is indicative of a more proximal obstruction.

49. **C.** The wall filter control eliminates the low frequency shift component of the spectral waveform.

50. **A.** Monophasic flow is seen proximal to a low-resistance bed. Multiphasic and reversal of flow are more commonly seen in high-resistance flow patterns. Respiratory phasicity is usually seen in venous flow.

Chapter 5

1. **C.** Although some labs may have semiannual preventative maintenance (PM), annual PMs are usually the standard.

2. **D.** The Doppler phantom uses a moving belt, vibrating string or a fluid pump to simulate fluid moving through the body.

3. **B.** The pins on a phantom for the dead zone tests the ability of reflectors to be accurately imaged within the first centimeter of the sound beam. If an area of interest likes within the dead zone, a stand off pad may be needed.

4. **B.** Vertical depth calibration uses pins within a phantom that lie parallel to the beam to evaluate the distance from the transducer or the depth of reflectors.

5. **D.** The report of malfunctioning equipment to a service engineer should be done immediately. Equipment that is not operating appropriately should be removed from service.

6. **D.** Cardiovascular Credential International (CCI) offers certification exams in cardiac and vascular testing.

7. **B.** Accreditation, or lab accreditation, is a voluntary process that acknowledges an organization's competency and credibility according to standards and essentials set forth by a reliable source.

8. **C.** Sensitivity is the ability of a system to display low-level echoes.

9. **A.** Slice-thickness errors occur when the elevational plane of the transducer is wider is not razor thin. Any tissue in the elevational plane will cause artificial echoes to appear within a cystic structure.

10. **A.** Vertical distance indicates the maximum depth of visualization.

11. **C.** Preventative maintenance is a methodical way of evaluating equipment's performance on a routine basis to ensure proper and accurate equipment function and should be part of a lab's QA program.

12. **D.** The sonographer plays a vital role in the maintenance of equipment and quality of care.

13. **B.** Axial resolution is the ability to accurately identify reflectors that are arranged front to back and parallel to the ultrasound beam.

14. **C.** Another name for range resolution is depth calibration.

15. **D.** The slice-thickness phantom is test object (phantom) that evaluates the elevation resolution, or the thickness portion, of the sound beam perpendicular to the imaging plane.

16. **A.** The system's ability to place echoes in the proper location horizontally and perpendicular to the sound beam describes horizontal calibration.

17. **C.** The test object that mimics the acoustic properties of human tissue and is used to ensure proper equipment performance is the tissue-equivalent phantom.

18. **B.** Doppler test objects are used to evaluate the flow direction, the depth capability or penetration of the Doppler beam, and the accuracy of sample volume location and measured velocity.

19. **B.** The American Registry for Diagnostic Medical Sonography is not an accreditation body, but a credentialing body. The parent company for the ARDMS is Inteleos.

20. **D.** The American Institute of Ultrasound in Medicine is not a certification granting body.

21. **B.** The true positive rate (sensitivity) describes how many patients were found to have disease. If ultrasound found that 90 tests were positive, the true positive rate is 90.

22. **D.** Sensitivity is the True Positive rate, which is the ability of a test to find that disease is present.

23. **B.** Populate the Chi square to answer this question:

	+	−
+	TP (A) = 90	FP (B) = 20
−	FN (C) = 10	TN (D) = 80

Recall that specificity = D / (B+D). Therefore, specificity = 80/100.

24. **C.** Quality improvement (QI) is important to ensure that staff have adequate training and feedback so the lab can provide the best patient care possible. QI is not about the equipment necessarily, but the staff.

25. **A.** Negative predictive value (NPV) is the ability of a test to determine that disease is not present. In other words, if a study says the exam is normal, NPV predicts how many patients with a normal result will not have the disease.

Chapter 6

1. **C.** The American Institute of Ultrasound in Medicine (AIUM) recommends the utilization of the ALARA principle: As Low As Reasonably Achievable. This term relates the amount of exposure time for the sonographer and the patient during a diagnostic ultrasound examination.

2. **B.** Verifying the patient's wristband information for identifying markers, which includes the patient's name, medical record number, and date of birth, is an essential part of patient care.

3. **C.** If a patient does not speak English, or national language, the sonographer should obtain an interpreter. This practice will ensure that the patient is completely informed about the procedure prior to the procedure taking place.

4. **D.** There is increased heating at a soft-tissue to bone interface, so keeping the transducer in one spot increases the risk of thermal bioeffects.

5. **A.** Pallor describes the skin being pale, rubor is too red, cyanosis is blue, and jaundice is yellow.

6. **A.** Contrast ultrasound is possible because the microbubbles produce harmonic signals in the presence of ultrasound waves.

7. **B.** Cavitation is the action of an acoustic field within a fluid to generate bubbles. There are two types of cavitation: stable and transient. Stable cavitation produces bubbles that oscillate, or fluctuate, in size but do not rupture. Transient cavitation, also referred to as collapse, has the potential of causing the most biologic damage.

8. **A.** Streaming is when acoustic fields cause motion of fluids.

9. **D.** The thermal index is the calculation used to predict the maximum temperature elevation in tissues as a result of attenuation of sound.

10. **B.** The maximum heating of tissue is related to the sound beam's spatial pulse temporal average (SPTA).

11. **D.** HIPAA does not attempt to deal with cleanliness in the healthcare setting.

12. **C.** Radiation forces are exerted by a sound beam on an absorber or reflector that can alter structures.

13. **C.** Transient cavitation, also referred to as inertial cavitation, or collapse, has the potential of causing the most biologic damage. With transient cavitation, larger bubbles are produced and subsequently rupture. The rupture of these bubbles produces a shock wave and an increase in tissue temperature in that area. This increase in temperature has been associated with biologic effects.

14. **B.** The mechanical index was developed to assist in evaluating the likelihood of cavitation to occur.

15. **D.** Cardiogenic shock is failure of the heart to pump the proper amount of blood to the vital organs. It can be caused by myocardial infarction, cardiac tamponade, dysrhythmias, or other cardiac pathology.

16. **A.** A nosocomial infection is best described as a hospital-acquired infection.

17. **C.** Anaphylactic shock is a subcategory of distributive shock that results from an exaggerated allergic reaction, leading to vasodilation and pooling in the peripheral blood vessels. It can be caused by medications, iodinated contrast agents that are often used in x-ray procedures, and insect venoms.

18. **C.** A urinary tract infection is a common infection acquired during a hospital stay.

19. **D.** A reservoir is needed for an infectious agent to initially survive.

20. **A.** The TIB is the thermal index user after 10 weeks, which assumes fetal bones at the focal point. After 10 weeks the fetal bones are more calcified and more likely to cause thermal bioeffects related to absorption.

21. **D.** Image orientation does not have to be removed from the image.

22. **C.** Tuberculosis is an airborne disease found in the lungs, and possibly other organs, of an infected person. The TB bacteria are released from an infected individual most often when that person coughs, sneezes, speaks, or sings.

23. **D.** The FDA has set the maximum mechanical index (MI) at 1.9. This value is the same as the maximum MI for tissues without existing gas bodies.

24. **B.** When ignoring the effects of attenuation, the highest intensity is where the area is the smallest, which assuming an hourglass-shaped beam, is at the focal point.

25. **C.** Elastography is using the push-force of ultrasound to measure stiffness in the tissue. The two types of elastography are strain and shear wave.

26. **C.** The machine and table placement should be optimized to bring the sonographer closer to the patient and minimize reaching. The LCD display should be placed to minimize straining of the sonographer's neck, but not directly over the patient's head.

27. **A.** The root *hepa-* is liver (from the Greek word *hepar*), and *-itis* is inflammation.

28. **D.** Obstructive shock results from pathologic conditions that interfere with the normal pumping action of the heart. It can be caused by pulmonary embolism, pulmonary hypertension, arterial stenosis, and possibly tumors that obstruct normal blood flow to the heart.

29. **D.** Absorption, the creation of heat with sound propagation in tissue, is the main contributor to attenuation. The law of energy conservation says that if heat is created, the energy of the beam must decrease.

30. **B.** The maximum allowable increase in temperature is 2 °C. If the temperature does not exceed 2 °C, soft tissue can be insonated without a time limit.

31. **A.** A "gas body" is something that has air or gas within it. Liver tissue does not normally contain air or gas unless contrast agents are administered or there is pathology.

32. **B.** Diabetic ketoacidosis occurs when a patient has insufficient insulin, resulting in excess glucose production by the liver. The patient may have sweet smelling breath.

33. **A.** In tissues that contain well-defined gas bodies, for example, lung, no effects have been observed for in situ peak rarefactional pressures below approximately 0.4 MPa or mechanical index values less than approximately 0.4.

34. **D.** The suggested position of the scanning arm is no more than a 30° angle of abduction. The sonographer should also place the patient as near to him or her as practical, because this situation will also reduce the amount of reach needed to perform most examinations. Intensities below 1 W/cm^2, or thermal index values of less than 2.

35. **B.** Lumason, also known as sulfur hexafluoride, is FDA approved for focal liver lesions and other limited uses in humans.

36. **C.** Releasing protected health information (PHI) to an unauthorized person is a violation of HIPAA.

37. **A.** It is not appropriate to reach across the sterile field as something may inadvertently drop onto the sterile field.

38. **B.** HIV is not spread through a handshake, but by blood and body fluids.

39. **D.** *Tachy-* means swift or rapid, and *-cardia* means heart, so tachycardia is an abnormally fast heart rate.

40. **B.** Alcohol-based hand rubs should never take the place of proper hand washing when the hands are visibly soiled.

41. **C.** The carotid pulse should be evaluated in the nonresponsive patient.

42. **B.** Glutaraldehyde-based solutions may be used to sterilize sonographic equipment, not act as personal protective equipment.

43. **D.** Intravascular ultrasound, or IVUS, is the insertion of a small transducer mounted onto a catheter to view the inside of vessels.

44. **C.** An accidental needle stick would be the most likely means of transmission of HIV from a patient to a sonographer.

45. **D.** Tuberculosis is an airborne disease.

46. **B.** Nonthermal mechanisms may also be referred to as mechanical mechanisms.

47. **C.** Iatrogenic injuries are caused incidentally from a medical procedure, like hemorrhage or a pseudoaneuyrsm.

48. **A.** No independently confirmed adverse effects caused by exposure from present diagnostic ultrasound instruments have been reported in human patients in the absence of contrast agents.

49. **B.** The use of gloves should never replace proper hand washing.

50. **D.** Transient cavitation, also referred to as inertial cavitation or collapse, has the potential of causing the most biologic damage. With transient cavitation, larger bubbles are produced and subsequently rupture.

Glossary

- Items marked with an asterisk (*) are not specifically mentioned on the September 2023 ARDMS SPI content outline but may be on other credentialing examinations. Be sure to check the content outlines of your credentialing exam.

13 μs rule—the rule that states that it takes 13 μs for a sound to propagate to a depth of 1 cm in soft tissue and return to the transducer

absorption—the conversion of sound energy to heat

acoustic cavitation—the production of bubbles in a liquid medium

acoustic radiation force impulse (ARFI) imaging—uses acoustic radiation force to compress the soft tissue and provides a qualitative measurement of stiffness without requiring pressure input from the sonographer

acoustic speckle—the interference pattern caused by scatterers that produces the granular appearance of what is called "parenchyma" on a sonographic image

acoustic variables—changes that occur within a medium as a result of sound traveling through that medium

ALARA—as low as reasonably achievable; the principle that states one should always use the lowest power and shortest scanning time possible to reduce the potential for bioeffects

aliasing—the wraparound of the spectral or color Doppler display that occurs when the frequency shift exceeds the Nyquist limit; occurs only with PW Doppler

A-mode—amplitude mode; ophthalmology-specific mode in which the height of the spike on the image is related to the strength (amplitude) of the echo generated by a reflector

amplification—the part of the receiver that increases or decreases the received echoes equally, regardless of depth

amplitude—the maximum (positive or negative) deviation of an acoustic variable from the average value of that variable; the strength the sound wave

amplitude mode—*see* the key term "A-mode"

analog-to-digital (A-to-D) converter—the part of the digital scan converter that converts the analog signals from the receiver to binary signals for processing by the computer

anechoic—without echoes or black

angle-correction—the Doppler tool used to inform the machine what the angle of flow is so that velocities can be accurately calculated

aperture—the diameter of the piezoelectric element(s) producing the beam

apodization—the technique that varies the voltage to the individual elements to reduce grating lobes

array—the transducer with multiple active elements

artifacts—echoes on the screen that are not representative of actual anatomy, or reflectors in the body that are not displayed on the screen

attenuation—a decrease in the amplitude and intensity of the sound beam as sound travels through tissue (in dB)

attenuation coefficient—the rate at which sound is attenuated per unit depth (in dB/cm)

autocorrelation—the color Doppler processing technique that assesses pixels as stationary or in motion

automatic external defibrillator*—a portable device that is used to detect and treat abnormal heart rhythms with electrical defibrillation

automatic scanning—same as real-time ultrasound

axial resolution—the ability to accurately identify reflectors that are arranged parallel to the ultrasound beam (in mm)

backing material—the damping material of a transducer assembly that reduces the number of cycles produced in a pulse

backscatter—scattered sound waves that make their way back to the transducer and produce an image on the display

bandwidth—the range of frequencies present within the beam

BART—the acronym used to describe color Doppler scale: "blue away, red toward"

baseline—the operator-adjustable dividing line between positive frequency shifts and negative frequency shifts on spectral and color Doppler (also called the *zero-flow baseline*)

beam uniformity ratio—the ratio of the center intensity to the average intensity across the transducer face; also referred to as the SP/SA factor or beam uniformity coefficient

Bernoulli's principle—the principle that describes the inverse relationship between velocity and pressure

B-flow imaging—a non-Doppler technology that offers real-time imaging of blood flow while scanning in grayscale

binary system—the digital language of zeros and ones

bistable—purely black-and-white image

bit—the smallest unit of memory in a digital device

B-mode—brightness mode; the brightness of the dots is proportional to the strength of the echo generated by the reflector

boundary layer—the stationary (or near-stationary) layer of blood cells immediately adjacent to the vessel wall

brightness—the term describing the intensity or luminance of the color Doppler display

brightness mode—*see* the key term "B-mode"

byte—8 bits of memory

calf muscle pump—the muscles in the calf that, upon contraction, propel venous blood toward the heart

capacitance—the ability of veins to store blood

capacitive micromachined ultrasound transducers—technology used to create comparable transducer technology to piezoelectric materials

cathode ray tube (CRT)—obsolete display that uses an electron gun to produce a stream of electrons toward a phosphor-coated screen

channel—a pulse delay and its corresponding piezoelectric element

clutter—acoustic noise in the color and/or spectral Doppler signal

coded excitation—a way of processing the pulse to improve contrast resolution and reduce acoustic speckle

collateral blood vessels—accessory vessels that dilate to permit blood flow in the presence of an obstruction in the main blood vessel

color Doppler imaging—Doppler shift information presented as a color (hue) superimposed over the grayscale image

color priority—the setting for color Doppler that allows the operator to select the frequency shift threshold; it determines whether color pixels should be displayed preferentially over grayscale pixels

comet tail—a small reverberation artifact caused by small reflectors (ie, surgical clips)

compensation—the function of the receiver that changes the brightness of the echo amplitudes to compensate for attenuation that occurs with depth

compression (in a medium)—an area in the sound wave of high pressure and density

compression (receiver)—the function of the receiver that decreases the range of signal amplitudes present within the machine's receiver; opposite of the dynamic range

connector—the part of a transducer cable that connects to the ultrasound machine

constructive interference—occurs when in-phase waves meet; the amplitudes of the two waves are added to form one large wave

continuity equation—the equation that describes the change in velocity as the area changes in order to maintain the volumetric flow rate

continuous wave—sound that is continuously transmitted

continuous-wave Doppler—non-imaging Doppler device that consists of two elements: one element is used by the system to constantly transmit sound and the other is used to constantly receive sound

contrast-enhanced ultrasound (CEUS)—type of imaging in which an ultrasound contrast agent containing microscopic gas bubbles is used to improve the visualization of structures or blood flow

contrast resolution—the ability to differentiate tissues with similar shades of gray

critical stenosis—the point at which a stenosis is hemodynamically significant with a drop in pressure or volume flow distal to the stenosis

crystal—a synonym for the active element of a transducer, the piezoelectric part of a transducer assembly that produces sound

Curie point—the temperature at which an ultrasound transducer will gain its piezoelectric properties and also the temperature at which a transducer will lose the ability to produce sound if heated again above this temperature

curved sequenced array—a transducer commonly referred to as a curvilinear or convex probe

damping—the process of reducing the number of cycles of each pulse in order to improve axial resolution

damping material—the same as the backing material; the part of the transducer assembly that reduces the number of cycles produced in a pulse

decibels—a unit that establishes a relationship or comparison between two values of power, intensity, or amplitude

demodulation—the function of the receiver that makes the signal easier to process by performing the functions rectification and smoothing; also called detection

density—mass per unit volume

depth ambiguity—the inability to determine the depth of the reflector if the pulses are sent out too fast for them to be timed (also called *range ambiguity*)

destructive interference—occurs when out-of-phase waves meet; the amplitude of the resultant wave is smaller than either of the original waves

diabetes mellitus*—a group of metabolic diseases that result from a chronic disorder of carbohydrates metabolism

diabetic ketoacidosis (DKA)*—a complication of diabetes that results from the severe lack of insulin

diastole—the relaxation of the cardiac ventricles following contraction

digital-to-analog (D-to-A) converter—part of the digital scan converter that converts the binary signals from computer memory to analog for display and storage

digitizer—*see* the key term "pulser"

directly related—relationship that implies that if one variable decreases, the other also decreases, or if one variable increases, the other also increases; also referred to as directly proportional

distance—how far apart objects are; may also be referred to as vibration or displacement

divergence—spreading of the beam that occurs in the far zone

Doppler effect—the change in the frequency of the received signal related to the motion of a reflector

Doppler equation—the equation that explains the relationship of the Doppler frequency shift (F_D) with the frequency of the transducer (f), the velocity of the blood (ν), the angle of blood flow (cos θ (in °)), and the propagation speed (c)

Doppler phantom—the test object used to evaluate the flow direction, the depth capability or penetration of the Doppler beam, and the accuracy of the sample volume location and measured velocity

dropout—defect in image that appears as a shadow emanating from the very top of the image

duplex—real-time two-dimensional imaging combined with the spectral Doppler display

duty factor—the percentage of time that sound is actually being produced

dwell time—the length of time the ultrasound transducer remains stationary over a volume of tissue

dynamic range—the range of echo amplitudes present within the signal, which corresponds to the shades of gray available

echogenic—a medium that has the ability to produce return echoes

echogenicity—a measure of relative brightness compared to adjacent structures

echotexture—measure of the relative "smoothness" of a structure imaged on B-mode ultrasound

edge shadowing—refraction artifact caused by the curved surface of the reflector

effective resistance—the sum of the individual resistances when multiple vessels are connected in series

elasticity—*see* the key term "stiffness"

elastography—a sonographic technique used to evaluate the stiffness of a mass or tissue

electrical interference—arc-like bands that occur when the machine is too close to an unshielded electrical device

element—the piezoelectric part of the transducer assembly that produces sound

elevational plane—*see* the key term "slice-thickness plane"

elevational resolution—the resolution in the third dimension of the beam; the slice-thickness plane

enhancement—an artifact of increased brightness in the tissue deep to a structure caused by sound passing through an area of lower attenuation

ensemble length—the number of pulses per scan line in color Doppler; also referred to as packet size

ergonomics—the scientific study of creating tools and using equipment effectively in order to help the human body adjust to the work environment

extrinsic pressure—pressure applied from the outside of an object

far zone—the diverging part of the beam distal to the focal point

fast Fourier transform—a mathematical process used for analyzing and processing the Doppler signal to produce the spectral waveform

fill-in interpolation—places grayscale pixels based on adjacent scan lines, where there is no signal information; also referred to as pixel interpolation

flash artifact—a motion artifact caused by the movement of tissue when using power Doppler

focal depth—the depth of the focal point/focal zone. It is the same as the depth of one near-zone length

focal point—the area of the beam with the smallest beam diameter

footprint—the size of the face of the transducer; the portion of the transducer that is in contact with the patient's skin

four-dimensional ultrasound—three-dimensional ultrasound in real time

frame—one complete ultrasound image

frame rate—the number of frames per second (in FPS or Hz)

Fraunhofer zone—*see* the key term "far zone"

frequency—the number of cycles per second (in Hz)

frequency compounding—averages the frequencies across the image to improve contrast resolution and reduce acoustic speckle

frequency shift—the difference between the transmitted and received frequencies

Fresnel zone—*see* the key term "near zone"

friction—a form of resistance, caused by two materials rubbing against each other, thereby converting energy to heat

fundamental frequency—the operating or resonating frequency emitted by a transducer

fusion imaging*—technology that provides the ability to view alternate imaging modality (eg, CT or MRI) during real-time sonography; also referred to as hybrid imaging

gold standard—the test that all other tests are compared to for statistical analysis. Considered to be the "best test" for that type of exam

grating lobes—an artifact caused by the extraneous sound that is not located along the primary beam path; occurs with arrays; reduced or eliminated by apodization, subdicing, and tissue harmonics

half-intensity depth—the depth at which sound has lost half of its intensity (in cm)

half-value layer thickness—*see* the key term "halfintensity depth"

harmonics—the harmonic signal produced by the patient's tissue and that is a multiple of the fundamental frequency

Health Insurance Portability and Accountability Act (HIPAA)—US law that, among many goals, upholds patient confidentiality and requires the use of electronic medical records

hemodynamically significant stenosis—*see* the key term "critical stenosis"

hemodynamics—the study of blood flow through the blood vessels of the body

hepatitis*—inflammation of the liver

hertz—a unit of frequency

horizontal calibration—the ability to place echoes in the proper location horizontally and perpendicular to the sound beam

housing—the plastic outside of a transducer that holds the electronics of the transducer and electrical shielding/insulation

hue—a term used to describe displayed colors (eg, red, blue, and green)

Huygen's principle—waves are the result of the interference of many wavelets produced at the face of the transducer

hydrophone—a device used to measure the output intensity of the transducer

hydrostatic pressure—describes the relationship between gravity, density of the blood, and the distance between an arbitrary reference point

hyperechoic—displayed echoes that are relatively brighter than the surrounding tissue

hypoechoic—displayed echoes that are relatively darker than the surrounding tissue

hypoglycemia*—a lower-than-normal blood sugar level

impedance—the resistance to the propagation of sound through a medium (in rayls)

inertia—Newton's first law of motion stating that an object at rest stays at rest and an object in motion stays in motion, unless acted on by an outside force

innervated—supplied with nerves

in-phase—waves whose peaks and troughs overlap

intensity—the power of the wave divided by the area over which it is spread; the energy per unit area (in W/cm^2 or mW/cm^2)

intensity reflection coefficient—the percentage of sound reflected at an interface

intensity transmission coefficient—the percentage of sound transmitted at an interface

interface—the dividing line between two different media

intravascular ultrasound—the technique that uses a miniature ultrasound transducer placed on a catheter and inserted into a circulatory system

inversely related—relationship that implies that if one variable decreases, the other increases, or if one variable increases, the other decreases; also referred to as inversely proportional

isoechoic—echogenicity that is identical to the surrounding tissue

kinetic energy—the energy form of flowing blood

lab accreditation—a voluntary process that acknowledges an organization's competency and credibility according to standards and essentials set forth by a reliable source

laminar flow—the flow profile represented by blood that travels in nonmixing layers of different velocities, with the fastest flow in the center and the slowest flow near the vessel walls

lateral resolution—the ability to accurately identify reflectors that are arranged perpendicular to the ultrasound beam (in mm)

law of conservation of energy—the total amount of energy in a system never changes, although it might be in a different form from which it started

lead zirconate titanate—the man-made ceramic of which many transducer elements are made; abbreviated PZT

linear sequenced array—a transducer commonly referred to as a linear probe or transducer

liquid crystal display (LCD)—display that uses the twisting and untwisting of liquid crystals in front of a light source; also called a flat panel

longitudinal waves—waves in which the molecules of the medium vibrate back and forth in the same direction that the waves are traveling

luminance—the brightness of the color Doppler image

master synchronizer—the timing component of an ultrasound machine that notes how long it takes for signals to return from reflectors (*see* the key term "range equation")

matching layer—the component of a transducer that is used to step down the impedance from that of the element to that of the patient's skin

matrix array transducer—a 2D array transducer that acquires real-time volumes utilizing over 90,000 elements compared with the 128 to 512 elements used in standard 1D array transducers

mechanical index (MI)—the calculation used to identify the likelihood that cavitation could occur

mechanical scanheads—transducers with a motor for steering the beam

medium—any form of matter: solid, liquid, or gas

mirror-image artifact—an artifact caused by sound bouncing off a specular reflector and causing a structure to appear on both sides of the reflector

mm Hg—millimeters of mercury; unit of pressure

M-mode—motion mode; used to display the motion of the reflectors

motion mode—*see* the key term "M-mode"

multipath—an artifact caused by the beam reflecting off several reflectors before returning to the transducer

near zone—the part of the beam between the element and the focal point

near-zone length—the length of the region from the transducer face to the focal point

noise—low-level echoes on the display that do not contribute to useful diagnostic information

nondirectional Doppler—a Doppler device that cannot differentiate between positive and negative frequency shifts

nonhemodynamically significant stenosis—a stenosis that has not reached a critical threshold for volume flow or pressure distal to the stenosis.

nonspecular reflectors—reflectors that are smaller than the wavelength of the incident beam

normal incidence—angle of incidence is 90° to the interface

nosocomial infection*—a hospital-acquired infection

Nyquist limit—the maximum frequency shift sampled without aliasing; equal to one-half of the pulse repetition frequency

oblique incidence—angle of incidence is less than or greater than 90° to the interface

Ohm's law—a law used in electronics in which flow (current, *I*) is equal to the pressure difference (Volts, *V*) divided by resistance (*R*)

oscillator—the component of a continuous-wave Doppler device that produces the voltage that drives the piezoelectric elements

out-of-phase—waves that are 180° opposite to each other; the peak of one wave overlaps the trough of the other and vice versa

output—output power; strength of sound entering the patient

overall gain—the receiver function that increases or decreases all echo amplitudes equally

packet size—the number of pulses per scan line; also called ensemble length

parameter—a measurable quantity

particle motion—the movement of molecules owing to propagating sound energy

path length—distance to the reflector

period—the time it takes for one cycle to occur (in μs)

persistence (color Doppler)—the averaging of color frames in order to display blood flow with a low signal-to-noise ratio

phase quadrature—the component of the Doppler device that determines positive opposed to negative frequency shifts and, therefore, the direction of blood flow

phased array—the transducer that uses phasing; shocking the elements in a pattern with small time differences, to steer and focus the beam

phasicity—in arteries, the phasicity describes the shape of the waveform based on the resistiveness of the distal bed (eg, multiphasic and monophasic); in veins, phasicity describes the flow pattern that results from respiratory variation (eg, respiratory phasicity)

phasing—the method of focusing and/or steering the beam by applying electrical impulses to the piezoelectric elements with small time differences between shocks

picture archiving and communication system—a type of display and storage device commonly used in sonography and other imaging modalities

piezoelectric—the ability to convert pressure into electricity and electricity into pressure

piezoelectric materials—a material that generates electricity when pressure is applied to it, and one that changes shape when electricity is applied to it; also referred to as the element or crystal

pixel (picture element)—the smallest component of a two-dimensional (2D) digital image

pixel interpolation—*see* the key term "fill-in interpolation"

plug flow—the flow profile represented by blood typically flowing at the same velocity

Poiseuille's law—the law that describes the relationship between the resistance, pressure, and flow

postprocessing—changes that can be made on a frozen image because the scan information has been stored in memory

potential energy—pressure energy created by the beating heart

power—the rate at which energy is transferred/transmitted (in W or mW)

power Doppler—a Doppler mode in which the signal is determined by the amplitude (strength) of the shift, not the shift itself; amplitude is directly proportional to the number of red blood cells; also referred to as amplitude Doppler

preamplification—increasing the weak incoming signal from the patient for easier processing by the machine

preprocessing—changes made before the scan information has been stored in memory (ie, while the image is live)

pressure—force per unit area or the concentration of force (in Pascals, Pa)

pressure gradient—the difference between pressures at two points of a blood vessel

preventative maintenance—a methodical way of evaluating equipment's performance on a routine basis to ensure proper and accurate equipment function

propagate—to transmit through a medium

propagation speed—the speed at which a sound wave travels through a medium (in m/s or mm/μs)

propagation speed errors—artifact that occurs because the actual propagation speed of the tissue is greater than or less than 1540 m/s, the machine places the reflector at the wrong location on the display

pulsatility—blood that flows in a pattern representative of the beating heart, with increases and decreases in pressure and blood flow velocity

pulsatility index—Doppler measurement used to determine how pulsatile a vessel is over time

pulse duration—the time it takes for sound to be transmitted; the "on" time (in μs)

pulse inversion technology—harmonic imaging technology in which the fundamental frequency is flipped 180°, which cancels out the fundamental frequency via destructive interference, leaving only the harmonic signal for processing

pulse repetition frequency—the number of pulses of sound produced in 1 s (in Hz or kHz)

pulse repetition period—the time taken for a pulse to occur, including the listening (or dead) time (in μs)

pulsed wave—sound that is sent out in pulses

pulsed-wave Doppler—the Doppler technique that uses pulses of sound to obtain Doppler signals from a user-specified depth

pulser—part of the beamformer that controls the amount of energy in the pulse (ie, the amplitude of the signal)

quality assurance program—a planned program consisting of scheduled equipment-testing activities that confirm the correct performance of equipment

quality factor (Q-factor)—a measure of beam purity; the operating frequency of the transducer divided by the bandwidth

quality improvement—a continuous process of evaluation, feedback, and skills development that occurs in the ultrasound lab

RABT—color scale set so that red is away from the transducer (negative Doppler shift) and blue is toward the transducer (positive Doppler shift)

radiation forces—forces exerted by a sound beam on an absorber or reflector that can alter structures

range equation—the equation used to calculate the distance to the reflector; in soft tissue, $d = 0.77t$, where "d" is the depth of the reflector and "t" represents the roundtrip time of the pulse

range gate—the gate placed by the operator in the region where Doppler sampling is desired; used with pulsed-wave Doppler

range resolution—the ability to determine the depth of echoes by timing how long it takes for the echoes to go from the transducer to the reflector and back; utilized by pulsed-wave devices

rarefaction—an area in the sound wave of low pressure

rate—the fixed quantity owed as the sound beam travels through tissue (related to attenuation)

Rayleigh scatterers—very small scattering reflectors, such as red blood cells

read zoom—the type of magnification performed in the D-to-A converter (postprocessing) that magnifies the image by enlarging the pixels

real time—live ultrasound, also known as automatic scanning

receiver—the component of the machine that processes the signals coming back from the patient

rectification—the part of the receiver that inverts the negative voltages to positive voltages

reflection—the echo; the portion of sound that returns from an interface

refraction—the change in the direction of the transmitted sound beam that occurs with oblique incidence angles and dissimilar propagation speeds

registration—the ability to place echoes in the correct location

rejection—the function of the receiver that is used to reduce image noise; sets a threshold below which the signal will not be displayed

resistance—the downstream impedance to flow determined by vessel length, vessel radius, and viscosity of blood

resistive index—Doppler measurement used to quantitate the resistiveness of the distal bed

resonate—the action of the crystal that produces sound

respirophasic flow—the characteristic waveform of peripheral veins; flow is determined by respiratory variations as a result of intrathoracic pressure changes (also called *respiratory phasicity*)

reverberation—an artifact caused by the beam bouncing between two strong reflectors

Reynolds number—the formula used to quantitate the presence of turbulence; Reynolds numbers greater than 2000 typically indicate turbulence

ring-down—an artifact caused by the vibration of air bubbles

sample volume—the area within the range gate where Doppler signals are obtained

saturation—the amount of white added to a hue; the more white is there, the less saturated the color

scale—the spectral Doppler and color Doppler tool that controls the number of pulses transmitted per second to obtain the Doppler information; also known as pulse repetition frequency in spectral Doppler and color Doppler

scan converter—the part of the ultrasound machine that processes the signals from the receiver; consists of an A-to-D converter, computer memory, and a D-to-A converter

scan line—created when one or more pulses of sound return from the tissue containing information related to the depth and amplitude of the reflectors

scattering—the phenomenon that occurs when sound waves are dispersed into different directions because of the small reflector size compared with the incident wavelength

section-thickness plane—*see* the key term "slice-thickness plane"

sensitivity—the ability of a system to display low-level or weak echoes

sequenced array—transducer elements in an array that are shocked in sequence to steer the beam; contrasts with the key term "phased array"

shadowing—an artifact caused by the failure of sound to pass through a medium with increased attenuation

shear waves—the transverse waves that emanate within the tissue perpendicular to the beam

shear-wave elastography (SWE)*—the elastography technique that uses shear-wave information to analyze the stiffness of tissue

shock*—the body's pathologic response to illness, trauma, or severe physiologic or emotional stress

side lobes—an artifact caused by extraneous sound that is not found along the primary beam path; occurs with single-element transducers

signal processor—part of the machine that includes the

slice-thickness artifact—artifact that occurs as a result of the beam not being razor-thin; thus, unintended echoes may appear in the image as the beam slices through structures adjacent to intended reflectors; also known as the elevational plane artifact or partial volume thickness artifact

slice-thickness phantom—the test object that evaluates the elevational resolution, or the thickness portion, of the sound beam perpendicular to the imaging plane

slice-thickness plane—the "third dimension" of the beam

smoothing—part of the demodulation component of the receiver; an "envelope" is wrapped around the signal to eliminate the "humps" or "ripples"

Snell's law—law used to describe the angle of transmission at an interface based on the angle of incidence and the propagation speeds of the two media

soft tissue—made-up of a medium whose propagation speed is the average of propagation speeds of various tissues found in the human body

sound—a traveling variation in pressure

spatial compounding—a technique that eliminates edge shadowing and reduces acoustic speckle because the object is imaged from different angles

spatial pulse length—the length of one pulse (in mm)

spatial resolution—the ability of the system to distinguish between closely spaced objects; refers to axial, lateral, contrast, and elevational resolution

speckle reduction—the algorithm used in signal processing to reduce the amount of acoustic speckle and to make the image appear smoother

speckle tracking—the method used to obtain the strain information

spectral broadening—the filling of the spectral window

spectral window—the area underneath the envelope on the spectral display

specular reflections—reflections that occur when the reflector is larger than the size of the wavelength of the incident beam. Assumes a 90° angle of incidence

specular reflectors—large, flat, smooth boundaries that cause reflection

stable cavitation—nonthermal bioeffect in which bubbles are created in the tissue

stenosis—pathologic narrowing of a blood vessel

stiffness—the ability of an object to resist compression and relates to the hardness of a medium

strain—the changing of the shape of the muscle as it lengthens and contracts

strain elastography (SE)*—operator dependent type of elastography that measures the change in tissue as a result of compression

strain reliever—flexible sheath that connects the cable to the transducer and is a potential shock hazard if damaged

streaming—when acoustic fields cause motion of fluids

subdicing—dividing the piezoelectric elements into very small pieces to reduce grating lobes

summer—creates the scan line on the receive end by adding together the received signals

sweep speed—the operator-adjustable spectral Doppler control that increases or decreases the number of heartbeats visualized on the spectral display

systole—the time period of the cardiac cycle when the ventricles of the heart are contracting

tachycardia*—rapid heart rate; a rate that exceeds the normal rate for the person's age

tardus parvus—an arterial waveform shape with a delayed peak systolic upstroke that indicates proximal obstruction (also called *parvus et tardus* and, more recently, *dampened*)

temporal resolution—ability to display moving structures in real time; also known as the frame rate

thermal index (TI)—the calculation used to predict the maximum temperature elevation in tissues

three-dimensional ultrasound—allows the user to see width, height, and depth; may also be referred to as volume scanning and multiplanar scanning

thrombus—combination of platelets, red blood cells, and fibrin that make up a blood clot

time-gain compensation—time-gain compensation; *see* the key term "compensation"

tissue Doppler imaging—the color Doppler imaging technique using a low-pass filter to document wall motion and eliminate the signal from flowing blood

tissue-equivalent phantom—the test object that mimics the acoustic properties of human tissue and is used to ensure proper equipment performance

total attenuation—the total amount of sound (in dB) that has been attenuated at a given depth

transducer—any device that converts one form of energy into another; may also refer to the part of the ultrasound machine that produces sound

transient cavitation—nonthermal bioeffect in which bubbles are created in the tissue but collapse violently potentially causing cell damage

transmit/receive switch—ensures the electrical signals travel in the correct direction

transmitter—*see* the key term "pulser"

transmural pressure—the difference in pressure inside a vessel compared with the pressure outside of the vessel

transverse waves—type of wave in which the molecules in a medium vibrate at 90° to the direction of travel

triplex—the ability to visualize real-time grayscale, color Doppler, and spectral Doppler simultaneously

tungsten—component of the backing material

tunica adventitia—the outer layer of a blood vessel

tunica intima—the inner layer of a blood vessel that is closest to the flowing blood

tunica media—the middle, muscular layer of a blood vessel

turbulent flow—chaotic, disorderly flow of blood cells in which they may move in any direction, not necessarily downstream

ultrasound—sound waves of frequencies exceeding the range of human hearing

variance mode—the color Doppler scale with mean velocities displayed vertically on the scale in shades of red or blue, and turbulence displayed horizontally in green

vasa vasorum—a network of small blood vessels that supply blood to the walls of arteries and veins

vasoconstriction—the narrowing of a blood vessel caused by the contraction of the vessel wall

vasodilatation—the widening of a blood vessel caused by the relaxation of the vessel wall

velocity mode—the color Doppler scale with mean velocities displayed vertically

vertical depth—the distance from the transducer

viscous energy—the energy loss caused by friction

volume flow—the volume of blood per unit time; typically measured in liter per minute or milliliter per second; represented by the symbol *Q*

voxel (volume element)—the smallest component of a three-dimensional (3D) image

wall filter—the operator control that eliminates low-frequency, high-amplitude signals caused by wall or valve motion; also called the high-pass filter

wavefront—the leading edge of a wave that is perpendicular to the direction of the propagating wave; formed as a result of Huygen's principle

wavelength—the length of a single cycle of sound (in mm)

wavelet—a small wave created as a result of Huygen's principle

write zoom—the type of magnification performed in the A-to-D converter (preprocessing) that magnifies the image by redrawing it before it is stored in memory

***x*-axis**—the plane that is perpendicular to the beam path (ie, horizontal)

***y*-axis**—the plane that is parallel to the beam path (ie, vertical)

***z*-axis**—the brightness, or amplitude, of the dots on the display

zero-flow baseline—*see* the key term "baseline"

Figure Credits

Chapter 1

Figure 1-4. Reprinted with permission from Bear MF, Connors BW, Parasido, MA. *Neuroscience: Exploring the Brain.* 4th ed. Wolters Kluwer; 2015. Figure 11-1.

Figure 1-11. Reprinted with permission from Armstrong WF, Ryan T. *Feigenbaum's Echocardiography.* 8th ed. Wolters Kluwer; 2019. Figure 2-1.

Figure 1-15. Reprinted with permission from Sanders R, Hall-Terracciano B. *Clinical Sonography: A Practical Guide.* 5th ed. Wolters Kluwer; 2015. Figure 1-3.

Figure 1-20. Reprinted with permission from Armstrong WF, Ryan T. *Feigenbaum's Echocardiography.* 8th ed. Wolters Kluwer; 2019. Figure 2-19.

Figure 1-22. Reprinted with permission from Armstrong WF, Ryan T. *Feigenbaum's Echocardiography.* 8th ed. Wolters Kluwer; 2019. Figure 2-2b.

Figure 1-23. Courtesy of Dr. Asbjorn Stoylen. Available at: http://folk.ntnu.no/stoylen/strainrate/Ultrasound/

Figure 1-25. Reprinted with permission from Beggs I. *Musculoskeletal Ultrasound.* Wolters Kluwer; 2013. Figure 2-13.

Chapter 2

Figure 2-2. Reprinted with permission from Penny SM. *Introduction to Sonography and Patient Care.* 2nd ed. Wolters Kluwer; 2021. Figure 12-25.

Figure 2-5. Reprinted with permission from Topol EJ, Califf RM. *Textbook of Cardiovascular Medicine.* 3rd ed. Wolters Kluwer; 2006. Figure 46-9.

Figure 2-6. Reprinted with permission from Feigenbaum H. *Feigenbaum's Echocardiography.* 6th ed. Wolters Kluwer; 2005. Figure 2-4.

Figure 2-7. Reprinted with permission from Bushberg JT, Seibert JA, Leidholdt EM, Boone JM. *The Essential Physics of Medical Imaging.* 4th ed. Wolters Kluwer; 2020. Figure 14-26.

Figure 2-9. Reprinted with permission from Sanders R. *Clinical Sonography: A Practical Guide.* 5th ed. Wolters Kluwer; 2016. Figure 2-6.

Figure 2-10. Reprinted with permission from Bushberg JT, Boone JM, Leidholdt EM, Seibert JA. *The Essential Physics of Medical Imaging.* 3rd ed. Wolters Kluwer; 2012. Figure 14-11.

Figure 2-14. Reprinted with permission from Armstrong WF, Ryan T. *Feigenbaum's Echocardiography.* 8th ed. Wolters Kluwer; 2019. Figure 2-20.

Figure 2-16. Reprinted with permission from Brant W. *Ultrasound.* Wolters Kluwer; 2001:2.

Figure 2-20. Reprinted with permission from Sanders R. *Clinical Sonography: A Practical Guide.* 5th ed. Wolters Kluwer; 2016. Figure 2-14.

Figure 2-21. Reprinted with permission from Brant W. *Ultrasound.* Wolters Kluwer; 2001:2.

Figure 2-22. Reprinted with permission from Savage RM, Aronson S, Shernan SK. *Comprehensive Textbook of Perioperative Transesophageal Echocardiography.* 2nd ed. Wolters Kluwer; 2010. Figure 1-13.

Figure 2-23. Reprinted with permission from Armstrong WF, Ryan T. *Feigenbaum's Echocardiography.* 8th ed. Wolters Kluwer; 2019. Figure 2-10A.

Figure 2-25. Reprinted with permission from Armstrong WF, Ryan T. Feigenbaum's Echocardiography. 8th ed. Wolters Kluwer; 2019. Figure 2-10B.

Figure 2-26. Photograph courtesy of GE Healthcare, Wauwatosa, WI.

Figure 2-27. Reprinted with permission from Sanders R. *Clinical Sonography: A Practical Guide.* 5th ed. Wolters Kluwer; 2016. Figure 5-1.

Figure 2-29. Reprinted with permission from Bushberg JT, Seibert JA, Leidholdt EM, Boone JM. *The Essential Physics of Medical Imaging.* 4th ed. Wolters Kluwer; 2020. Figure 14-40A.

Figure 2-31. Reprinted with permission from Shernan SK. *Comprehensive Atlas of 3D Echocardiography.* Wolters Kluwer; 2012. Figure 1-2.

Figure 2-34. Reprinted with permission from Armstrong WF, Ryan T. *Feigenbaum's Echocardiography.* 8th ed. Wolters Kluwer; 2019. Figure 2-14.

Figure 2-37. Reprinted with permission from Cosby KS. *Practical Guide to Emergency Ultrasound.* 2nd ed. Wolters Kluwer; 2014. Figure 2.5.

Figure 2-38. Reprinted with permission from Bushberg JT, Boone JM, Leidholdt EM, Seibert JA. *The Essential Physics of Medical Imaging.* 3rd ed. Wolters Kluwer; 2012. Figure 14-21.

Figure 2-39. Reprinted with permission from Bushberg JT, Boone JM, Leidholdt EM, Seibert JA. *The Essential Physics of Medical Imaging.* 3rd ed. Wolters Kluwer; 2012. Figure 14-14A.

Figure 2-41. Reprinted with permission from Bushberg JT, Boone JM, Leidholdt EM, Seibert JA. *The Essential Physics of Medical Imaging.* 3rd ed. Wolters Kluwer; 2012. Figure 14-19B.

Figure 2-42. Reprinted with permission from Bushberg JT, Seibert JA, Leidholdt EM, Boone JM. *The Essential Physics of Medical Imaging.* 4th ed. Wolters Kluwer; 2020. Figure 14-23.

Figure 2-43. Reprinted with permission from Bushberg JT, Boone JM, Leidholdt EM, Seibert JA. *The Essential Physics of Medical Imaging.* 3rd ed. Wolters Kluwer; 2012. Figure 14-34.

Chapter 3

Figure 3-1. Courtesy of Wills Eye Hospital, Philadelphia, PA.

Figure 3-4. Reprinted with permission from Penny SM. *Introduction to Sonography and Patient Care.* Wolters Kluwer; 2015. Figure 3-7.

Figure 3-5. Reprinted with permission from Bushberg JT, Boone JM, Leidholdt EM, Seibert JA. *The Essential Physics of Medical Imaging.* 3rd ed. Wolters Kluwer; 2012. Figure 14-29.

Figure 3-7. Reprinted with permission from Bushberg JT, Seibert JA, Leidholdt EM, Boone JM. *The Essential Physics of Medical Imaging.* 4th ed. Wolters Kluwer; 2020. Figure 14-24A.

Figure 3-16. Reprinted with permission from Perrino AC, Reeves ST. *Practical Approach to Transesophageal Echocardiography.* 2nd ed. Wolters Kluwer; 2008. Figure 21-2.

Figure 3-18. Reprinted with permission from Perrino AC, Reeves ST, Glas K. *Practice of Perioperative Transesophageal Echocardiography: Essential Cases.* Wolters Kluwer; 2010. Figure 23-5.

Figure 3-23. Courtesy of Wikimedia Commons.

Figure 3-25. Courtesy of Wikimedia Commons

Figure 3-26. Reprinted with permission from Daffner RH. *Clinical Radiology: The Essentials.* 3rd ed. Wolters Kluwer; 2008. Figure 1-4.

Figure 3-27. Reprinted with permission from Daffner RH. *Clinical Radiology: The Essentials.* 3rd ed. Wolters Kluwer; 2008. Figure 1-5.

Figure 3-28. Reprinted with permission from Brant W. *Ultrasound.* Wolters Kluwer; 2001:15.

Figure 3-29. Reprinted with permission from Cosby KS. *Practical Guide to Emergency Ultrasound.* 2nd ed. Wolters Kluwer; 2014. Figure 2-9B.

Figure 3-30. Reprinted with permission from Brant W. *Ultrasound.* Wolters Kluwer; 2001:15.

Figure 3-31. Reprinted with permission from Brant W. *Ultrasound.* Wolters Kluwer; 2001:16.

Figure 3-32. Reprinted with permission from Shirkhoda A. *Variants and Pitfalls in Body Imaging.* 2nd ed. Wolters Kluwer; 2010. Figure 8-34b.

Figure 3-33. Reprinted with permission from Sanders R. *Clinical Sonography: A Practical Guide.* 5th ed. Wolters Kluwer; 2016. Figure 6-5.
Figure 3-34. A: Reprinted with permission from Sanders R. *Clinical Sonography: A Practical Guide.* 5th ed. Wolters Kluwer; 2016. Figure 2-23. **B:** Image courtesy of GE healthcare, Milwaukee, WI.
Figure 3-36. Reprinted with permission from Sanders R. *Clinical Sonography: A Practical Guide.* 5th ed. Wolters Kluwer; 2016. Figure 6-18A.
Figure 3-37. Reprinted with permission from Doubilet PM, Benson CB. *Atlas of Ultrasound in Obstetrics and Gynecology.* 2nd ed. Wolters Kluwer; 2011: Figure 28-3.4.
Figure 3-38. Reprinted with permission from Sanders R. *Clinical Sonography: A Practical Guide.* 5th ed. Wolters Kluwer; 2016. Figure 6-3.
Figure 3-39. Reprinted with permission from Sanders R. *Clinical Sonography: A Practical Guide.* 5th ed. Wolters Kluwer; 2016. Figure 6-22.

Chapter 4

Figure 4-1. Reprinted with permission from Oatis CA. *Kinesiology.* 3rd ed. Wolters Kluwer; 2017. Figure 48-23.
Figure 4-3. Reprinted with permission from Kupinski AM. *Diagnostic Medical Sonography: The Vascular System.* 3rd ed. Wolters Kluwer; 2022. Figure 5-3.
Figure 4-4. Asset provided by Anatomical Chart Co.
Figure 4-10. Reprinted with permission from Hashemi RH, Lisanti CJ, Bradley WG. *MRI: The Basics.* 3rd ed. Wolters Kluwer; 2018. Figure 26-1d.
Figure 4-13. Reprinted with permission from Porth CM. *Pathophysiology.* 7th ed. Wolters Kluwer; 2004. Figure 23-3.
Figure 4-14. Reprinted with permission from Preston RR, Wilson T. *Lippincott Illustrated Reviews: Physiology.* 3rd ed. Wolters Kluwer; 2024. Figure 18-11.
Figure 4-15. Reprinted with permission from Kupinski AM. *Diagnostic Medical Sonography: The Vascular System.* 3rd ed. Wolters Kluwer; 2022. Figure 7-30a.
Figure 4-25. Reprinted with permission from Casserly IP, Sachar R, Yadav JS. *Practical Peripheral Vascular Intervention.* 2nd ed. Wolters Kluwer; 2011. Figure 3-5.
Figure 4-28. Reprinted with permission from Armstrong WF, Ryan T. *Feigenbaum's Echocardiography.* 8th ed. Wolters Kluwer; 2019. Figure 2-34.
Figure 4-31. Reprinted with permission from Topol EJ, Califf RM. *Textbook of Cardiovascular Medicine.* 3rd ed. Wolters Kluwer; 2006. Figure 46-14.
Figure 4-58. Reprinted with permission from Armstrong WF, Ryan T. *Feigenbaum's Echocardiography.* 7th ed. Wolters Kluwer; 2009. Figure 7-17.
Figure 4-61. Reprinted with permission from Armstrong WF, Ryan T. *Feigenbaum's Echocardiography.* 7th ed. Wolters Kluwer; 2010. Figure 6-54.
Figure 4-62. Reprinted with permission from Shirkhoda A. *Variants and Pitfalls in Body Imaging.* 2nd ed. Wolters Kluwer; 2010. Figure 8-34c.

Chapter 5

Figure 5-10. Courtesy of ATS Laboratories.
Figure 5-11. Courtesy of ATS Laboratories.
Figure 5-12. Courtesy of ATS Laboratories.
Figure 5-13. Courtesy of ATS Laboratories.
Figure 5-14. Courtesy of ATS Laboratories.

Chapter 6

Figure 6-1. Adapted from Murphy D. Infectious microbes and disease: general principles. *Nurs Spectr.* 1998;7(2):12–14.
Figure 6-2. Reprinted with permission from Lynn PB, Bartlett JL. *Fundamentals of Nursing.* 10th ed. Wolters Kluwer; 2022. Figure 25-2.
Figure 6-4. Reprinted with permission from Siegel MJ. *Pediatric Sonography.* 4th ed. Wolters Kluwer; 2010. Figure 1-23.
Figure 6-6. Reprinted with permission from Sanders R. *Clinical Sonography: A Practical Guide.* 5th ed. Wolters Kluwer; 2016. Figure 2-27.
Figure 6-8. Reprinted with permission from Kawamura D, Lunsford B. *Diagnostic Medical Sonography: Abdomen and Superficial Structures.* 3rd ed. Wolters Kluwer; 2012. Figure 5-36.
Figure 6-9. A: Reprinted with permission from Penny SM. *Introduction to Sonography and Patient Care.* Wolters Kluwer; 2015. Figure 3-42a. **B:** Courtesy of Philips Ultrasound.
Figure 6-10. Reprinted with permission from Penny SM. *Introduction to Sonography and Patient Care.* Wolters Kluwer; 2020. Figure 3-46.
Figure 6-11. Reprinted with permission from Cohen B, Hull K. *Memmler's The Human Body in Health and Disease.* 13th ed. Wolters Kluwer; 2015.

Index

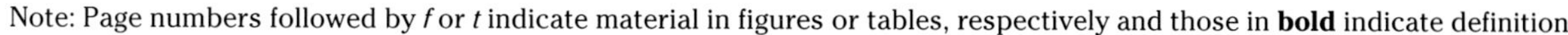

Note: Page numbers followed by *f* or *t* indicate material in figures or tables, respectively and those in **bold** indicate definition.